Cosmetic Microbiology

A Practical Approach

Third Edition

Edited by
Philip A. Geis

Geis Microbiological Quality, Affiliated with
Advanced Testing Laboratory,
The Villages, Florida

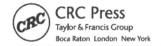

CRC Press
Taylor & Francis Group
Boca Raton London New York

CRC Press is an imprint of the
Taylor & Francis Group, an **informa** business

Third edition published 2021
by CRC Press
6000 Broken Sound Parkway NW, Suite 300
Boca Raton, FL 33487-2742

and by CRC Press
2 Park Square, Milton Park, Abingdon, Oxon OX14 4RN

© 2021 Taylor & Francis Group, LLC

CRC Press is an imprint of Taylor & Francis Group, LLC

ISBN: 978-1-138-73357-2 (hbk)
ISBN: 978 0 429 11369 7 (ebk)

Contents

To parents Bob and Virginia, mentors Flavin and Paul—and to Carol.

Preface

In the context of corporate entities, the cosmetic industry was born in the early 20th century with companies such as the California Perfume Company (Avon) and the Safe Hair Dye Company of France (L'Oreal). Concern for microbiological quality followed soon after with efforts to reduce contamination risks using preservative parabens and benzoic acid as well as product pasteurization. Formaldehyde preservation was applied largely in the 1930s with the development of synthetic shampoos. Though attention to the quality of the cosmetic product category in the United States was addressed in the Federal Food, Drug, and Cosmetic Act of 1936, cosmetic microbiological quality received little regulatory attention until after World War II. At that time, manufacturing quality and preservation were clearly insufficient to ensure microbiological quality in the context of greatly ramped-up production to satisfy the demands of post-war economies. Shelf surveys in the United States and Europe found that up to 40% of the products on shelves were heavily contaminated with bacteria and fungi. With the additional realization of consumer contamination of products during use came heightened regulatory attention, including development by the FDA (Food and Drug Administration) of methods for preservative testing.

Through the latter half of the 20th century, the cosmetic industry prioritized microbiological quality. Hygienic manufacturing guidelines and methods for finished product quality and preservative efficacy testing and package design were developed and codified in compendia such as the CTFA (Cosmetics, Toiletries, and Fragrance Association) Guidelines. Development and application of new preservatives profoundly expanded the stable of useful chemicals during this period with the introduction of organic alcohols, formaldehyde releaser, and isothiazolinone preservatives. These critical quality elements were developed, documented, and applied by a small group of industrial microbiologists whose arcane expertise established decades of excellent microbiological quality and consumer safety as recognized by industry and regulators.

With the dawn of the 21st century came increasing consumer interest and demand for "green" products. This growing category niche is characterized by rejection of traditional preservative systems, including parabens and formaldehyde preservatives, and conversion to alternative preservative systems, especially the so called natural preservatives. These alternative preservative systems have been applied often without adequate understanding of accompanying contamination risks. In recent years, this lack of understanding of risk has led to compromised product quality. Although major marketers invested efforts in the development of compliant products and found alternative systems to be feasible, most found the accompanying compromise in preservative efficacy insufficient to satisfy business demands and risk assessment protocols especially as applied to short-cycle product development and high-speed, high-volume manufacturing demands. However, many small- and medium-sized companies targeted this consumer demand. Production in the context of lesser expertise in product quality demands resulted in increased microbiological contamination-based recalls of cosmetics to levels not seen for many decades. Examination of relevant enforcement reports typically finds these microbiological quality excursions among smaller companies pursuing alternative preservative or preservative-free systems. Regulatory attention to these quality concerns has confirmed risks associated with application of alternative systems.

The third edition of this series brings the 21st-century understanding of microbiology and the critical applied elements of cosmetic microbiological quality. Progress in the context of regulatory controls and human safety understanding, effective development and application of conventional and alternative preservative systems in this field since the last edition of this book was published is also discussed. Testing protocols too are updated and expanded to include rapid method, and hygienic manufacturing is discussed both as a quality concept and in its application and monitoring.

Philip A. Geis

About the Editor

Philip A. Geis is a native Texan who earned bachelor and doctor of philosophy degrees in microbiology from the University of Texas. His career in microbiology began in the US Army, which awarded him the Army Medal of Commendation for his service to its 45th Field Hospital. Geis subsequently worked in commercial media production and joined the Procter & Gamble Company (P&G) following graduate school.

Through three decades with P&G, Geis managed global preservative and disinfectant development, studies of household and skin microbial ecologies, and hygienic manufacturing. He was the first recipient of P&G's namesake award—Dr. Philip Geis Microbiology Quality Award. While at P&G, he also carried responsibilities for state and federal regulatory compliance and policy matters as well as formulation and product development for which he is co-inventor for a number of domestic and international products. Geis published, lectured, and represented P&G's technical interests on subjects of applied microbiology and environmental policy. He edited the second edition of *Cosmetic Microbiology: A Practical Handbook* and served as trustee of the Ohio Academy of Science, chairing its Science Policy Committee.

In 2011, Geis retired from P&G, establishing Geis Microbiological Services in affiliation with Advanced Testing Laboratory. His domestic and international clients range from the French Ministry of Culture to Dow 50 companies. He currently serves as the editor of the journal *International Biodeterioration and Biodegradation* journal and as instructor at the Microbiology and Cell Science department at the University of Florida.

Dr. Geis possesses unique global expertise and experience in diverse regulatory, manufacturing, and product quality disciplines and knowledge of consumer preferences for a broad range of products from OTC (over-the-counter) drugs to fabric softeners to dog food and cultural/historic properties.

Contributors

Terry L. Amoroso, PhD, Director, Corporate Quality Assurance, The Procter & Gamble Co., Mason Business Center, Mason OH

Donald L. Bjerke, PhD/DABT, Global Product Stewardship, The Procter & Gamble Co., Mason Business Center, Mason, OH

Laura M. Clemens, BS, Regional Industrial Microbiologist, The Procter & Gamble Co., Swisher, IA

Corie A. Ellison, PhD, The Procter & Gamble Co., Cincinnati, OH

Donald J. English, MS, Donald J. English Microbiological Quality Consulting LLC, Florham Park, NJ

Peter J. King, PhD, College of Natural Sciences, University of Texas at Austin, Austin, TX

Neil J. Lewis, BS, Global Technical Leader, Microbiology Delivery, The Procter & Gamble Co., Mason Business Center, Mason, OH

Michael J. Miller, PhD, Microbiology Consultants, LLC, Lutz, FL

Alhaji U. N'jai, PhD, Department of Pathobiological Sciences, School of Veterinary Medicine, University of Wisconsin-Madison, Madison WI

Steven F. Schnittger, MS, Vice President, Global Microbiology and Fermentation, The Estée Lauder Companies Inc., Melville, NY

Harry L. Schubert, BS, Retired, Sardinia, OH

David C. Steinberg, BS, MBA, FRAG, Steinberg & Associates, Inc., Pompton Plains, NJ

Scott V.W. Sutton, PhD, deceased

1

Basic Microbiology

Peter J. King

Introduction to Microbiology

This chapter will serve as a primer for those new to microbiology and as an updated reference for those familiar with the science. The discipline of microbiology has advanced rapidly since the refinement of Galileo's light microscope by Van Leeuwenhoek (1674), the disproving of spontaneous generation by Pasteur (1861), the elucidation of the links between specific microbes and human diseases by Koch (1876), and the discovery of viruses by Ivanovsky and Beijerinck (1892). The rate of discovery since the early 1800s represents a mirror of the development of the microbiological techniques used to culture, identify, and characterize microorganisms of all classes. Collectively, the combination of microbiologic techniques and the resulting description of the properties of microbes led to the evolution of impactful techniques of detection of microbes and development of methods for the prevention and treatment of human infectious diseases. While modern microbiology focuses on bacteria (living prokaryotic organisms) and viruses (non-living biologic entities), prions (infectious proteins), protozoa (unicellular eukaryotes), fungi (unicellular and multicellular eukaryotes), and helminths (multi-cellular eukaryotic worms) are generally studied under the microbiology umbrella. This chapter will focus on bacteria and fungi and the methods to detect the presence of bacterial and fungal organisms.

The Prokaryotes

All living cells on the planet can be separated into having either a eukaryotic or a prokaryotic cell structure. Prokaryotes ("before the nucleus") have a simple cell structure comprising a cell membrane and an internal fluid environment called the cytosol. Eukaryotic cells ("true nucleus") have these components as well as multiple membrane-enclosed "organelles" evolved for specific functions just like the nucleus. While eukaryotes can be subdivided into plant-like and animal-like cell types, extant prokaryotes can be classified into two major phylogenetic groups based on genomic sequencing, specifically that of 16S ribosomal RNA (rRNA) genes (Figure 1.1) (1). The first prokaryotic group, which appears to have given rise evolutionarily to eukaryotic cells, belongs to the domain *Archaea*, the archaebacteria. These organisms appear to represent more ancient forms of prokaryotic cells, many of which evolved to occupy extreme niches such as hydrothermal vents and extreme acid and alkali environments. Although these organisms are fascinating due to their mechanisms of adaptation to these environments and their

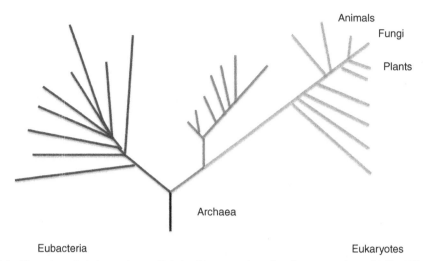

FIGURE 1.1   The universal phylogenetic tree. Relationship comparisons based on comparison of 16S rRNA sequences where the longer the line and spacing, the more distant the evolutionary relationship. Only certain lineages are depicted.

similarity to eukaryotes, and have proven useful in biotechnology, no known human pathogens fall into this group, and therefore, they will not be emphasized in this chapter. The second phylogenetic group of extant prokaryotes is within the domain *Bacteria*, the eubacteria. The group ("true bacteria") reflects their perceived position as the more recently evolved and are the most commonly studied prokaryotes, including all known human pathogenic prokaryotes. *Archaea* and *Bacteria* are commonly referred to collectively as prokaryotes although more modern approaches have led most to suggest that the archaebacteria and eubacteria are different enough, that grouping them together is not scientifically accurate, and that the term "prokaryote" should be replaced with the term "bacteria", referring to the domain *Bacteria* exclusively. The eubacteria comprise 5,000 known species with new species being discovered almost daily, including those found as cosmetic contaminants. The common structures, genetics, metabolism, growth, and diversity of eubacteria will be discussed in detail in this chapter and the terms eubacteria and bacteria will be used interchangeably.

The Bacteria

Summarizing the observed types of bacterial shapes and sizes is difficult due to the far-ranging diversity of the bacteria. However, in general eubacterial species range from very small (nanobacteria, 0.05 mm– 0.2 mm in diameter) to very large (*Epulopiscium fisheloni*, 600 mm × 80 mm). An "average-sized" bacterium such as *Escherichia coli* is 1.5 mm × 2.6 μm. The most basic morphologies observed in bacteria are the coccus (pl. cocci) and the bacillus or "rod" (pl. bacilli) (Figure 1.2). In addition, the cocci and bacilli can associate in characteristic arrangements such as in pairs of two or four, chains, or filaments and clusters. Many bacteria can be identified by these characteristic arrangements such as *Staphylococcus* (grape-like clusters of cocci) and *Streptococcus* (chains of cocci) species. Several bacteria are characterized by a spiral or corkscrew morphology such as the *Vibrio*, the Spirilla, and the Spirochetes. An additional "morphology" observed in bacteria is amorphic or pleomorphic where consistent regular morphologies are not observed usually due to the lack of a rigid cell wall as observed in the genus *Mycoplasma*.

Bacterial Cell Structure

The bacteria share several common structural characteristics with eukaryotic cells such as an outer cell membrane and an internal cytosol. In bacteria, together these are referred to as the "protoplast". However,

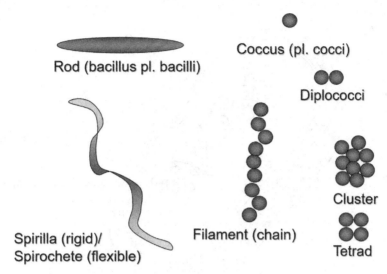

FIGURE 1.2 Common bacterial morphologies. Representative bacterial morphologies are shown. Note that all possible morphologies are not depicted including pleomorphic.

whereas eukaryotic cells have internal membrane-bound organelles (e.g., the nucleus), bacteria lack these internal organelles and hence the moniker "prokaryotes", reflecting a common belief that eukaryotic cells evolved from such progenitors. Several observable bacterial cell structures as well as their composition and function(s) are listed in the section that follows (see Figure 1.3). Special attention is given to the bacterial cell wall.

> ***Plasma membrane***—A phospholipid bilayer which creates a semi-permeable barrier and delineates the boundaries of the cell. This is the location of many important membrane-associated proteins including receptors and enzymes as well as transport proteins designed to internalize desired extracellular components and to extrude cellular contents such as waste.
>
> ***Nucleoid***—Although bacteria do not have a membrane-bound nucleus where DNA is contained, the bacteria do organize and compartmentalize their DNA. The nucleoid is a DNA-rich region within the bacteria cell where DNA has been compacted to allow it fit within the cell. Rather than being haphazardly condensed, bacterial nucleoids have specific sequences contained within specific areas of the nucleoid to optimize the use of DNA.
>
> ***Inclusions and vacuoles***—These very small membrane-bound structures represent micro-organization of nutrients and waste for storage and transport. In the case of gas vacuoles, some bacteria in aqueous environments use these for buoyancy.
>
> ***Ribosomes***—Observable under the microscope, these macro-protein RNA molecular machines are the protein synthesis apparatus of the cell.
>
> ***Capsules and slime layers***—These are extracellular layers of carbohydrates that are well organized and firmly attached to the cell (capsule) or disorganized and loosely attached to the cell (slime layer) that are utilized for attachment to surfaces and sometimes to avoid host immune responses.
>
> ***Fimbriae***—These are fine hair-like projections from the cell that are often found in large numbers and are used to attach to surfaces and for "twitching" motility.
>
> ***Pili***—Also called "sex pili", these are found in smaller numbers that fimbriae (1 or 2 per cell). Pili are large-diameter proteinaceous "tubes" used for conjugation among bacteria where DNA is transferred between members of the same species or even between different species.
>
> ***Flagella***—These large proteinaceous machines are anchored to the bacterial membrane and cell wall structures and are "spun" to create swimming or swarming motility for those species that possess them. The flagella with its whip-like structure help motile bacteria to swim toward or away from certain substances by "chemotaxis".

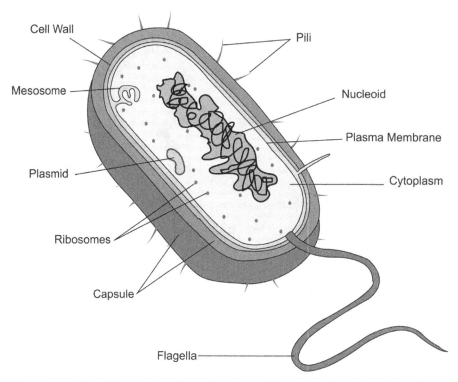

FIGURE 1.3 Common intracellular structures observed in bacteria. Note that not all structures described in the text are depicted.

Endospore—In a few genera, bacteria can internally generate this protective structure by a process termed "sporulation" usually induced by unfavorable conditions. The endospore is an environmentally resistant, metabolically inert structure which contains, at the least, the bacterial DNA, some proteins, calcium, and dipicolinic acid. Upon the return of favorable conditions, the endospore can reproduce the growing form of the bacteria by "vegetation" or outgrowth. Few genera contain spore-forming bacteria, most notably the *Clostridium* and *Bacillus* genera form spores.

S-layer—Some bacteria have an external covering comprising glycoproteins, which is part of bacterial cell wall components. S-layers provide structural integrity as well as facilitate adhesion to surfaces and in some cases help avoid host immune responses.

Bacterial Cell Wall

Free-living bacteria require protection against osmotic stresses. Osmotic stress is encountered when bacteria enter hypotonic or hypertonic environments depending on the concentration of solutes within the cell. This can lead water to cross the plasma membrane by osmosis in an attempt to normalize solute concentrations across the membrane. Excess gain of water can cause the bacteria to lyse or explode due to cellular swelling whereas excess loss of water can cause membrane rupture by excessive shrinkage (plasmolysis). Most bacteria utilize a carbohydrate-based cell wall in order to provide resistance to osmotic forces. The basis of the cell wall is a macromolecular complex unique to bacteria called "peptidoglycan" or murein (Figure 1.4). The basic repeating structure of peptidoglycan is a disaccharide comprising N-acetylglucosamine (NAG) linked to N-acetylmuramic acid (NAM). This disaccharide is repeated hundreds of times to build long carbohydrate chains that are linked together by short peptides (called stem peptides) that contain unusual amino acids, some not found in proteins. These long chains appear to be wound into helices first and then cross-linked to other helices to form the peptidoglycan structure (2).

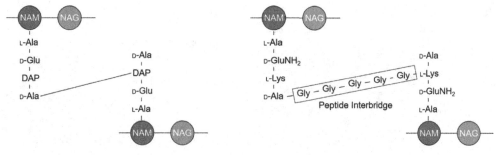

FIGURE 1.4 A simple depiction of peptidoglycan chemical structure. The structure of peptidoglycan as observed in Gram-negative (left) and Gram-positive (right) bacteria. Abbreviations: N-acetylmuramic acid (NAM), N-acetylglucosamine (NAG), L-Alanine (L-Ala), D-Glutamate (D-Glu), Diaminopimelic acid (DAP), D-Alanine (D-Ala), D-Glutamate modified with NH_2 (D-GluNH$_2$), L-lysine (L-Lys), Glycine (Gly). Solid lines represent covalent bond.

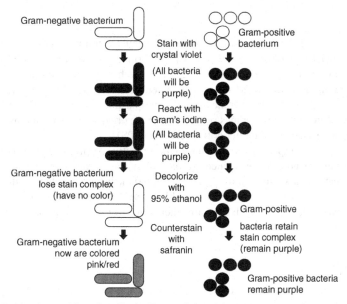

FIGURE 1.5 The Gram stain procedure. Steps in the Gram staining procedure along with the color state of the bacteria at each stage.

The peptidoglycan is attached firmly to the cell membrane by lipoproteins. Although bacteria have proteins that determine the overall morphology of the cell, the peptidoglycan reinforces that morphology.

In bacteria there are two general peptidoglycan-containing cell wall arrangements that can be differentiated by the "Gram stain" (Figure 1.5). This is a staining/microscopic procedure invented in 1884 by the Danish physician Christian Gram to differentiate bacteria based on the characteristics of their cell wall structures.

> *Gram-positive cell wall structure*—In Gram stain positive cells, a thick layer (20–80 nm) of peptidoglycan is attached to the plasma membrane with very little "periplasmic space" between the peptidoglycan and the membrane (Figure 1.6a). The membrane and peptidoglycan are also decorated with teichoic acids (peptidoglycan) and lipoteichoic acids (membrane) that are unique to Gram-positive bacteria. Overall, peptidoglycan contributes 90% of the wet weight of Gram-positive organisms.

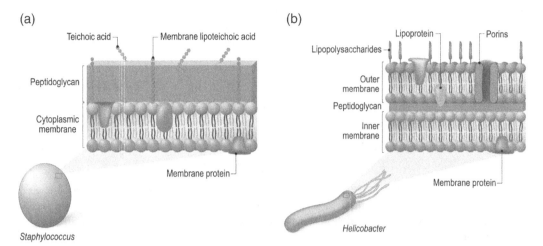

(a) (b)

Teichoic acid — Membrane lipoteichoic acid

Lipoprotein — Porins

Lipopolysaccharides

Peptidoglycan

Outer membrane

Peptidoglycan

Cytoplasmic membrane

Inner membrane

Membrane protein

Membrane protein

Staphylococcus

Helicobacter

FIGURE 1.6 Basic structures of bacterial cell walls. Shown are representative structures for Gram-positive (a) and Gram-negative (b) bacteria.

Gram-negative cell wall structure—In Gram-negative cells, a thin layer (2–7 nm) of peptidoglycan is found sandwiched within a periplasmic space formed by the presence of two complete cell membranes (Figure 1.6b). The periplasmic space is much larger in Gram-negative organisms perhaps contributing as much as 20–40% of their total cell volume. Many enzymes and transport proteins are found in both membranes and the periplasmic space to facilitate metabolism. The outer bilayer of the outer membranes of Gram-negative organisms also contains a polymer unique to Gram-negative species called lipopolysaccharide (LPS).

Other—Although many important bacteria have Gram-positive or Gram-negative cell wall structures, not all bacteria are able to be stained by the Gram stain procedure due to various chemical differences that block Gram staining. Several important bacteria including those of the genera *Mycobacterium* and *Nocardia* are not susceptible to the Gram stain. In addition, the species of the genus *Mycoplasma* lack peptidoglycan altogether which results in these species being pleomorphic and osmosensitive.

Bacterial Genetics

The chromosome of most bacteria is a closed circle of double-stranded DNA although a few species have linear genomes. Most bacteria are haploid, containing only one copy of the genome per cell. Genome sizes vary by species but are considered small for the most part when compared to eukaryotic genomes. Bacteria do not in general contain "junk" DNA sequences such as intronic sequences, removing the necessity for RNA splicing, but rather their protein-coding sequences are concentrated when compared to eukaryotic genomes. As mentioned previously, bacterial DNA is too large to fit within cells unless it is compact and organized, often in conjunction with contact with the plasma membrane into the nucleoid.

Bacteria also contain plasmid DNAs which are smaller circular double-stranded DNAs that exist "episomally" (outside of the genome) and are usually replicated independently of the bacterial genome. Copy number control sequences within the plasmid control the number of copies of the plasmid within the cell that can vary from one per cell to many thousands of copies per cell. It is rare for the genes encoded on plasmids to be essential for the life of the bacteria but rather plasmids appear to confer advantageous characteristics to the bacteria that harbor them. Several characteristics of groups of plasmids are listed in the section that follows.

"F" or conjugation plasmids—Confer the ability for bacteria to generate sex pili to transfer DNA between members of the same species or to different species.

"R" or resistance plasmids—Contain genes that confer antimicrobial resistance to bacteria that harbor them. Often these genes are efflux pumps or degradative enzymes that remove antimicrobials from the cell or degrade the antimicrobial to an inactive form.

"Col" plasmids—Contain genes that allow for the production of bacteriocins. These are substances that kill un-related species of bacteria and confer a competitive advantage on the bacteria that produce them.

Metabolic plasmids—Allow bacteria to utilize unique environmental resources that cannot be utilized by bacteria without the plasmid.

Virulence plasmids—Contain genes that, when present, allow bacteria to more easily infect or to increase the pathogenicity of the diseases that they cause.

DNA Transfer in Bacteria

Vertical Gene Transfer

Like all living organisms, bacterial cells generate progeny cells by cell division wherein the genomic DNA is replicated, and copies of the genome are passed on to each progeny cell. While eukaryotic cells undergo cell division by mitosis, or in some cells meiosis, bacterial cell division occurs by a simpler process called "binary fission", a mechanism of asexual division (Figure 1.7). Simply put, the genome is replicated and the cell enlarges by synthesis of membrane and peptidoglycan and is partitioned into two equal parts each containing one copy of the bacterial genome. Therefore, as with eukaryotic cells, daughter cells inherit DNA sequences which confer phenotypes common to the parental cell.

Horizontal Gene Transfer

Unlike eukaryotic cells, bacteria can transfer DNA sequences between individuals that are not of the same lineage. This can occur between members of the same species or between different species. The three main mechanisms that bacteria use to perform horizontal gene transfer are listed here.

Transformation—DNA found within the extracellular environment of the bacteria is actively taken up into the bacteria and is used either in its native state, such as with plasmids, or incorporated into the genome, as with chromosomal DNA sequences. The utilization of these sequences can often confer drastic new phenotypes on the bacteria that harbor those sequences.

Transduction—Viruses that are present, incorporated into the chromosome of a bacterium, exit the infected bacteria to infect new host cells. In the process, they remove small portions of the

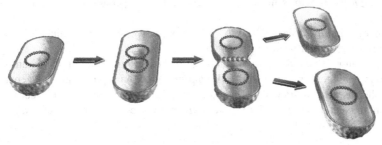

FIGURE 1.7 Binary fission in bacteria. Asexual reproduction in bacteria involves (1) replication of the genome; (2) increases in cell membrane, cell wall, cell volume, and intracellular contents; (3) creation of a "septum" between putative daughter cells to create separate cell chambers; and (4) separation of daughter cells.

chromosome of the infected bacteria. In the new host, these sequences are integrated into the new host genome.

Conjugation—As mentioned previously, bacteria that are able to conjugate by producing sex pili can transfer DNA sequences across the pili and lead to incorporation of new chromosomal sequences within the other mating bacteria.

The Genetics of Bacterial Antimicrobial and Preservative Resistance

Given the operation of natural selection, in an environment that contains antimicrobial agents or preservatives, bacteria that develop resistance to these agents by any means will become overrepresented in any population. Bacteria can gain resistance genes by any of the means described earlier. The transformation of plasmids containing resistance genes can occur with most bacteria even between species. Genes conferring resistance can likewise be spread by intra- or inter-species transfer via transduction or conjugation, and hereditary transfer of resistance genes confers the advantageous resistance phenotype from parent cells to daughter cells by vertical gene transfer. Given the benefit of resistance to the survivability of the offspring, antimicrobial and preservative resistance can quickly spread and expand in any bacterial population where resistance genes exist and antimicrobial agents or preservatives are present.

Bacterial Metabolism

Like all other living cells, bacteria must perform both anabolic (building up) and catabolic (breaking down) metabolic reactions. And like all cells, bacteria require food sources that can be metabolized via catabolic reactions to provide energy to fuel their anabolic reactions required for building proteins, cell division, and so on. Bacteria also require macronutrients and micronutrients that serve as the "building blocks" for their anabolic reactions. However, bacteria have evolved to acquire their metabolic requirements by a wide variety of mechanisms with a diversity that is not observed in eukaryotic cells. These metabolic adaptations probably reflect a variety of ecological niches that existed during bacterial evolution as well as a metabolic plasticity that was allowed early in evolution.

Temperature—As the bacteria evolved, they survived in a wide variety of niches irrespective of the temperature. Therefore, their membranes and enzymes evolved to optimize function under those temperature conditions. This is evident as extant species display optimal growth temperatures that reflect those niches. "Cardinal" temperatures for any species can be experimentally defined and represent the minimum, maximum, and optimal temperatures for the growth of that species.
- *Psychrophiles* grow optimally at very low temperatures: 0–20°C (15°C optimal).
- *Mesophiles* are active at more moderate temperatures: 20–45°C (20–40°C optimal). These species include those that colonize and infect mammals.
- *Thermophiles* growth is most effective at warmer temperatures: 45°C and higher (55–65°C optimal).
- *Hyperthermophiles* have evolved to exist in extremely warm environments with optimal temperature of 90°C and above.

pH—As with temperature, alkalinity or acidity of niches during evolution led extant species to display varying preferences regarding pH. *Acidophiles* growth is optimal in acidic environments (pH 0–5.5) whereas *neutrophiles*, which include organisms that colonize and infect mammals, grow best at more neutral pH (pH 5.5–8). *Alkalophiles* (pH 8.5–11.5) and *extreme alkalophiles* grow best in basic environments.

All bacteria have common requirements for metabolism which are highlighted here along with common bacterial mechanisms for satisfying these requirements.

Carbon—As most biological macromolecules such as proteins, DNA, carbohydrates, and lipids are "organic" molecules (i.e., they are based largely on carbon), bacteria require a constant influx of carbon from the environment if those are to survive. Two main strategies have evolved for bacteria to acquire carbon.

- *Autotrophs*—These bacteria acquire carbon for their metabolism from the environment as carbon dioxide (CO_2). This is advantageous as CO_2 is abundant in the atmosphere and water due to the photosynthetic activity of organisms such as plants and algae.
- *Heterotrophs*—These bacteria must ingest and metabolize other carbon-containing compounds in order to acquire carbon. For bacterial cosmetic contaminants, preservatives can often be metabolized and used as a source of carbon.

Other atoms—Hydrogen, oxygen, phosphorous, nitrogen, sulfur, potassium, calcium, magnesium, and iron are other atoms used in large amounts to create biological macromolecules or necessary for critical biochemical processes; therefore, bacteria must obtain these elements along with carbon. Usually, heterotrophic bacteria harvest these atoms from the same organic molecules they utilize for obtaining carbon. However, autotrophic bacteria must have strategies in place to additionally harvest these atoms.

Micronutrients—A number of elements are required in small amounts for bacterial growth and although the amounts necessary are lesser than the "macroelements" previously described, these "trace elements" are no less important than macroelements and bacteria must have strategies to ensure they are absorbed. These include manganese, zinc, cobalt, molybdenum, nickel, and copper.

Energy sources—As mentioned previously, like all other living organisms bacteria must fuel their energy-requiring anabolic processes. Inevitably, the source of this energy comes from catabolic processes that oxidize organic (or inorganic) molecules to provide energy for anabolism. The source of these organic molecules can differ by the type of bacteria involved.

- *Chemotrophs*—In the case of many bacteria (as with humans) these compounds are ingested from the environment. These molecules are the anabolic products of other organisms or less commonly are inorganic compounds found in the environment.
- *Phototrophs*—For photosynthetic bacteria (as with plants) energy from sunlight is utilized to produce ATP (Adenosine Triphosphate). That ATP can also be used to generate organic molecules such as glucose by anabolic processes which can then be oxidized to provide energy for other anabolic processes within the cell.

Electrons—High-energy electrons are required to produce ATP which serves as the universal energy "currency" within the cell. Generation of ATP serves as the common reaction and all catabolic harvesting of energy within the cell is funneled such that a single energy currency can be utilized to fuel all metabolic processes. The electrons required to produce ATP are necessary as "oxidative respiration" is the process that has evolved to be most efficient in the production of ATP. Bacteria have two main mechanisms to obtain these electrons.

- *Organotrophs*—These organisms remove electrons from organic molecules, either those that have been ingested by chemotrophs or synthesized via photosynthesis for phototrophs.
- *Lithotrophs*—Less commonly reduced inorganic molecules are utilized for electron harvesting. The literal translation of lithotroph is "rock eater", indicating that these organisms can utilize inorganic sources.

Oxygen—Aerobic respiration has evolved in fungal, plant, and animal cell as the most efficient process for harvesting energy and electrons from organic molecules for the purpose of producing ATP. Given the name of this process, it is obvious that aerobic respiration requires oxygen to function. However, aerobic respiration is not the only ATP-generating process observed in bacterial species and as such many species differ in their requirements for the presence (or absence) of oxygen. These diverse mechanisms probably exist as bacteria have evolved under a variety of environmental conditions including periods of time on earth when oxygen was completely absent or present in smaller amounts. Therefore, bacteria can be characterized by their relationships to oxygen.

- *Obligate aerobes*—Like almost all multicellular organisms, these bacteria are completely dependent on atmospheric oxygen (O_2) for respiration.
- *Microaerophiles*—These bacteria require O_2 but are damaged by atmospheric concentrations of O_2 (20%) and require lower O_2 concentrations (2–10%) for growth.

- *Facultative anaerobes*—These species grow optimally in the presence of atmospheric O_2 but have adapted other mechanisms (primarily fermentation) to carry out ATP production in the absence of O_2. Fermentation is described below.
- *Aerotolerant anaerobes*—These species do not require O_2 to generate optimal amounts of ATP as they evolved in an atmosphere devoid of O_2. These bacteria have evolved alternative respiratory pathways that do not require O_2 but are unaffected by the presence of O_2.
- *Obligate anaerobes*—Like aerotolerant anaerobes, these bacteria possess alternative respiratory mechanisms for producing ATP that do not require O_2. However, for these organisms O_2 is toxic and exposure to atmospheric O_2 results in their death.

Fermentation

Facultative anaerobes have evolved mechanisms to produce ATP (although in smaller amounts) by breaking down sugars when O_2 is absent. Collectively referred to as fermentation, these mechanisms produce ATP along with a number of interesting byproducts depending on the species. Many of these byproducts are important commercially. The mechanisms of fermentation are categorized based on the major acid or alcohol byproducts that are produced.

Homolactic fermentation—Produces lactic acid exclusively as a byproduct of fermentation.
Heterolactic fermentation—Produces lactic acid in addition to ethanol and CO_2.
Alcoholic fermentation—In this mechanism, ethanol is the primary byproduct in addition to CO_2.
Mixed acid fermentation—Produces multiple byproducts including acetic acid, lactic acid, succinic acid, and formic acids as well as ethanol.
Butanediol fermentation—In this mechanism, butanediol and ethanol are produced in large amounts along with lactic acid.

Major Nutritional Types of the Bacteria

Given the mechanisms available to acquire carbon, the ultimate source of energy in the cell and the different sources available to harvest electrons, bacteria have evolved satisfying these requirements by combinations of the mechanisms described. By combining the roots of the terms described, bacteria can be placed into five different nutritional types.

Photolithoautotrophs—These bacteria are also referred to as "photoautotrophs" including the purple and green sulfur bacteria, cyanobacteria, and diatoms. They harvest carbon from atmospheric CO_2, are photosynthetic, and utilize inorganic molecules as electron sources such as hydrogen, hydrogen sulfide, and elemental sulfur.
Photoorganoheterotrophs—There are a few known photosynthetic bacteria in this group including the purple non-sulfur bacteria and green non-sulfur bacteria. Although they utilize light as their primary energy source, they acquire carbon and electrons from organic sources.
Chemolithoautotrophs—The bacteria of this type—including the sulfur-oxidizing bacteria, hydrogen-oxidizing bacteria, methanogens, nitrifying bacteria, and iron-oxidizing bacteria—obtain energy and electrons from reduced inorganic sources such as iron or sulfur compounds and harvest carbon from atmospheric CO_2.
Chemolithoheterotrophs—These bacteria, including a few sulfur-oxidizing bacteria, utilize organic sources for carbon and inorganic sources for energy and electrons.
Chemoorganoheterotrophs—These organisms (like humans) fulfill all their requirements by the consumption of organic material from other living cells. These organic materials provide carbon, energy, and electrons for their metabolism. This large group of bacteria contains most non-photosynthetic bacteria including nearly all human pathogens and most bacterial cosmetic contaminants.

The Fungi

Fungi are within the domain Eukarya (see Figure 1.1) indicating that their cells are of eukaryotic type. Fungi are a diverse group of species that contain both unicellular and multicellular organisms. No organisms within this group are photosynthetic because as chemoorganoheterotrophs, all fungal species absorb their nutrients from the environment, a process termed "osmotrophy". Although members of Fungi are beneficial in the ecosystem, economically, well over 5,000 fungal species are known to be pathogenic to humans, animals, or plants with 20 new human pathogens discovered each year.

Fungal Structure

Fungal cells are eukaryotic, containing membrane-bound intracellular organelles, but also possess cell walls. However, rather than peptidoglycan (bacterial) or cellulose (plants), the fungal cell wall is composed of glucans, mannans, glycoproteins, trehalose, and chitin (a strong and flexible polysaccharide). Single-celled microscopic fungi are referred to as "yeasts" and contain a single nucleus and ovoid morphology. Yeasts are commonly larger than bacteria and lack extracellular fibers like flagella or fimbriae. Multicellular fungal forms are called "molds" comprising long branching filaments called hyphae with many individual cells where the cytoplasm in the hyphae are contiguous with neighboring cells. The hyphae of molds generally form a tangled mass called a mycelium. "Dimorphic" fungi are those that can alternate between yeast and mold forms depending on environmental conditions. For example, *Histoplasma capsulatum* grows in the environment as a mold but upon infection of the lung grows exclusively as a yeast form (3).

Fungal Reproduction

Fungal species can undergo either asexual division (as with binary fission in bacteria) or sexual division where gametes are formed and fused to create genetically novel zygotes.

Asexual reproduction—Asexual reproduction of fungi can occur by several mechanisms. Most simply, a single fungal cell (such as a yeast) can undergo a single cycle of mitosis by copying the genome and segregating the reproduced DNA to each putative daughter cell, generating new membrane and cell wall material as well as other intracellular elements and create two clonal daughter cells. This appears very similar to binary fission in bacteria. In addition, "budding", observed especially in yeast, involves production of daughter cells that, while clonal, are produced as much smaller cells that must develop into larger cells after being separated from the precursor cell. Such "spores" can be produced in large numbers from fungi through the mechanism called dispersal in the environment but should not be confused with bacterial endospores as their composition is different and, although they are environmentally resistant, are not as stress resistant as bacterial endospores.

Sexual reproduction—Sexual reproduction of fungi involves production of gametes containing compatible nuclei which fuse to form zygotes. Some fungi are self-fertilizing and produce compatible gametes from the same mycelium. Other species require out-crossing involving production of gametes from compatible "mating types" represented by separate sexually compatible mycelia. These gametes are also referred to as spores and display the same environmentally resistant properties as spores produced by asexual reproduction.

Both—Many species of fungi can perform both asexual and sexual reproduction.

Fungal Divisions

Although diversity is tremendous within the fungal species, they can be grouped into six divisions by the structure of their cells, their mechanisms of reproduction (specifically how spores are produced), and spore morphology. As with grouping bacteria by nutritional type, the fungi can be categorized under multiple phylogenetic groups.

Chytridiomycetes—These fungi, commonly referred to as "chytrids", are free-living or parasites of plants and insects. They are characterized by both asexual and sexual production of spores that possess a single flagellum that allow motility to the spore.

Zygomycetes—The species in this group are either free-living or parasitic and are common on surfaces of decaying matter such as the bread mold *Rhizopus stolonifer*. They extend hyphae into the decaying material to absorb nutrients as well as above the substrate producing numerous black spores by asexual reproduction giving the mold a characteristic black color. These species can also reproduce by sexual reproduction when food source becomes limiting.

Glomeromycota—This group contains important symbiont of plants. These species are also called "*Arbuscular mycorrhizal* fungi" that grow in proximity to plant roots and provide important resources to the plant in return for carbohydrates produced by photosynthesis. They produce large spores by asexual reproduction and have flat hyphae called appressoria that facilitate their interaction with plant cells.

Ascomycota—These fungi are commonly referred to as "sac fungi" due to the characteristic reproductive structure. They produce a structure (ascus) which contains their spores (ascospores). Some species are just yeast whereas others alternate between yeast and mold forms. A well-known yeast formed from this group is the baker's *Saccharomyces cerevisiae* and cosmetic contaminants such as the *Ascomyetous* fungi of genera *Candida, Aspergillus,* and *Penicilium*.

Basidiomycota—This group, also called the "club fungi", contains the mushrooms as well as some plant parasites. They are named for a characteristic structure, the basidium, which is involved in sexual reproduction of these species. The basidium is usually club shaped leading to the common name for this group, and cosmetic contaminants such as the *Basidiomycetous* fungi of the genus *Rhodotorula* belong to this group.

Microsporidia—This group contains species that are obligate intracellular organisms, which mean that their life cycle must occur within the intracellular space of a living cell. Although their inclusion into the domain Fungi is controversial, it is based largely on 16S rRNA sequencing and the composition of the cell wall of these species (4). Their structures, however, are not characteristic of fungi, yet they do produce spores. They are important parasites of animals including humans with deficient immune responses.

Common Contaminants in the Cosmetics Industry

Given the scope of this text, it is pertinent to reflect on the general biology of the bacteria and fungi in respect to the microbes most commonly found as contaminants in cosmetics. A complete list of possible microbial contaminants is found elsewhere in this text.

Bacteria

Burkholderia cepacia—This species is found with the phylum Proteobacteria which contains eight classes of Gram-negative organisms. *B. cepacia* is placed within the class Betaproteobacteria containing about 400 different species that have bacilli morphology, are obligate aerobes, chemoorganoheterotrophs, and most are motile due to the presence of polar flagella. *B. cepacian* is a common inhabitant of soil and water and can cause fatal human infections in individuals who are immunocompromised and/or have pre-existing lung disease such as cystic fibrosis. In these individuals, pneumonia leading to rapid lung failure is the most common and severe form of disease.

Pseudomonas aeruginosa—The "pseudomonads" are members of the phylum Proteobacteria and the genus *Pseudomonas*. The almost 200 species in this genus are all Gram-negative rods and display great metabolic diversity as a group but are all chemoorganoheterotrophs. An important pseudomonad, *P. aeruginosa*, is a species found in water and soil, is motile with polar flagella and is encapsulated by exoploysaccharides which allow *P. aeruginosa* to effectively colonize a wide variety of surfaces of natural and man-made origin. Although considered strictly anaerobic, *P. aeruginosa* is tolerant to a variety of low oxygen conditions which allows it to participate in "biofilms" in which multiple species are present in a large biomass attached to a surface (5). This species causes problematic infections, mostly in immunocompromised individuals, as it displays multiple drug resistance.

"Enteric" bacteria—The family *Enterobacteriaceae* contains 50 genera and over 200 species of chemoorganoheterotrophic Gram-negative bacilli with diverse metabolic capacities. Most species are flagellated and motile and produce fimbriae which make them attach to surfaces. The family was named so as many of the organisms present in this group colonize the intestines of animals (including humans). The majority of species in this group are facultative anaerobes and display diverse mechanisms of fermentation. A number of pathogenic bacteria are found in this group, and the several genera which are common cosmetics contaminants are mentioned here.

- *Klebsiella*—This genus contains *K. pneumoniae* and *K. oxytoca*. *Klebsiella* are common colonizers of the intestines and skins of humans and intestines of animals and are also ubiquitous in soil and water. They are heavily encapsulated and cause opportunistic infections of the respiratory and urinary tracts of immunocompromised individuals.
- *Escherichia*—The most prominent member of this genus is *E. coli* which is a widely studied bacteria in nature. *E. coli* is a "coliform" bacteria. The coliforms are intestinal bacteria with common characteristics that are present in feces and, therefore, their presence or absence is used as a measure of water quality. Many *E. coli* isolates are innocuous, but in the presence of virulence factors *E. coli* can cause water- and food-borne infections, some of which can be severe or fatal.
- *Enterobacter*—Members of this genus include *E. cloacae* and *E. aerogenes*. These species are also intestinal colonizers and members of the coliform group. They commonly cause infections in immunocompromised individuals of the urinary and respiratory tracts.

Staphylococcus aureus—This Gram-positive coccus arranges in grape-like clusters and is a facultative anaerobe assigned to the phylum Firmicutes. *S. aureus* is a normal colonizer of the skin and mucous membranes of humans and commonly causes the pyogenic (pus-forming) infections of skin. Certain isolates of *S. aureus* possess virulence factors and can cause serious infections of skin and deeper tissues including necrotizing fasciitis. Increasing drug resistance in *S. aureus* has become a serious problem for hospitals and clinics (6).

Fungi

Candida albicans—This species of the division Ascomycota is dimorphic and a common colonizer of the human mouth and intestines. *C. albicans* is often found in microbial biofilms that also contain bacteria in a biomass attached to surfaces both natural and man-made. *C. albicans* commonly causes opportunistic infections in immunocompromised individuals that can rapidly become life-threatening. Although the yeast form seems ideal for spreading during infection, the ability to produce hyphae and switch to filamentous form is considered a virulence factor for *C. albicans* (7).

Rhodotorula—This genus contains organisms from the division Basidiomycota which are pigmented unicellular yeast. Species in the genus include *R. mucilaginosa*, *R. glutinis*, and *R. minuta* which are known to cause diseases in humans. These species are normally present in soil and water but can attach to medical surfaces and cause blood-borne infection in the immunosuppressed.

Cladosporium—Members of this genus of the division Ascomycota include some of the most common outdoor molds. *Cladosporium* spores are well dispersed in air and although their spores serve as allergens, they are rarely associated with invasive diseases in humans.

Fusarium—This genus contains a large number of filamentous species of the division Ascomycota. Many of these species are abundant participants in soil communities. Most species pose no threat to humans and are common colonizers of human skin. However, species within the *Fusarium solani* complex can cause life-threatening infections in the immunocompromised. *Fusarium* species can also cause disease in immunocompetent individuals of the nails and cornea.

Penicillium—Although the most famous member of this genus is *P. notatum*, the original source of penicillin, the members of this genus from the division Ascomycota are common filamentous molds that cause food spoilage and are ubiquitous in soil in cool and moderate climates. These species are abundant in the air and dust of indoor environments and several, including *P. marneffei,* are known to infect immunocompromised individuals.

REFERENCES

1. Pace N. 1997. A Molecular View of Microbial Diversity and the Biosphere. *Science.* **276**:734–740.
2. Vollmer W, Blanot D, Pedro MAD. 2008. Peptidoglycan Structure and Architecture. *FEMS Microbiol Rev.* **32**:149–167.
3. Maresca B, Kobayashi GS. 1989. Dimorphism in *Histoplasma capsulatum*: A Model for the Study of Cell Differentiation in Pathogenic Fungi. *Microbiol Rev.* **53**:186–209.
4. Hibbett D, Binder M, Bischoff J, Blackwell M, Cannon P, Eriksson O, Huhndorf S, et al. 2007. A Higher-Level Phylogenetic Classification of the Fungi. *Mycol Res.* **111**:509–547.
5. Høiby N, Ciofu O, Bjarnsholt T. 2010. *Pseudomonas aeruginosa* Biofilms in Cystic Fibrosis. *Future Microbiol.* **5**(11):1663–1674.
6. Calfee DP. 2011. The Epidemiology, Treatment, and Prevention of Transmission of Methicillin-Resistant Staphylococcus aureus. *J Infus Nurs.* **34**(6): 359–364.
7. Jiménez-López C, Lorenz MC. 2013. Fungal Immune Evasion in a Model Host–Pathogen Interaction: Candida albicans versus Macrophages. *PLoS Pathog.* **9**:e1003741.

2

Preservatives and Preservation

Philip A. Geis

Introduction

Effective and appropriate preservation of cosmetics is an arcane and complex technology. Unlike drug preservation, it enjoys neither the highly controlled aseptic manufacturing systems nor the disciplined application of products in the hands of clinicians. The microbiological safety of foods is ensured by additional protective elements of refrigeration and consumer experience and perception alerting spoilage. Similarly, cosmetics must be made microbiologically stable for years through consumer use and reasonably foreseeable misuse. Further, cosmetic microbiological failure typically offers no obvious signal to consumers alerting to risk. The cosmetic microbiologist is additionally challenged by the complexity of products in this category. By statutory definition (1), cosmetics are articles intended to be rubbed, poured, sprinkled, sprayed on, introduced into, or otherwise applied to the human body for cleansing, beautifying, promoting attractiveness, or altering the appearance. The diversity by which industry functionally serves these broad objectives can be seen in products uniquely composed of tens to hundreds of ingredients marketed as solutions, suspensions, emulsions, creams, pastes, powders, and solids and packaged in tubes, bottles, jars, aerosol cans, some with applicators, to be applied daily to skin and even intimate body surfaces.

Concerns for cosmetic safety drove this product category's inclusion in the 1936 Food Drug and Cosmetic Act (2). Though not recognized at that time, subsequent and recent medical and technical literature as well as FDA enforcement records clearly indicate microbiological contamination presents the greatest safety risk to consumers (3). The path to microbiologically safe cosmetics involves a number of critical elements, the most essential of which is preservation that provides protection in the context of appropriate good manufacturing practices (GMPs) and even more importantly under normal and reasonably foreseeable conditions of consumer use (4).

Scope of Preservations and Microbiological Targets of Preservation

On the basis of FDA enforcement and recall reporting data, the primary concerns for cosmetics are ingredient safety, especially for color additives, and microbiological adulteration (3). Clearly, the latter has been and continues to be the most significant and increasing risk in recent years (3,5). Most infections resulting from exposure of healthy individuals to contaminated cosmetics would be expected to be transient, superficial and limited unless damaged skin was exposed (6,7). However, much more serious issues have been reported especially among those considered immunocompromised. Wilson and Ahearn reported serious eye infections, including blindness resulting from the use of contaminated mascaras (8). Here the compromising factor was found to be physical disruption of corneal surface by careless use of mascara wands. Some authors have reported serious and even fatal infection traced to contaminated cosmetic products (9–12). These risks were associated with systemically immunocompromised population, a group estimated to compose over 25% of the US population (13). This includes those suffering chronic illnesses such as diabetes, cystic fibrosis, and AIDs, the very young and the very old, those undergoing immunocompromising therapeutic regimens for conditions ranging from cancer to rheumatoid arthritis and Crohn's disease, as well as those constrained by temporary those conditions such pregnancy, existing infection, and compromised skin.

The scope of microbial integrity relevant to preservation extends from raw material quality to the safety of the last product use by the consumer. In application, the objective of preservation is to ensure that consumers face minimal microbiological risk through foreseeable and typical product use. Although manufacturing hygiene and package protection are critical to cosmetic microbiological integrity, product preservation as determined in a relevant challenge test is perhaps the most commonly cited and utilized measure of cosmetic microbial safety assessment. Preservation in its broadest meaning is the central, pivotal element of this quality effort, controlling risks associated with nonsterile, in-process manufacturing as well as consumer contamination risks associated with reasonable consumer use. This dual role is not functional for all products. For example, products such as aerosol mousse packaged in pressurized barrier containers are not subject to contamination in use, leaving the objective of their chemical preservatives focused only on in-process contamination.

Elements of manufacturing processes and materials and packaging certainly can both contribute to preservative efficacy as well as compromise the stability and efficacy of the product preservative. This chapter will focus primarily on finished product chemical preservation and will also consider cosmetic preservation in the broader context as the application of chemical, physical, procedural, and energetic means to establish and maintain microbiological quality of finished products, manufacturing intermediates, and raw materials.

Targets of Preservation

Potential microbial contaminants, the ultimate targets of product preservation, are numerous (Table 2.1; see also Refs. 6,9,11,14,15,16,17,18–21) and include a wide range of Gram-positive and Gram-negative bacteria and fungi. Manufacturing and consumer-derived contaminants generally overlap, with little difference in the range of microorganisms. *Burkholderia cepacia* and *Pseudomonas aeruginosa* are most commonly encountered as manufacturing contaminants (22,23) with the former very rarely reported as a consumer contaminant (24). Less frequently reported consumer contaminants include skin and oral microbes *Staphylococcus*, *Streptococcus*, and *Corynebacterium* spp. Apparently unique to manufacturing contaminants are microbes such as *Clostridium* spp. attributed to earth-derived materials such as talc (24). Microbial risks established in manufacturing are diverse and include those derived from contaminated raw materials, especially process water, poorly designed equipment, persistent dilute product that facilitates adaptation of microbes to preserved product, equipment that resists effective cleaning and sanitization, poor worker and facility hygiene, and lack of appropriate hygiene training and awareness (25).

Consumer contamination is diverse as a function of the various practices and microbiological exposures of global consumers. One of the few detailed reports describing the range of microbiological

TABLE 2.1

Microbiological contaminants of cosmetics and related materials and products

Gram-Positive Bacteria

Staphylococcus aureus	*Staphylococcus epidermidis*
Staphylococcus warneri	*Staphylococcus* spp.
Propionibacterium spp.	*Corynebacterium diphtheriae*
Clostridium tetani	*Clostridium perfringens*
Bacillus spp.	*Bacillus anthracis (historic)*

Gram-Negative Bacteria

Pseudomonas aeruginosa	*Burkholderia cepacia*
Burkholderia pickettii	*Stenotrophomonas maltophilia*
Acinetobacter spp.	*Moraxella* spp.
Escherichia coli	*Klebsiella pneumoniae*
Klebsiella oxytoca	*Citrobacter freundii*
Serratia marcescens	*Aeromonas* spp.
Salmonella spp.	*Proteus* spp.
Raoultella planticola	*Rhizobium radiobacter*
Achromobacter xylosoxidans	*Pantoea agglomerans*

Fungi

Candida albicans	*Candida lipolytica*
Saccharomyces cerevisiae	*Rhodotorula* spp.
Aureobasidium pullulans	*Paecilomyces variotii*
Aspergillus fumigatus	*Aspergillus niger*
Scopulariopsis spp.	*Penicillium* spp.

elements of consumer contamination is that of Brannan et al. (14). The authors placed shampoo and lotion products with differing preservative capacities (described as unpreserved, marginally preserved, and effectively preserved) in the hands of consumers and recovered products after extended consumer use. Microbiological examination of recovered products recovered a wide range of microorganisms including both bacteria and fungi. Contamination correlated in both number and type to the respective level of preservation, with unpreserved and marginally preserved categories most at risk.

For both manufacturing and consumer-derived contamination, Gram-negative bacteria provide the greatest risk due to their ubiquitous presence in aqueous environments (14,25,26) and propensity to adapt and grow in products and develop preservative resistance (15,27).

Rationale for Preservative Use

The rationale or objective of cosmetic preservation is to establish and maintain microbiological quality. Some degree of preservation is always required in nonsterile manufacturing; under GMPs, controls are intended to mitigate contamination risk (25). However, the primary objective of the cosmetic preservative is to protect the consumer during product use. Consequences of failure to serve this objective include loss of product esthetics and functionality, compromised consumer safety and the resulting regulatory intervention.

Esthetics and functionality. The classic consumer perception of a contaminated cosmetic is pigmented mold colony on the surface of a cream in an open jar (Figure 2.1). If consumers dared to sniff the moldy cream, they'd certainly perceive compromise of the product perfume to the great frustration of the perfumer whose artistic combination of hundreds of perfume components was wasted. A common odorant of mold spoilage odor is octen-3-ol whose threshold of olfactory detection is 2 ppb (28). Bacteria that contaminate cosmetics can produce hydrogen sulfide, indole, and skatole (3-methyl indole), compounds whose

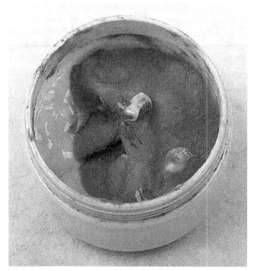

FIGURE 2.1   Reported cosmetic microbiological contaminants.

characteristic fecal odors can be perceived at ppb levels (29). Visual signals of contamination include microbial pigments such as prodigiosin from *Serratia marcescens* and pyoverdin from *Pseudomonas aeruginosa* (30). I have observed both general pigment-based discoloration as well as localized compromise at the surface of the product—red ring on the surface of a white liquid hand soap contaminated with *S. marcescens*. Both fungal and bacterial contamination can physically compromise a product with sediment production and breaking of emulsions (31). Unfortunately, microbial contamination more often presents no discernable effect, denying the consumer a signal that the product being used may offer a potential safety risk.

Human safety is clearly the most significant driver for preservation. Whereas topical application of contaminated product may result in only transient skin infection in healthy individuals (6), consumers with some degree of physical or immunocompromised system are certainly at much more significant risk (13). Very serious eye infections have been traced to the application of contaminated mascara (6). These individuals had been compromised by the misuse of mascara applicators brush resulting in scratched corneal surfaces. For some, infections resulted in blindness. Serious as this was, fatal infections have been attributed to contaminated cosmetics. Use of a regionally produced baby shampoo contaminated with *Serratia marcescens* in a children's ward in a hospital resulted in 15 cases of septicemia, one of which was fatal (11). Similarly, a report from MD Anderson Hospital traced serious infections, one fatal, of women under chemotherapy for breast cancer to a shampoo contaminated with *Pseudomonas aeruginosa* used in the hospital salon (12). The individuals had visited the salon and been shampooed before head shaving in anticipation of chemotherapy-associated alopecia.

On the basis of concerns for product safety, cosmetic microbiological quality is monitored by regulatory bodies around the world including the US FDA, Health Canada, Australia's Therapeutic Goods Administration, and the European Commission. Microbiological contamination is considered a significant risk for which recall from shelf is typically considered an appropriate action. Although such recalls of cosmetics are typically infrequent, microbiological contamination is by far the primary rationale for any regulatory action regarding cosmetic quality. In regulatory consideration of microbiological quality, it is recognized that cosmetics are not expected to be sterile, but detectable microbes should be very few in numbers and should not include objectionable microorganisms (32). Excessive numbers are interpreted as indicating unsanitary, filthy manufacturing processes and presence of objectionable, potentially pathogenic, "objectional" microorganisms is seen as a direct threat to consumer safety. Microbiological standards identified by the US FDA establish a total microbial limit of 500 CFU/g for eye-area products and 1000 CFU/g for all other cosmetics (32). An exclusive list of objectionable microorganisms that would be of concern if detected is difficult if not impossible to assemble but would be expected to include

Staphylococcus aureus, *Streptococcus pyogenes*, *Pseudomonas aeruginosa*, and *Klebsiella pneumoniae* (32). A recent unpublished survey found typical industry specification to establish 100 CFU/g and absence of detected *Candida albicans*, *Staphylococcus aureus*, and Gram-negative bacteria (as a group).

Chemical Preservatives

Microbiological safety of cosmetics relies on a number of factors, and chemical preservation is clearly the most compelling. Although some historic cosmetics may have included ingredients of antimicrobial potential, the realization of chemical preservation as a necessary formulation element was a 20th-century realization with initial application of phenolics, organic acid, formaldehyde, and parabens (33,34). As GMPs and quality control testing were not in evidence at that time, it is assumed that early efforts for preservation were directed at mold contamination that developed on the surfaces of relevant cosmetics. Postwar expansion of the cosmetics industry in the 1950s and early 1960s was not accompanied by increasing control of microbiological quality. Reports of significant levels of contaminated products in both America and Europe (35,36,37) as well as a pivotal publication (8) reporting serious eye infection and blindness from contaminated mascaras provoked substantial regulatory concern and proposed intervention (38). Industry response was extensive and included introduction of new and very effective preservatives, some of which were based on formaldehyde release (Table 2.2,39). Especially in combination with parabens, formaldehyde-releasing preservatives became the staple for effective preservation. Methylchloroisothiazolinone (MCIT) was introduced in the late 1970s and expanded in the following decade to become the primary global preservative for rinse-off products—shampoos, conditioners, body washes, and liquid hand soaps. Sensitization concerns prevented MCIT use in leave-on products (40). The minor component of marketed MCIT, methylisothiazolinone (MIT), was introduced as a stand-alone preservative in the late 1990s and was promoted for use with both leave-on and rinse-off products based on safety assessment (41). A controversial 2001 publication provocative to human safety concerns for parabens (42) drove considerable interest in parabens replacements, especially in leave-on products. Many formulators chose MIT and to a lesser extent phenoxyethanol as paraben replacements. However,

TABLE 2.2

Preservatives in descending frequency of use for 2014 per FDA voluntary reporting program, summarized by Steinberg

Phenoxyethanol
Caprylyl glycol
Ethylhexyl Glycerine
Benzoic Acid/Sodium Benzoate
Benzyl Alcohol
Sorbic Acid/Potassium Sorbate
Methylchloroisothiazolinone/Methylisothiazolinone
Methylisothiazolinone
Methyl Paraben
Hexane Diol
Dehydroacetic Acid/Potassium Dehydroacetate
Propyl Paraben
Pentylene Glycol
Chlophenesin
Diazolidinyl Urea
DMDM Hydantion
Imidazolidinyl Urea

reports of MIT sensitization provoked a ban of its use in this application (43). The pursuit of parabens replacements and growing consumer interest in natural, organic, and formaldehyde-free products after the turn of the century drove much greater diversity into cosmetic preservative use.

Commonly Used Cosmetic Preservatives

The most recent (2018) survey of cosmetic preservative use as reported to the US FDA was that of Steinberg (39), which is summarized in Table 2.2. This section addresses preservatives of greatest reported use.

Parabens. These are esters of para-hydroxy benzoic acid including methyl, ethyl, propyl, isopropyl, and benzyl parabens with methyl parabens being historically the most commonly used cosmetic preservative. The mechanism of action for parabens has been attributed to a number of factors, including disruption of proton motive force and inhibition of transport (44). Parabens historically have been used in combinations (composed of dual/multiple parabens) especially with a formaldehyde-releasing preservative to preserve emulsion, leave-on and fine and color cosmetics at total parabens concentrations up to 8000 ppm (24,45,46). Short chain parabens are more effective versus bacteria and longer chain parabens fungi with the latter used at lesser levels due to their limited aqueous solubility (47). Parabens are active through pH range 3–8 and are used most effectively against Gram-positive bacteria and fungi (23,45). They are commonly used with formaldehyde releasers or phenoxyethanol to address their lesser efficacy against Gram-negative bacteria (24). Parabens are formulated with the heated water phase pre-emulsion or as premix solution in solubilizing product ingredients such as propylene glycol (45). Preservatives are most effective when solubilized in water phase. As parabens possess significant lipid solubility, especially longer-chain parabens, for efficacy it is essential that emulsions formulation maintain these preservatives in the water phase (45,16). Parabens show decreased efficacy above pH 8 due to the formation of the phenolate anion (pKa = 8.4) and undergo hydrolysis in highly acidic and basic solutions (45,48). They are physically compromised by cyclodextrins and nonionic surfactants (especially polysorbates) resulting in mitigated efficacy (45,49–51). Loss of efficacy in the presence of nonionic surfactants can be reduced by formulation with butylene glycol (45). Parabens (esp. methyl paraben) can undergo transesterification in the presence of some sugars and polyols (52) and can be absorbed by some tubing materials (53).

Formaldehyde-releasing preservatives. Formaldehyde as a stand-alone preservative was phased out in the mid-20th century and replaced by the so-called formaldehyde releasers introduced through 1960s and 1970s. With parabens, these became and remain central to many effective preservative systems. Efficacy of these preservatives is attributed to persistent release of low levels of formaldehyde (54) though some activity of the parent molecule has been reported (55). The dominant molecules of this group are imidazolidinyl urea, DMDM Hydantoin, diazolidinyl urea, and hydroxymethyl glycinate and are typically used at levels up to 3000 ppm across a broad pH range of rinse-off and leave-on products and color cosmetics (24,45). Most effective against Gram-negative bacteria, they are often formulated with parabens or organic acids to address fungal contamination (24). These formaldehyde-releasing preservative molecules are sensitive to heat and should be formulated at less than 70°C and in the water phase of emulsions as they are not soluble in the lipid phase and may not be adequately distributed if added to completed product (45). Formulators should be aware of potential perfume and sunscreen interactions that limit efficacy as well as reaction with some free amino acids and protein hydrolysates with both free formaldehyde and parent molecules (24,56–58). Formaldehyde-releasing preservatives should not be used with dehydroacetic acid (DHA) as free formaldehyde will accelerate DHA degradation (57).

Isothiazolinones. This class of preservatives is thought to function by interaction with thiol and amine groups (59). Methylchloroisothiazolinone (MCIT) was introduced in the late 1970s and became the dominant preservative for rinse-off products—shampoos, conditioners, body washes, and liquid detergent hand "soaps" (24). Concerns for sensitization have prevented its application in leave-on cosmetic products (40). Typically used at concentrations up to 7.5 ppm in acidic and neutral pH products, MCIT is unstable at alkaline pH especially in the presence of amines (59,60). MCIT is most efficacious against bacteria and, though rinse-off surfactant-based products are generally less susceptible to fungal contamination, is often combined with additional preservatives such as benzoic acid to expand efficacy against yeasts and mold (24,45). As a cosmetic raw material, MCIT is stabilized in a magnesium salt solution. Premix dilution in deionized water should be avoided due to stability concerns (59). The molecule is unstable in the presence of pyrithione zinc and reducing and oxidizing agents (45,59). Residual reducing agents in some surfactants have proven problematic and some surfactants themselves can also compromise stability (59,61). Formulation temperatures should be less than 50°C due to MCIT heat sensitivity (45,59). Some protein hydrolysates can mitigate efficacy (45), and combination of MCIT with DHA should be avoided as the magnesium salt of MCIT ingredient accelerates DHA degradation (62).

The marketed ingredient MCIT includes a largely ineffective level of Methylisothiazolinone (MI). Though requiring greater concentration, MI is much more stable than MCIT especially at higher pH and can be used effectively with a co-preservative targeting fungus (45). As noted previously, MI was introduced as a stand-alone preservative in the late 1990s and found rapid application as parabens replacement in leave-on products. Sensitization issues in this application resulted in significant regulatory restraints for its use.

Organic acids. These are some of the oldest cosmetic preservatives and currently include benzoic, sorbic, and dehydroacetic acids. Mode of action is generally attributed to factors such as disruption of proton motive force and acidification of cytoplasm (63). As antimicrobial activity is associated with the protonated molecule, these are primarily effective at pH less than or approximating their pKas (45,63). Used at concentrations up to 8000 ppm, they are primarily effective against Gram-positive bacteria and fungi (45). However, benzoic acid has been used as an effective co-preservative versus Gram-negative bacteria at near-neutral pH in some rinse-off, surfactant-based cosmetics. Foster et al. recently reported the combination establishes a significant increase in apparent pKa through interaction with surfactant micelles (64).This phenomenon with resulting greater efficacy challenges the long-held industry assumption that the pKa of benzoic acid remains at a constant 4.2 in all aqueous systems. Again, in surfactant-based products, benzoic acid with benzyl alcohol can establish synergistic efficacy against Gram-negative bacteria. Smauqi et al. (65) reported unexpected efficacy of organic acid combinations in olive oil emulsion using a modified, novel preservative effectiveness test. However, to address general Gram-negative bacterial risk, organic acids are routinely combined with formaldehyde releasers, phenoxyethanol, or MCIT (24). Combination with other preservatives is also important as organic acids can serve as substrate for microbial metabolism (45,66,67). Organic acid preservatives are routinely formulated as their respective sodium (benzoate and dehydroacetic) or potassium (sorbate) salts as these are much more soluble at the pH of a conventional cosmetic product formulation (45). Benzoic acid, and perhaps other organic acids, may be removed from aqueous solution by cyclodextrin and absorption by clays such as montmorillinote and some flexible tubing materials (68–70). Sorbic acid can undergo degradation with some amino acids, glycerol, and some salts (70). Further care should be taken with sorbic acid as it is prone to auto-oxidation especially at higher (less acidic) pH (71), a phenomenon accelerated by EDTA (ethylene diamine tetraacetic acid), a commonly used chealtor (72). Dehydroacetic acid should not be combined with formaldehyde releasers or MCIT due to reaction with free formaldehyde of the former and the stabilizing magnesium ion of the latter (73,74).

Alcohols. Included in this group are ethyl, phenoxyethyl and benzyl alcohols. Ethanol at higher levels is considered to function via dehydration and enzyme denaturation. At preservative levels ethanol as well as phenoxyethanol and benzyl alcohol are thought to disrupt cytoplasmic membrane integrity and oxidative phosphorylation (75–78). Ethyl alcohol effectively offers complete preservative capacity at concentrations of 20%, and lower levels can have some limited effect that can be useful if combined with other preservatives (78). Phenoxyethanol is a commonly used preservative and has found significantly greater application in recent decades as a parabens replacement (42,45). At concentrations up to 8000 ppm, phenoxyethanol is used primarily as an antibacterial preservative, importantly against Gram-negative bacteria, and is often combined with preservatives such as benzoic acid targeting fungi (24).

Benzyl alcohol is similarly effective at levels up to 8000 ppm though less effective against Gram-negative bacteria (45). Benzyl alcohol is often formulated with antioxidants such as tocopherol to address potential autocatalytic oxidation (39,77,79). Organic alcohols are most appropriately formulated in emulsion water phase to control potential partitioning into the lipid phase of emulsions (80). Though effective as preservatives, organic alcohols are readily biodegradable if used at low levels so are most appropriately used in combination with other preservatives (45,81,82). As with some organic acids, organic alcohols may be absorbed by some tubing materials (69).

Glycols. Although necessary concentrations typically compromise cosmetic acceptability, propylene glycol possesses a degree of antimicrobial efficacy via modulation of water activity (83). Lower concentrations may serve to improve efficacy of preservative systems. Similarly, lower concentrations of butylene glycol may facilitate preservation, especially in raw materials. Long-chain 1,2-glycols including pentylene, hexylene, and caprylyl glycols possess unique preservative efficacy potential that exceed modulation of water activity (84–86). Largely effective against bacteria, these are used in cosmetic preservative systems at concentrations 1–5% often with an antifungal preservative to establish broad spectrum efficacy (45,85,86).

Chlorphenesin. Chlorphenesin is used primarily in makeup and color cosmetics at concentrations up to 3000 ppm (45,87). Largely an antifungal preservative of limited effect against bacteria, chlorphenesin is more often used in preservative systems as a co-preservative or adjunct (87,88). It should not be confused with the pharmaceutical muscle relaxant chlorphenesin carbamate.

Iodopropynyl butyl carbamate (IPBC). This is a poorly soluble antifungal preservative typically used at levels up to 100 ppm. It is used with other preservatives such as isothiazolinones and formaldehyde releasers in combinations, some of which are claimed to be synergistic in efficacy (89). Owing to its poor water solubility, it is combined with glycols or other solubilizing vehicles for incorporation (45).

Preservative Combinations

"Broad spectrum" is a term commonly offered in marketing of commercial cosmetic preservatives. Rarely is this claim found to be effective in practice. Suppliers are not advertising falsely, rather the broad-spectrum efficacy claim is based on testing under ideal conditions. In application, differential efficacies against the range of relevant bacteria and fungi as well as formula parameters drive formulators to multiple preservative systems (24). The combination of a formaldehyde-releasing preservative and two or more parabens and the chelator EDTA serves as a classic example. This system had been the mainstay of leave-on cosmetic microbiological quality for many decades (24). Though marketing and literature instructed that use concentrations of each should be broadly and individually effective against Gram-positive and Gram-negative bacteria and fungi (90–92), practical experience both in testing and manufacturing quality consistently drove to combinations that exploited the primary efficacy of each against their most susceptible microbial target group. Some report such combinations to establishing synergy (93,94). Although valid synergy has been demonstrated (95), this conclusion is often more subjective than quantitative (96). In use, preservative systems not only offer greater assurance of efficacy, but by establishing multiple chemical barriers to contamination, provide greater hurdles to the development of preservative resistance and facilitate elimination of resistant contaminants (24,97–99). Also compelling to preservative combinations is the rapid development cycle of major manufacturers. In some formulations, single preservatives may be apparently sufficient in challenge testing, but a dual system of appropriate human safety assessment assures with each new formulation greater confidence of rapid clearance to market without engaging in preservative development. Whereas the literature reports a number of combinations showing increased efficacy (100–102), those enjoying continued, reliable success are few. Table 2.3 lists composition of current preservative systems established in major brands sold in mass market context. Although systems were chosen to show diversity and complexity of preservatives systems between product categories and among products in categories, Table 2.3 likely provides a more accurate indication of systemic preservative application than voluntary submission of formula data reported in Table 2.2. Factors driving diversity in preservative systems include unique formulation and packaging, divergent individual and corporate chemical-use policies and risk assessments. Against historic preservative combinations (24), parabens and formaldehyde-releasers find increasingly limited application, whereas organic alcohols and acids and phenoxyethanol find common use across many categories as does the chelator EDTA. MCIT continues to be frequently used in rinse-off products such as hand and body washes, shampoos, and conditioners. Typical of color cosmetics, powders preservative systems are complex and variable and product preservative systems in this category are quite variable in composition.

Preservative Adjuncts/Helpers

Nominal product preservatives are the primary drivers to antimicrobial efficacy. However, specific ingredients and general product formulation can substantially magnify preservation capabilities, for example, formulation and formula characteristic such as pH, water activity, order and condition of ingredient addition, and specific ingredients (24,43,102,103). Many of these, often termed "dual functional" ingredients, also are used in their functional roles as cosmetic ingredients. These will be discussed in a later chapter and are addressed further in Chapter 4 of this text.

Within the range of cosmetic-acceptability, pH manipulation alone will not serve as a primary preservative function (24). However, as noted in a previous section, efficacy of some preservatives is very much pH driven. Similarly, cosmetic acceptability generally eliminates water activity as a stand-alone cosmetic preservative mechanism, but its management can contribute to contamination protection (104). Gram-negative bacteria generally are the most frequent microbial contaminants of cosmetic products and are also more sensitive to reduced water activity (43,105). Product formulation itself can facilitate preservation. Water-in-oil emulsions are reportedly more resistant to in-use contamination (106,107), and manipulation of droplet size has been reported to facilitate preservation (108). Fungal contamination of shampoos or body washes is a very rare occurrence presumably due to surfactant content.

Specific, purpose-added ingredients inadequate as preservatives are known to facilitate effective preservation. The chelator EDTA is very effective as preservative adjunct. Although it does not possess stand-alone efficacy, EDTA adds significantly to the efficacy of preservative systems and can be found in many cosmetic products. In this context, it is presumed not only to sequester divalent cations necessary for microbial stability and metabolism, but also to destabilize bacterial capsules and biofilm, allowing better access of the preservative to the biological active (17,109,110). Other chelators such as phytic acid (hinokitol) and gluconolactone presumably offer similar effect (111,112) though the literature offers no compelling data regarding impact on efficacy. Similarly, the efficacy of pyrithione antimicrobials is at least in part associated with divalent cation sequestration (113). In addition to chelators, ingredient such as anisic and levulinic acids, ethyl hexyl glycerine, essential oils, and low levels of ethanol are used as preservative adjuncts (76,114,115,116). General formulation elements contributing to mitigated microbiological risks are also detailed in the relevant ISO guideline (117).

Strategic combinations of specific ingredients with selected formula parameters can be organized into a preservation concept often referred to as the "Hurdle" approach to preservation (89). Adapted from food preservation, this considers establishment of a series of moderate impediments to microbial survival and growth that, in combination, establish effective preservation. Descriptions in the literature and technical press offer Hurdle as replacement for traditional cosmetic preservative systems (117). However, review of preservative systems in marketed products found no apparent application of this approach to preservation (Table 2.3).

TABLE 2.3

Cosmetic preservative systems from major marketers sold in mass market outlet in 2020

Product	Category Preservative System
Shampoo	MCIT*/Na Benzoate/NaEDTA**
	Gluconolactone/Na Benzoate/NaEDTA
	Phenoxyethanol/Na Benzoate/Benzyl alcohol MCIT/DMDM Hydantoin/IPBC***
Conditioner	MCIT/Benzyl alcohol/NaEDTA
	Phenoxyethanol/Chlorhexidine
	MCIT/DMDM Hydantoin/NaEDTA
	Benzyl alcohol/Phenoxyethanol
Lotion	Benzyl alcohol
	Na Anisate/Na Levinate/Benzyl alcohol/Caprylyl glycol
	Phenoxyethanol/Hexylene glycol/DMDM Hydantoin
	Methyl and Propyl parabens/IPBC/NaEDTA
	DMDM Hydantoin/Methyl parabens/IPBC/NaEDTA
Cream	Benzyl alcohol/Phenoxyethanol
	Benzyl alcohol/Methyl, Propyl, and Ethyl parabens/EDTA
	Phenoxyethanol/Ethylhexyl glycerine/Anisic acid/Benzyl alcohol/EDTA
	Phenoxyethanol/Caprylyl glycol/Chlorphenesin/EDTA
Sunscreen	Diazolydinyl urea/Methyl and Propyl parabens
	Phenoxyethanol/Caprylyl glycol/Methyl and Propyl Parabens
	Phenoxyethanol/Methyl and Propyl parabens
	Phenoxyethanol/Ethyl hexylene/NaEDTA
Mascara	Phenoxyethanol/Phenylethyl alcohol/NaEDTA
	Phenoxyethanol/Caprylyl glycol/Na Dehydroacetate/NaEDTA
	Propyl paraben/Phenoxyethanol/Methyl, Butyl, and Ethyl Parabens
	Phenoxyethanol/Ethylhexyl glycerine
Pressed powder	Phenoxyethanol/Ethylhexyl glycerine
	Caprylyl glycol
	Methyl paraben
	Methyl and Propyl paraben, Na Dehydroacetate

* MCIT = Methylchloroisothiazolinone/Methyl isothiazolinone (3:1).

** NaEDTA = Sodium ethylene diamine tetraacetate.

*** IPBC = Iodopropynyl butyl carbamate.

Packaging. Product package is clearly the dominant yet least-recognized controlling element of quality. As a mechanical, physical barrier, packaging limits microbial compromise from the external, contaminated world to a level the chemical preservative system can overcome. In its typical design, the primary source of packaging risk lies in its product dispensing mechanism (118). For example, wide mouth jars of creams offer product exposure to hand and air microbes providing a contamination opportunity that may result in microbiological failure (14). The same product in a pump dispenser would offer greatly mitigated risk (21). Whereas well-preserved products will overcome simple exposure to microbes in the user environment, exposure to tap water as a result of compromised packaging offers a much more significant risk. As observed with shampoo used and stored in showers (14,119), tap water exposure will dilute preservative systems. As tap water typically includes Gram-negative microorganisms, especially *Pseudomonas aeruginosa* of special concern microbiological quality (32), the resulting diluted, inoculated product is at significant microbiological risk. Serious disease and even death have been attributed to infection from tap-water-associated shampoo contamination (12). Such waterborne contamination risk can be somewhat mitigated by increasingly robust preservative systems (14) and more effectively prevented by use of dispensing mechanisms that reduce the potential of water ingress. Active dispensing mechanisms such as pump dispensers and even aerosol assemblages further mitigate risk, especially if designed to prevent suck back and pooling of externalized product within the dispensing mechanisms (89,119). Presumably maximizing physical controls, some packaging is promoted as allowing "preservative-free" formulations. One such design assumes aseptic production and filling in a package designed to filter makeup air that enters the package as product is pumped out, removing potential contaminants (120). These have not found extensive use in cosmetics though initial protocols have been proposed to address their qualification (121). Catovic et al. (122) recently offered an in vitro protocol intended to address in-use product package/dispenser risks in context of low-level and even "preservative free" products and protective packaging. The proposed method uses a single isolate in model bacteriostatic formula, and packages are assigned to categories based on levels of microbial recovery after treatment per protocol. Whereas protective packaging anticipated by authors may well require lesser levels of preservation to protect product in use, validation offered appeared to be limited. An in-use study of greater power such as that of Brannan et al. (14) expanded to address global diversity of consumer use would be appropriate for confirmation of validation. Further, lesser preservation reasonably demands aseptic production, an expensive capacity not readily available in the cosmetic category.

Preservation during Manufacturing

Microbiological quality of finished cosmetic products is traditionally considered as preservative-driven and assessed via preservative challenge testing with potential validation by in-use testing (24). However, this chapter addresses finished product and presumes adequate manufacturing control. As many preservatives are most effectively added late in the formulating process, control of risk during manufacturing requires effective process design, good manufacturing practices, and effective operation (25). Even with these established, the product formulator is responsible to design a making process that minimizes risk. Unpreserved premixes and captured intermediates as well as flow paths—tubes, piping, heat exchangers for unpreserved ingredient combinations—provide the greatest risks in the context of nonsterile manufacturing. Effective mitigation of such risks is accomplished by careful process design that establishes microbiological control throughout the manufacturing steps by control of pH, water activity, heat, order of addition, residence times, and tactical addition of preservatives (24).

Overview

Effective preservation is the most compelling element of cosmetic microbiological safety. In this role, the preservative serves the unique role as the only cosmetic ingredient added exclusively for a safety purpose. As biologically active chemicals, preservatives can potentially impact human safety and therefore are used at low concentrations establishing relative limited antimicrobial capacity. By comparison, cosmetic preservatives fail to achieve in a month efficacy required of a disinfectant in less than ten minutes. As even 70% ethanol and hospital-grade disinfectants can suffer microbial contaminated (18,123), it is clear that preservation alone cannot ensure quality in the context of all potential manufacture scenarios, for example, significant Gram-negative bacterial contamination of purified water systems. Similarly, effective in the context of relevant package and consumer use, preservation will not ensure quality if the product is abused such as dilution with bacteria-laden tap water. Despite these limitations, preservatives and preservation offer the single element for quantitative assessment, and every cosmetic should include an appropriate formulation. Industry best practice directs the use of systems composed of multiple preservatives effective against the range of microbes as well as a chelator.

Whereas continued understanding has identified alternative approaches including natural and alternative preservatives, the "Hurdle" concept and preservative-free packages, conventional preservatives remain the primary means to microbiological safety. New chemicals continue to be proposed for this purpose (124), but few if any provide the confidence in efficacy obtained by traditional preservatives. This is significantly driven by the dynamic nature of cosmetic industry in which application of traditional preservative combinations reliably and effectively satisfies the rapid development cycle and critical speed to market demanded by this competitive business.

REFERENCES

1. Federal Food Drug and Cosmetic Act. 21 US Code. Subchapter VI. Sections 361–364.
2. Cavers, DF. The Food, Drug, and Cosmetic Act of 1938: its legislative history and its substantive provisions. *Law & Contemp Probs* 1939;6:2–42.
3. www.fda.gov/safety/recalls/enforcementreports/default.htm.
4. www.cosmeticseurope.eu/files/3714/6407/8024/Guidelines_for_the_Safety_Assessment_of_a_Cosmetic_Product_-_2004.pdf.
5. Periz G., Misock J, Huang MCJ, et al. FDA 2014 survey of eye area cosmetics for microbiological safety. *Lett Appl Microbiol* 2018;67:32–38.
6. Leyden JJ, Stewart R, Kligman AM. Experimental inoculation of *Pseudomonas aeruginosa* and *Pseudomonas cepacia* on human skin. *J Soc Cosmet Chem* 1980;31:19–28.
7. Eissa ME. Risk of infection from application of two types of pharmaceutical creams. *Eur Med Health Pharma J* 2018;10:1–4.
8. Wilson LA, Ahearn DG. Pseudomonas-induced corneal ulcers associated with contaminated eye mascaras. *Am J Ophthalm* 1977;84:112–119.
9. Álvarez-Lerma F, Maull E, Terradas R, et al. Moisturizing body milk as a reservoir of *Burkholderia cepacia*: outbreak of nosocomial infection in a multidisciplinary intensive care unit. *Critical Care* 2008 Feb;12(1):R10.
10. Irwin AE, Price CS. More than skin deep: moisturizing body milk and *Burkholderia cepacia*. *Crit Care* 2008;12:15.
11. Madani TA, Alsaedi S, James L, et al.. *Serratia marcescens*-contaminated baby shampoo causing an outbreak among newborns at King Abdulaziz University Hospital, Jeddah, Saudi. *Arab J Hosp Inf* 2011;78:16–19.
12. Fainstein V, Andres N, Umphrey J, et al. Hair clipping: another hazard for granulocytopenic patients? *J Inf Dis* 1988;158:655–656.
13. Gerba CP, Rose JB, Haas CN. Sensitive populations: who is at the greatest risk? *Int J Fd Microbiol* 1996;30:113–123.
14. Brannan DK, Dille JC, Kaufman DJ. Correlation of in vitro challenge testing with consumer use testing for cosmetic products. *Appl Env Microbiol* 1987;53:1827–1832.
15. Périamé M, Pagès JM, Davin-Regli A. *Enterobacter gergoviae* adaptation to preservatives commonly used in cosmetic industry. *Int J Comet Sci* 2014;36:386–395.
16. Patel NK, Romanowski JM. Heterogeneous systems II: influence of partitioning and molecular interactions on in vitro biologic activity of preservatives in emulsions. *J Pharm Sci* 1970;59: 372–376.
17. Hacking AJ, Taylor IWF, Jarman TR, et al. Alginate biosynthesis by *Pseudomonas mendocina*. *Microbiol* 1983;129:3473–3480.
18. Nasser RM, Rahi AC, Haddad MF, et al. Outbreak of *Burkholderia cepacia* bacteremia traced to contaminated hospital water used for dilution of an alcohol skin antiseptic. *Inf Cont Hosp Epidem* 2004;25:231–239.
19. Weber DJ, Rutala WA, Sickbert-Bennett EE. Outbreaks associated with contaminated antiseptics and disinfectants. *Antimic Ag Chemoth* 2007;51:4217–4224.
20. Garcia-San Miguel L, Sáez-Nieto JA, Medina MJ, Hernández SL, Sánchez-Romero I, Ganga B, Asensio Á. Contamination of liquid soap for hospital use with *Raoultella planticola*. *J Hospit Infec* 2014;86:219–220.
21. Braide W, Nwosu IL, Offor EIU, Popgbara LB, Awurum IN. Microbial quality of some topical pharmaceutical products sold in Abia state, Nigeria. *Int J Pharm and Therapeutics* 2012;2:26–37.
22. Wong S, Street D, Delgado SI, et al. Recalls of foods and cosmetics due to microbial contamination reported to the US Food and Drug Administration. *J Fd Protect* 2000;63:1113–1116.

23. Sutton S, Jimenez L. Microbiology – a review of reported recalls involving microbiological control 2004–2011 with emphasis on FDA considerations of "objectionable organisms". *Am Pharma Rev* 2012;15:42.

24. Geis PA, Preservation strategies. In Geis PA, ed. *Cosmetic Microbiology: A Practical Handbook*, 2nd edn. New York; Taylor & Francis 2006:163–180.

25. Mulhall R, Schmidt E, Brannan DK. Microbial environment of the manufacturing plant. In Geis PA, ed. Cosmetic Microbiology: A Practical Handbook, 2nd edn. New York; Taylor & Francis:73–96.

26. Van der Kooij D, Oranje JP, Hijnen WA. Growth of *Pseudomonas aeruginosa* in tap water in relation to utilization of substrates at concentrations of a few micrograms per liter. *Appl Env Microbiol* 1982;44:1086–1095.

27. Berkelman RL, Anderson RL, Davis BJ, et al. Intrinsic bacterial contamination of a commercial iodophor solution: investigation of the implicated manufacturing plant. *Appl Environ Microbiol* 1984;47:752–756

28. Schnürer J, Olsson J, Börjesson T. Fungal volatiles as indicators of food and feeds spoilage. *Fungal Gen Biol* 1999;27:209–217.

29. Stotzky G, Schenck S, Papaviza GC. Volatile organic compounds and microorganisms. *Crit Rev Microbiol* 1976:4:333–382.

30. Moss M. Bacterial pigments. *Microbiologist* 2002;3:10–12.

31. Spooner DF. Hazards associated with the microbiological contamination of cosmetics, toiletries and non-sterile pharmaceuticals. In Baird RM, Bloomfield SF, eds. *Microbial Quality Assurance in Pharmaceuticals, Cosmetics, and Toiletries*. New York; Taylor & Francis 1996:9–27.

32. FDA. Bacteriological Analytical Manual. Chapter 23.Microbiological Methods for Cosmetics. www.fda.gov/Food/FoodScienceResearch/LaboratoryMethods/ucm565586.htm.

33. Curry JC, Brannan DK, Geis PA. History of cosmetic microbiology. In Geis PA, ed. *Cosmetic Microbiology: A Practical Handbook,* 2nd edn. New York; Taylor & Francis 2006:3–18.

34. Orth DS, Garrett AW. A history of cosmetic microbiology in the United States. In Orth DS, Kabara JJ, Denyer SP, et al. eds. *Cosmetic and Drug Microbiology.* New York; Taylor & Francis 2006:33–44.

35. Smart R, Spooner DF. Microbiological spoilage in pharmaceuticals and cosmetics. *J Soc Cosmet Chem* 1972;23:721–737.

36. Dunnigan AP, Evans JR. Report of a special survey: microbiological contamination of topical drugs and cosmetics. *TGA Cosmet J* 1970;Winter:39–41.

37. Baker JH. That unwanted cosmetic ingredient: bacteria. *J Soc Cosmet Chem* 1959;10:133–143.

38. FDA draft monograph regulation – FDA questions adequacy of preservation of eye area cosmetics. Fed Reg October 11, 1977 (42 FR 54837).

39. Steinberg DC. Preservative update. Frequency of preservative use through 2018. *Cosmet Toiletries* 2019;134:69–74.

40. Heid SE, Kanti A, McNamee PM, et al. Consumer safety considerations of cosmetic preservation. In Geis PA, ed. *Cosmetic Microbiology: A Practical Handbook*, 2nd edn. New York; Taylor & Francis 2006:193–214.

41. Basketter DA, Rodford R, Kimber I, et al. Skin sensitization risk assessment: a comparative evaluation of 3 isothiazolinone biocides. *Cont Derm* 1999;40:150–154.

42. Darbre PD. Underarm cosmetics are a cause of breast cancer. *Eur J Cancer Prev* 2001;10:389–393.

43. European Commission. 2016. Commission Regulation (EU) 2016/1198 of 22 July 2016. Official J Europ. Union. https://eur-lex.europa.eu/legal-content/EN/TXT/?uri=CELEX%3A32016R1198.

44. Maillard JY. Bacterial target sites for biocide action. *J Appl Microbiol* 2002;92:16S–27S.

45. Steinberg DC, ed. *Preservatives for Cosmetics*, 2nd ed. Carol Stream, IL; Allured 1996:1–137.

46. Charnock C, Finsrud T. Combining esters of para-hydroxy benzoic acid (parabens) to achieve increased antimicrobial activity. *J Clin Pharm Therap* 2007;32:567–572

47. Giordano F, Bettini R, Donini C, et al. Physical properties of parabens and their mixtures: solubility in water, thermal behavior, and crystal structures. *J Pharm Sci* 1999;88:1210–1216.

48. Morteza PH, Reza FM, Nasrin S, et al. Deterioration of parabens in preserved magnesium hydroxide oral suspensions. *J Appl Sci* 2007;7:3322–3325.

49. Parker MS, Barnes M, Bradley TJ. The use of the Coulter counter to detect the inactivation of preservatives by a non-ionic surface-active agent. *J Pharm Pharmacol* 1966;18:103S–106S.

50. Chin YP, Mohamad S, Abas MRB. Removal of parabens from aqueous solution using β-cyclodextrin cross-linked polymer. *Int J Molec Sci* 2010;11:3459–3471.

51. Shimamoto, T, Mima H. Effect of polyols on the interaction of p-hydroxybenzoic acid esters with polyoxyethylene dodecyl ether. *Chem Pharma Bull* 1979;27:2602–2607.

52. Hensel A, Leisenheimer S, Müller A, et al. Transesterification reactions of parabens (alkyl 4-hydroxybenzoates) with polyols in aqueous solution. *J Pharma Sci* 1995;84:115–118.

53. Bahal SM, Romansky JM. Sorption of parabens by flexible tubings. *Pharm Dev Technol* 2001;6:431–440.

54. Lv C, Hou J, Xie W, et al. Investigation on formaldehyde release from preservatives in cosmetics. *Int J Cosmet Sci* 2015;37:474–478.

55. Kireche M, Peiffer JL, Antonios D, et al. Evidence for chemical and cellular reactivities of the formaldehyde releaser bronopol, independent of formaldehyde release. *Chem Resear in Toxicol* 2011;24:2115–2128.

56. Tome D, Naulet N. Carbon 13 nuclear magnetic resonance studies on formaldehyde reactions with polyfunctional amino acids. *Chem Biol Drug Design* 1981;17:501–507.

57. Rassat F, Gonzenbach H, Pittet GH. Use of sunscreen and vitamins in daily-use cosmetics. *Drug Cosmet Ind* 1997;December:16–20.

58. Kireche M, Gimenez-Arnau E, Lepoittevin JP. Preservatives in cosmetics: reactivity of allergenic formaldehyde-releasers towards amino acids through breakdown products other than formaldehyde. *Cont Derm* 2010;63:192–202.

59. Law AB. Kathon CG: a new single component, broad spectrum preservative for cosmetics and toiletries. In Kabara JJ, ed. *Cosmetics and Drug Preservation Principles and Practices*. New York; Marcel Dekker 1984:129–141.

60. Barman BN, Preston HG. The effects of pH on the degradation of isothiazolone biocides. *Tribol Int* 1992;25:281–287.

61. Ferm DJ, Griffin TS. Studies on the stability of Kathon® CG/ICP microbicide in alpha olefin sulfonate-based systems. *J Am Oil Chem Soc* 1990;67:116–122.

62. Bennassi CA, Semenzato A, Lucchiari M, et al. Dehydroacetic acid sodium salt stability in cosmetic preservative mixtures. *Int J Cosmet Sci* 1988;10:29–32.

63. Brul S, Coote P. Preservative agents in foods: mode of action and microbial resistance mechanisms. *Int J Fd Microbiol* 1999;50:1–17.

64. Foster S, Farrell B, Pippine K, Stokes R, Blankenship J, Yarnell A. Using Surfactants and Sodium Benzoate to Elevate Product Performance and Improve Preservation Efficacy. Society Cosmetic Chemists Technical Conference, New York, December 2019.

65. Smaqui S, Hlima HB, Kadri A. Effects of three acidic preservatives. *Household Pers Care Today* 2013;8:24–29.

66. Razika B, Abbes B, Messaoud C, et al. Phenol and benzoic acid degradation by *Pseudomonas aeruginosa*. *J Water Res Protect* 2010;2:788–791.

67. Melnick D, Luckmann FH, Gooding CM. Sorbic acid as a fungistatic agent for foods. VI. Metabolic degradation of sorbic acid in cheese by molds and the mechanism of mold inhibition. *J Fd Sci* 1954;19:44–58.

68. Yariv S, Russell JD, Farmer VC. Infrared study of the adsorption of benzoic acid and nitrobenzene in montmorillonite. *Israel J Chem* 1966;4:201–213.

69. Bahal SM, Romansky JM. Sorption of benzoic acid, sorbic acid, benzyl alcohol, and benzalkonium chloride by flexible tubing. *Pharma Dev Technol* 2002;7:49–58.

70. Huang MJ, Watts JD, Bodor N. Theoretical studies of inclusion complexes of α-and β-cyclodextrin with benzoic acid and phenol. *Int J Quantum Chem* 1997; 65:1135–1152.

71. Arya SS. Stability of sorbic acid in aqueous solutions. *J Ag Fd Chem* 1980;28:1246–1249.

72. Campos CA, Rojas AM, Gerschenson LN. Studies of the effect of ethylene diamine tetraacetic acid (EDTA) on sorbic acid degradation. *Fd Res Int* 1996;29:259–264.

73. Bennassi CA, Semenzato A, Lucchiari M, et al. Dehydroacetic acid sodium salt stability in cosmetic preservative mixtures. *Int J Cosmet Sci* 1988;10:29–32.

74. Benassi CA, Bettero A, Manzini P, et al. Interaction between dehydroacetic acid sodium salt and formaldehyde: structural identification of the product. *J Soc Cosmet Chem* 1998;39:85–92.

75. Lucchini JJ, Corre J, Cremieux A. Antibacterial activity of phenolic compounds and aromatic alcohols. *Res Microbiol* 1990;141:499–510.
76. Kalathenos P, Russell NJ. Ethanol as a food preservative. In *Food Preservatives*. Boston, MA; Springer 2003;196–217.
77. Lowe I, Southern J. The antimicrobial activity of phenoxyethanol in vaccines. *Lett Appl Microbiol* 1994;8:115–116.
78. Bandelin FJ. Antibacterial and preservative properties of alcohols. *Cosmet Toilet* 1977;92:59–70.
79. Abend AM, Chung L, Bibart RT, et al. Concerning the stability of benzyl alcohol: formation of ben-zaldehyde dibenzyl acetal under aerobic conditions. *J Pharma Biomed Anal* 2004;34:957–962.
80. Puschmann J, Herbig ME, Müller-Goymann CC. Correlation of antimicrobial effects of phenoxyethanol with its free concentration in the water phase of o/w-emulsion gels. *Eu J Pharmac Biopharm* 2018;131:152–161.
81. Frings J, Schink B. Fermentation of phenoxyethanol to phenol and acetate by a homoacetogenic bac-terium. *Archiv Microbiol* 1994;162:199–204.
82. Basu A, Dixit SS, Phale, PS. Metabolism of benzyl alcohol via catechol ortho-pathway in methylnaphthalene-degrading Pseudomonas putida CSV86. *Appl Microbiol Biotech* 2003;62:579–585.
83. Kinnunen T, Koskela M. Antibacterial and antifungal properties of propylene glycol, hexylene glycol, and 1, 3-butylene glycol in vitro. *Acta Derm Venereol* 1991;71:148–150.
84. Shin KH, Kwack IY, Lee SW, et al. Effects of polyols on antimicrobial and preservative efficacy in cosmetics. *J Soc Cosmet Sci Korea* 2007;33:111–115.
85. Roden K. A rational approach to the preservative conundrum: preservatives. *S African Pharma Cosmet Rev* 2015;42:20–22.
86. Lawan K, Kanlayavattanakul M, Lourith, N. Antimicrobial efficacy of caprylyl glycol and ethylhexylglycerine in emulsion. *J Health Res* 2009;23:1–3.
87. Schnittger S. Introduction to the preservation of makeup type products. In Orth DS, Kabara JJ, Denyer SP, et al. eds. *Cosmetic and Drug Microbiology.* New York; Taylor & Francis 2006:145–154.
88. Roden K. Preservatives in personal care products. *Microbiol Australia* 2010;31:195–197.
89. Papageorgiou S, Varvaresou A, Tsirivas E, Demetzos C. New alternatives to cosmetics preservation. *J Cosmet Sci* 2010:61:107.
90. Rosen WE, Berke PA. Germall 115: a safe and effective preservative. In Kabara JJ, ed. *Cosmetic and Drug Preservation.* New York; Marcel Dekker 1984:191–208..
91. Haag T, Loncrini DF. Esters of para-hydroxybenzoic acid. In Kabara JJ, ed. *Cosmetic and Drug Preservation.* New York; Marcel Dekker 1984:63–77.
92. Hall AL. Cosmetically acceptable phenoxyethanol. In Kabara JJ, ed. *Cosmetic and Drug Preservation.* New York; Marcel Dekker 1984:79–108.
93. Neza E, Centini M. Microbiologically contaminated and over-preserved cosmetic products according Rapex 2008–2014. *Cosmetics* 2016;3:3–14.
94. Elder T, Lindstrom S, Ravita T. Diazolidinyl urea and iodopropynyl butylcarbamate: A synergistic blend. *Cosmetics and Toiletries* 1997;112:73–81.
95. Denyer SP, Hugo WB, Harding VD. Synergy in preservative combinations. *Int J Pharma* 1985;25:245–253
96. Lintner K, Genet V. A physical method for preservation of cosmetic products. *Int J Cosmet Sci* 1998;20:103–115.
97. Richards RME. Inactivation of resistant Pseudomonas aeruginosa by antibacterial combinations. *J Pharma Pharmacol* 1971;23:136S–140S.
98. Toler JC. Preservative stability and preservative systems. *Int J Cosmet Sci* 1985;7:157–164.
99. Rushton L, Sass A, Baldwin A, et al. A key role for efflux in the preservative susceptibility and adaptive resistance of *Burkholderia cepacia* complex bacteria. *Antimic Ag Chemother* 2013;57:2972–2980.
100. Ziosi P, Manfredini S, Vandini A, et al. Caprylyl glycol/phenethyl alcohol blend for alternative preser-vation of cosmetics. *Cosmet Toilet* 2013;128:538–551.
101. Lawan K, Kanlayavattanakul M, Lourith N. Antimicrobial efficacy of caprylyl glycol and ethylhexylglycerine in emulsion. *J Health Res* 2009;23:1–3.
102. Denyer SP, King RO. Development of preservative systems. In Baird RM, Bloomfield SF, eds. *Microbial Quality Assurance in Cosmetics, Toiletries and Non-sterile Pharmaceuticals*, 2nd edn. London; Taylor & Francis 1996:133–147.

103. Orth DS, Lutes-Anderson CM, Smith DK, et al. Synergism of preservative system components: use of the survival curve slope method to demonstrate anti-Pseudomonas synergy of methyl paraben and acrylic acid homopolymer/copolymers in vitro. *J. Soc. Cosmet. Chem* 1989;40:347–365.

104. Enigl DC, Sorrells KM. Water activity and self-preserving formulas. In Kabara JJ, ed. *Preservative-Free and Self-Preserving Cosmetics and Drugs: Principles and Practices.* New York; Marcel Dekker 1997:45–74.

105. Grant WD. Life at low water activity. Phil Trans Royal Soc. London B: *Biol* Sci 2004;359:1249–1267.

106. Schnittger S, Sabourin J, King D. Preservation of water-in-silicone emulsions. *J Cosmet Sci* 2002;53:78–80.

107. Varvaresou A. Papageorgiou S, Tsirivas E, et al. Self-preserving cosmetics. *Int J Cosmet Sci* 2009;31:163–175.

108. Fang B, Yu M, Zhang W, Wang F. A new alternative to cosmetics preservation and the effect of the particle size of the emulsion droplets on preservation efficacy. *Int J Cosmet Sci* 2016;38:496–503.

109. Lambert RJW, Hanlon GW, Denyer SP. The synergistic effect of EDTA/antimicrobial combinations on *Pseudomonas aeruginosa. J Appl Microbiol* 2004;96:244–253.

110. Kabara JJ. Chelating agents as preservative potentiators. In Kabara JJ, ed. *Preservative-Free and Self-Preserving Cosmetics and Drugs: Principles and Practices.* New York; Marcel Dekker 1997:209–226.

111. Nassar RI, Nassar M. Antimicrobial effect of phytic acid on *Enterococcus faecalis. Int Arabic J Antimic Ag* 2017;6:1–7.

112. Kornhauser A, Coelho S, Hearing V. Applications of hydroxy acids: classification; mechanisms; and photoactivity. *Clin Cosmet Investig Dermatol* 2010;20: 35–142.

113. Khattar MM, Salt WG, Stretton RJ. The influence of pyrithione on the growth of micro-organisms. *J Appl Bacteriol* 1988;64:265–272.

114. Papageorgiou S, Varvaresou A, Tsirivas E, et al. New alternatives to cosmetics preservation. *J Cosmet Sci* 2010;61:107–123.

115. Langsrud S, Steinhauer K, Lüthje S, et al. Ethylhexylglycerin impairs membrane integrity and enhances the lethal effect of phenoxyethanol. *PloS one* 2016 Oct 26;11(10):e0165228.

116. Siegert W. Preservative trends in wet wipes. *SOFW Journal* 2011;137:44–51.

117. International Standards Organization. ISO 29621:2017. Cosmetics — Microbiology — Guidelines for the risk assessment and identification of microbiologically low-risk products.

118. Kabara JJ. Hurdle Technology: are biocides always necessary for product protection? *J Appl Cosmet* 1999:17:102–109.

119. Brannan DK. The role of packaging in product preservation. In Kabara JJ, ed. *Preservative-Free and Self-Preserving Cosmetics and Drugs: Principles and Practices.* New York; Marcel Dekker 1997:227–243.

120. Brannan DK, Dille JC. Type of closure prevents microbial contamination of cosmetics during consumer use. *Appl Environ Microbiol* 1990:56:1476–1479.

121. Marx D, Birkhoff M. Multi-Dose Container for Nasal and Ophthalmic Drugs: A Preservative-Free Future? In Chris R, ed. *Drug Development – A Case Study Based Insight into Modern Strategies* 2011 Dec 7. ISBN: 978-953-307-257-9, In-Tech, DOI: 10.5772/27767.

122. Catovic C, Martin S, Desaint S, et al. Development of a standardized method to evaluate the protective efficiency of cosmetic packaging against microbial contamination. *AMB Express* 2020 Dec;10(1):1–10.

123. Devlieghere F, De Loy-Hendrickx A, Rademaker M, et al. A new protocol for evaluating the efficacy of some dispensing systems of a packaging in the microbial protection of water-based preservative-free cosmetic products. *Int J Cosmet Sci* 2015;37:627–635.

124. Wesgate R, Menard-Szczebara F, Khodr A, et al. Hydroxyethoxy phenyl butanone, a new cosmetic preservative, does not cause bacterial cross-resistance to antimicrobials. *J Medic Microbiol* 2020 Mar 18:jmm001147.

3

Natural Preservatives

Terry L. Amoroso

Introduction

In developing a preservation system, the goal of the R&D microbiologist is to ensure the microbial integrity of the product throughout its life cycle. Microbial integrity means that the product, as manufactured and during intended consumer use, should remain safe for use and be adequately resistant to loss of product stability/function. Strong advocacy can be found for both natural and synthetic preservation approaches. Consumers tend to embrace natural materials as part of their product consumption world, because it allows for a more connected perspective to the already complex ingredient labeling on many products. R&D microbiologists may be more enthusiastic for synthetic preservatives, given their historical vetting, very predictable application, proven efficacy, and product compatibility compared to natural materials.

Numerous factors may impact the overall strategy in establishing a sustainable preservation system, as shown in Figure 3.1. These factors will be in a constant and, hopefully, healthy tension. Some factors (e.g., safety, preservative efficacy, regulatory compliance) represent baseline requirements and expectations of responsible cosmetic manufacturing. Other factors (e.g., cost, consumer perception, marketing strategy) may have a wider flexibility. This chapter will not attempt to position whether using natural preservatives, synthetic preservatives, or a combination of the two is best in achieving microbial integrity. Rather, the intent of this chapter is to provide perspective on some of the challenges in the application of natural preservatives in cosmetics (using botanical extracts as a primary lens for the discussion), and to give a very brief survey of some current and potential natural preservative approaches.

The Need for Cosmetic Preservation

Responsible cosmetic manufacturers operate facilities which have undergone appropriate qualifications and validations (e.g., cleaning and sanitization). These facilities are well controlled and continually monitored to ensure an appropriate manufacturing environment. Cosmetics are not required to be produced in a sterile environment, nor are the starting materials used to batch the product required to

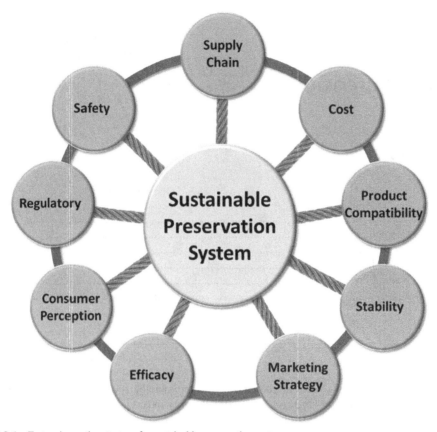

FIGURE 3.1 Factors impacting strategy for sustainable preservation systems.

be sterile. Even under highly controlled conditions, cosmetic formulations may be exposed to transient, low level contaminations during their life cycle. For many cosmetic products, this type of exposure will routinely occur via ongoing human-mediated contamination as a normal part of consumer habits and practices (CHPs) during product application (e.g., hand dispensing and application) and storage (e.g., in humid, warm environments like bathrooms). Preservative systems are central to ensuring the microbial integrity of cosmetic products during intended CHPs.

There are many ways a robust preservative system can be established in a cosmetic product. The approach may range from a single hostility driver (e.g., an added preservative), to a synergistic combination of added preservative chemistry/potentiator/intrinsic hostility (e.g., preservative, chelator, and low pH), to a highly integrated hurdle-based combination of added preservative chemistry, intrinsic hostility, potentiator, packaging, and processing.

Compared to the foods product category, cosmetics have a more complex and uncharacterized set of preservation drivers. Preservation approaches for the cosmetic industry have historically converged toward a strong reliance on a limited number of synthetic, well-defined preservative chemistries. Several factors related to the nature of cosmetics versus foods or pharmaceuticals tend to drive cosmetic preservation toward favoring synthetic chemistries (Figure 3.2).

Many of the recent mainstream cosmetic preservative chemistries—parabens, formaldehyde donors, and isothiazolinones—are regarded as high-profile ingredients (HPI), based on their continuing regulatory, scientific, and public scrutiny. Some of these evaluations have been scientifically based, well-vetted, and critically reviewed and credentialed; others have not. The result from a consumer standpoint can be a complex and often highly conflicting set of perspectives. This confusion, in turn, has positioned the role and concept of preservation itself, which on its face should be a highly desirable product aspect, to a relatively negative perspective.

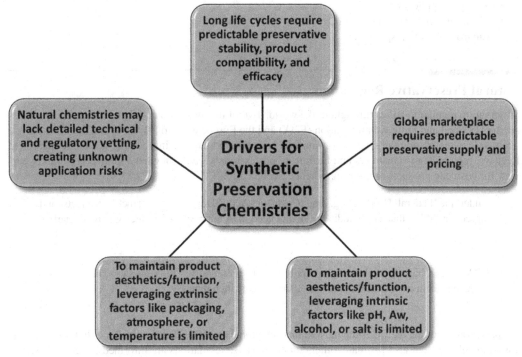

FIGURE 3.2   Drivers for synthetic chemistries in cosmetics.

Consequently, consumer interest has grown for natural preservation to help eliminate some of the concerns of synthetic preservatives, both real and perceived, and to get a better grounding into the myriad of ingredients typically found in the cosmetic products they use on a daily basis.

Consumer Perspective

Public scrutiny of preservation and the ability to access information and opinion on current preservation practices in food, cosmetic, and drug products have reached unprecedented levels, driven by the ever-broadening communication highway of the internet, combined with the vibrant information-push aspects of social media. Much of this content is unfiltered, with regulatory bodies, regulatory influencers, trade associations, companies, entrepreneurs, governmental organizations, non-governmental organizations (NGOs), health professionals, and individuals each adding to the message. The basis of these perspectives ranges from highly vetted and credentialed peer-reviewed scientific studies to personal opinions via a blog or a website. Given the often widely conflicting positions on the numerous aspects of preservation, the consumer has a difficult task in sifting through all the inputs to come to a well-grounded conclusion. The confusion can be further propagated within the scientific community, where different parties with well-regarded expertise may analyze the same studies and datasets, yet offer widely differing conclusions on the safety and appropriate application of preservatives.

Both natural and synthetic materials are carved from the same set of elements and each category can claim its share of great successes and great failings. While companies and marketing organizations often advocate for "natural" components as a trustworthy and safe approach, they are also subject to the tensions in Figure 3.1 when developing products. Consumers generally have a strong advocacy for natural ingredients, fostered by decades in which "synthetic chemicals" have been portrayed as undesirable (often deserved) and based on the following factors and perceptions:

- More trustworthy
- Greater understanding as to the constituents of the product

- Safety of application
- Limiting exposure to harmful ingredients
- Environmentally responsible.

Natural Preservative Regulation

Preservation regulation varies throughout the world. Two of the most influential global regulatory bodies are the US Food and Drug Administration (FDA) and the European Union (EU). While the FDA plays a strong role in monitoring the safety of on-market cosmetic products (via inspections, Cosmetic Ingredient Reviews, reports from consumers and healthcare professionals, etc.), they have limited pre-market purview for cosmetic products or their ingredients. Specifically:

> Under the Federal Food, Drug, and Cosmetic Act (FD&C Act), cosmetic products and ingredients, other than color additives, do not need FDA approval before they go on the market.
>
> ...
>
> FDA doesn't have special rules that apply only to preservatives in cosmetics. The law treats preservatives in cosmetics the same as other cosmetic ingredients.

(1)

For preservative usage, the EU is the most influential global regulator. This is true not only for the nations within its alliance, but also for many other countries whose regulations are informed by EU policy. The EU has established Annex V, of Regulation (EC) No 1223/2009 ("Cosmetics Regulation"), with a list of allowable preservatives. While Annex V lists over 50 preservatives, a much smaller subset of the chemistries are considered practical by manufacturers for broad product and geographical application. The most commonly used chemistries, namely parabens, formaldehyde donors, the isothiazolinones, and alcohols, have been under consistent pressure for either reducing or eliminating their use. Even when chemistries are deemed safe for use at efficacious levels, the underlying negative perception of preservation in general, may limit their application from a consumer and marketing acceptance viewpoint.

The current preservation option dynamic has also driven interest in the use of multifunctional ingredients. Multifunctionals have a primary product functionality (e.g., emollience), while also providing a potentially significant contribution to product preservation. With the current focus on ingredient/function transparency, and the cosmetics industry eager for consumers to more readily embrace preservation as beneficial, there has been vibrant discussion on how best to leverage multifunctionals within an appropriate regulatory framework. Overall, the current gamut of uncertainties on preservatives and their regulation has been a major driving force in directing focus on natural preservatives as an alternative approach to traditional preservation systems.

With this brief background to the dynamics of natural preservatives versus synthetic preservatives, the following sections address aspects for the use of natural preservatives, as well as some common current and potential approaches. The section on botanical extracts is the most expansive in terms of perspective for use, application, and management, given the long history and prevalence of their use. The principles of this perspective may also have application for other categories of natural preservatives.

Categories of Natural Preservatives

Botanical Extracts

Introduction

Life forms have defense mechanisms to help compete in their ecology and ensure survival and proliferation. For plants, mechanisms have evolved to defend against numerous potential threats, including animal, insect, and microbial invasion. One strategy that plants use to counter microbial invasion is the production of a wide variety of compounds which have antimicrobial activity (2) against a broad array of organisms. As a result, botanical extracts have played a large part in the very first applications of antimicrobials:

- Serving as the first crude medicinal preparations to fight infections and playing a strong role in drug discovery efforts for antimicrobial compounds.
- Serving as a major means of preserving foods; spices in particular have served dual roles of imparting desirable flavor while also providing protection from microbial decay.

Perspectives on Use

Historically, the initial application of material with some observed or proposed activity (e.g., antimicrobial, medicinal) has been via a relativity undefined form—an extract, a solution, or a mixture. Modern science has provided the means to better understand identification of the active and mechanism of action at the molecular level. Molecular-level understanding has provided the basis for evaluating modern human concerns for safety, allergenicity, toxicity, and so on, as well as modern market concerns for availability, consistency, compatibility, and cost. For cosmetics, this approach has fostered the use of very defined preservation chemistries, and the basis for a working knowledge on how to best use them to complement intrinsic (e.g., pH, Aw) and extrinsic (e.g., packaging) product properties. The following section addresses the challenges of using natural preparations or source materials, such as spices and botanical extracts, for the purposes of preservation.

Sustainable Application

The preservative efficacy of a product must be established to ensure that it will remain microbially robust throughout its product life cycle. One of the primary challenges associated with using botanical extracts as preservatives is the consistency, predictability, and stability of its preservative capacity.

Preservative preparations derived from natural materials will have inherent variations in their compositions based on geographic, seasonal, and species variations. Even with a consistent starting material, further variation may be introduced by the processes used to concentrate and isolate active materials. Methods as diverse as solvent extraction, supercritical fluid extraction, steam distillation, and solid phase extraction may be used. Process conditions can affect the efficiency of the active(s) extraction, final concentrations of various extract components, and the presence and concentration of other components aside from the active.

Use of botanically derived materials is further complicated in that the specific hostility driver(s) may either be unknown or may only been generally be partially characterized or understood. This lack of understanding results in several challenges not usually issues with highly characterized preservative chemistries:

- Assays/metrics to measure the nature and range of seasonal/varietal/geographic variations may be difficult to establish.
- The mechanism of action (MOA) may not be understood, limiting the ability to leverage intrinsic properties of the product to optimize preservation compared to highly characterized preservatives (e.g., adjusting pH toward pKa values for organic acids to optimize activity).
- The impact of processing conditions (whether those used to prepare the extract or as part of product batching) on preservation capacity may be difficult to assess.
- Stability of the hostility drivers may be difficult to establish.
- Variable levels or undefined hostility factors could potentially call into question whether the product release method is suited to purpose for detecting microbial bioburden.

Just as it may be difficult to manage preservative capacity, there may be other factors which can create complexity in using natural extracts. These include:

- It may also be difficult to fully predict how other ingredients within the extract may introduce artifacts or other concerns. These include ingredients which may affect or degrade key product aesthetics (appearance, color, odor, phase stability, and texture). The potential for unintended effects may be particularly relevant with natural extracts, since they are often needed at higher concentrations than synthetic preservatives to be sufficiently effective.
- Compatibility with specific product function.
- Compatibility of the active(s) to the manufacturing process.
- Supply sufficiency since global or high-volume products require a supply chain which can sustainably provide sufficient supply of active preservative, regardless of seasonal supply or unforeseen agricultural outages (3).
- Achieving a defined preservative effectiveness using extracts typically cost more based on the price of raw materials and the higher levels of usage required.

Application of natural extracts as a primary or supplementary means of product preservation presents challenges for consistent use and sustainability across the product life cycle. In this respect, using a botanical extract for preservation would require a more deliberate integration into the product design, with far less latitude than synthetic preservatives to "drop in" once the product components and aesthetics have already been established.

Similarly, developing an ideal cosmetic preservative from natural materials can also be an arduous process (4), consisting of a number of time- and resource-intensive phases. These would include identifying appropriate and sustainable source materials, establishing an appropriate extraction process and activity assay, identifying actives, establishing compatibility in product matrices, and ensuring that the extract will comply with necessary safety and regulatory requirements. Appreciation for these steps provides a calibration for the time, investment, and commercial risk that companies and preservative houses must assume in hopes that an effective and commercially viable natural preservative may be developed and marketed.

Effective Concentrations

Most literature on the antimicrobial activity of preservatives, including natural preservatives, will provide detail on the spectrum of effectiveness (bacterial, fungal, viral, etc.,), inhibitory or cidal concentrations/ranges, and the methodology used to establish these concentrations. The two major methods for quantifying activity are some form of either a disc/well diffusion on an agar plate or a dilution in a nutrient broth. Even with defined single synthetic molecules there can be considerable variation in determining the minimum inhibitory concentration (MIC). Sources of this variability include analyst technique, inherent variations in microbial strains and culture preparation, media choice and preparation, data interpretation, and so on.

Establishing consistent and predictable inhibitory/cidal concentrations for botanical extracts is even more difficult given the innate variability of the extracts themselves. In their review of literature on tea tree oil, Carson et al (2006) reported MICs for a given bacterial species varied routinely by tenfold, with the highest MIC variation spanning a more than a three hundredfold difference (5). The reported variation in MIC against a single species provides insight into the difficulty for an R&D microbiologist trying to establish a sustainable preservative capacity appropriate in a complex product against a potentially broad spectrum of bacteria and fungi.

For these reasons, this chapter will not attempt to provide guidance on target concentrations for a given type of botanical extract. Such guidance would inevitably provide only a narrow slant of the available scientific literature, and would be biased based on technique, botanical preparation, biological variation, product effects, and so on. The preservation practitioner is encouraged to thoroughly vet the literature for initial guidance and to collaborate with preservative suppliers and developers to establish the correct scientific approach on feasibility of application and credentialing of preservation sustainability. As with more defined and traditional preservative approaches, the qualification of a preservation system based on botanical extracts will necessitate an understanding of the starting material product and process variables, a clear and definitive preservative strategy and success criteria, and the development of solid data to establish confidence in the microbial integrity for the marketed product.

Major Drivers of Antimicrobial Activity

Although there is an incredibly broad range of compounds produced by plants, two broad categories which are particularly prominent in driving the antimicrobial activity associated with botanical extracts are the terpenes and the phenolic compounds.

Terpenes/Terpenoids

Terpenoids represent a diverse class of molecules and are a primary constituent of essential oils. Terpenoids are variations on terpenes $(C_5H_8)_n$, where methyl groups have been replaced with additional functional groups such as alcohols, ketones, or aldehydes. Common terpenes with antimicrobial activity include limonene, terpinen-4-ol (5), geraniol (6), and menthol (Figure 3.3). Most terpenoids are colorless, and many have characteristic odors which must be accommodated for in the final product form. They tend to have low solubility in water and are commonly soluble in alcohols and other organic solvents.

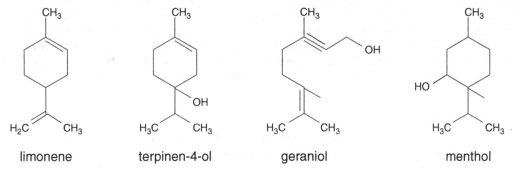

FIGURE 3.3   Terpenes with antimicrobial activity commonly found in botanicals.

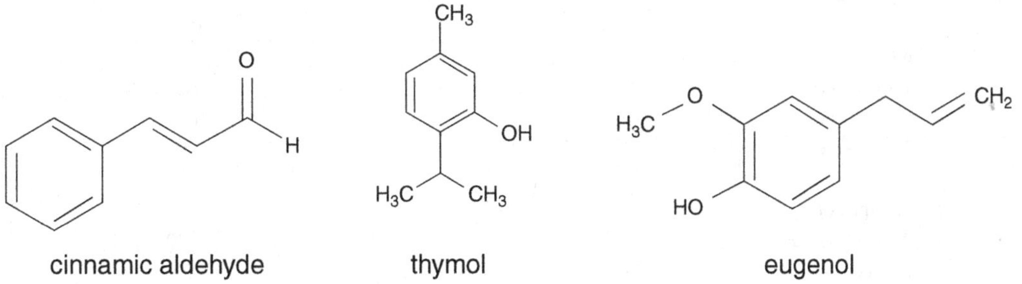

FIGURE 3.4   Phenolics with antimicrobial activity commonly found in botanicals.

Phenolics

Phenolic compounds are a second major class responsible for driving antimicrobial activity in botanical extracts (Figure 3.4). They contain one or more aromatic rings which bear one or more hydroxy groups. The simplest of these compounds is phenol which consists of a single aromatic ring and one hydroxy group. Complex phenolics may contain multiple ring structures, creating complex polymer structures. Common examples of phenolics with antimicrobial activity include thymol, cinnamic acid, and eugenol.

Selected Botanical Extracts

Tea Tree Oil

Tea tree oil (TTO) is an essential oil extracted by steam distillation of the leaves of *Melaleuca alternifolia*, the tea tree, native to Australia. TTO is a straw-colored mixture, consisting of a complex mixture of compounds. Depending on the initial source, there may be more than a hundred components (7). Batch-to-batch variation may be considerable. In an effort to bring some degree of consistency in its manufacture and composition, the International Organization for Standardization (ISO) has established a standard definition for TTO, listing 14 components and their concentration minimums, making TTO a relatively standardized extract (Table 3.1) (8). Numerous studies have been conducted demonstrating the antibacterial and antifungal activity of TTO (5). The antimicrobial activity is driven by the presence of terpenes and their associated alcohols (9). The majority of antimicrobial activity is attributed to terpinen-4-ol, the highest concentration component of TTO. Other components, in particular the terpenes, undoubtedly contribute to the overall antimicrobial activity, but the degree of contribution is complex, and leveraging potential synergy requires further study.

Formulating products using TTO presents challenges, including understanding the concentration, activity, and stability of its components, miscibility of the extract into aqueous-based products, minimizing potential integration of TTO into packaging components, and integrating the characteristic turpentine-like odor. As with many extracts, considerably higher doses of TTO (typically in the range of several %) are necessary to approach the antimicrobial activity demonstrated by synthetic preservative chemistries (typically in the 0.1% range or lower). A query of the Mintel Global New Product Database demonstrated application of TTO in products ranging from hand lotions to shaving preps.

TABLE 3.1

Components and their minimum levels in tea tree oil as defined by ISO

Component	Minimum %
α-Pinene	1.00
Sabinene	Traces
α-Terpinene	6
Limonene	0.5
p-Cymene	0.5
1,8-Cineole	Traces
γ-Terpinene	14
Terpinolene	1.5
Terpinen-4-ol	35
α-Terpineol	2
Aromadendrene	0.20
Ledene	0.10
δ-Cadinene	0.2
Globulol	Traces
Viridiflorol	Traces

Neem Oil

Neem oil is extracted from the fruit and seeds of the neem tree (*Azadirachta indica*), commonly found in India. The extract has a number of terpene and phenolic species which account for its antimicrobial activity. Of particular interest is the association of chewing neem sticks or bark for enabling the inhibition of colonization of Streptococcus mutans on tooth surfaces (10). Depending on the part of the plant used for the preparation, there may be well over a 100 compounds in a given extract (11). The compounds responsible for antimicrobial activity have been attributed to nimbidin and azadirachtin, with nimbinin (12) the primary activity being directed toward Gram-positive organisms (13).

Usnic Acid

A secondary metabolite derived from lichen, usnic acid has been reported to have antimicrobial activity against Gram-positive bacteria and yeast (14), as well as being a potential disrupter of biofilms.

Spice/Herbal Extracts and Essential Oils

There are numerous spices and herbs that contain compounds with antimicrobial activity (2,15–17) (Table 3.2). As noted, there are a variety of antimicrobial compounds such as terpenes, phenolics, and flavonoids present in these materials which may contribute to the observed inhibition. Each of these will have specific aspects of application, spectrum of activity, effectiveness, and so on. There are numerous suppliers of extracts and essential oils, both as blends and single-source materials. The practitioner should vet the scientific literature, technical information and specification from vendors, and regulatory/safety source materials as part of the due diligence to applying botanical extracts to product formulation and in establishing the framework for labelling.

There is widely varying information available for most botanical extracts, reflecting the various aspects of extracts sourcing and manufacturing as mentioned earlier. It is contingent on the practitioner to ensure these materials are credentialed appropriately to establish a robust preservative system. Some of these materials have a fairly strong foundation of efficacy, and there has been sufficient scientific vetting to establish confidence for use. Other materials may be more questionable. For example, grapefruit seed extract has had a particular challenging path for scientific validation. Several studies have concluded that the observed antimicrobial activity comes from materials (e.g., benzethonium chloride) other than those which would be found naturally in the source material (18). With all of these extracts, confidence in use as natural preservatives will be increased via in-depth detail on actives and mechanism of action.

Organic Acids

The use of acids as antimicrobials is among the most ancient of practices, with fermentation being one of the very first mechanisms of preservation. Once the nature of the microbial membrane was elucidated as being a lipid bilayer carrying a negative charge and that the interior of the cell maintained a pH relatively

TABLE 3.2

Some spices and herbs containing antimicrobial compounds

Almond	Fennel	Licorice	Paprika
Anise	Garlic	Mace	Pepper
Basil	Ginger	Marjoram	Peppermint
Cardamom	Horseradish	Mustard	Rosemary
Cinnamon	Lavender	Onion	Sage
Clove	Lemon	Oregano	Thyme
Coriander	Lime	Orange	Turmeric

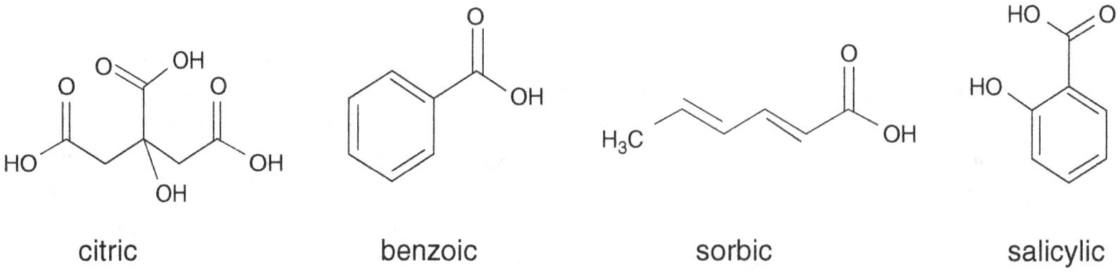

FIGURE 3.5 Organic acids commonly used as preservatives in cosmetics.

neutral to the surrounding media, the relationship between pH and the efficacy of organic acid became clear. To be effective, acids must gain the interior of the microbial cell where subsequent acidification of the cytoplasm can then elicit inhibitory and lethal effects. Thus, conditions which favor the undissociated form of the acid are the most effective for antimicrobial activity since the acid molecule can readily pass through the cell membrane. Therefore, systems which approach the pKa of the acid species increase the efficacy of the organic acid. In addition, longer chain acids can more readily integrate into the cell membrane due to their greater lipophilic nature. However, higher lipophilic nature of the acid will limit solubility in the product matrix. While the antimicrobial quality of acids can prove detrimental to many species, they are particularly effective as antifungal agents.

Many of the organic acids found their first major applications in foodstuffs. However, a wide variety of acids are also in use in cosmetics, including benzoic acid (pKa 4.2), citric acid (pKa 6.4, 4.8, 3.1), sorbic acid (pKa 4.8), and salicylic acid (pKa 3.0) (Figure 3.5). These are frequently added to the product via the appropriate salt in order to aid solubility. While each of these acid species is produced synthetically, each is also found in natural materials.

Citric acid can be found in citrus extracts. Citric acid is widely used as an acidulent in creams and gels. It also has chelating activity, which may contribute some portion of its antimicrobial activity. Benzoic acid occurs naturally in many plants and is found in many berries, particularly cranberries. Benzoic acid and its salts and esters find usage in the formulation of oral products, including toothpastes, mouthwashes and dentifrices. It is also used in creams and lotions when these products are formulated with a sufficiently low pH to elicit antimicrobial activity. Sorbic acid was first isolated from the berries of *Sorbus aucuparia* (the Rowan tree), from which it derives its common name. Salicylic acid is found in a number of plant materials. Its most prominent natural source is willow bark extract.

Enzymes

Introduction

Enzymes are most often thought of as key components for enabling rapid and selective reactions needed for cell metabolism, energy generation, and reproduction. However, they can also play a key role in organism defense. While a number of hydrolytic (e.g., lysozyme, subtilisins) and oxidative (e.g., superoxide dismutase) enzymes have been shown to elicit antimicrobial activity either by direct enzymatic effect or through the products of their enzymatic reaction, relatively few enzymes systems have been commercialized for use in consumer products. Although they can be highly effective, their cost is relatively high and product/process must be tailored to maintain enzyme activity. In addition, their potential to elicit allergic reactions must be vetted as part of their application. To date, the cosmetic industry's primary focus for enzymatic-based preservation has been on the lactoperoxidase/glucose oxidase system.

Lactoperoxidase and Glucose Oxidase

Lactoperoxidase belongs to the peroxidase family of enzymes and has been established as a key component of a broader system in nature which yields natural antibacterial components as part of the body's

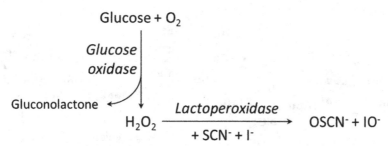

FIGURE 3.6 Reaction catalyzed in the lactoperoxidase system.

defense. The lactoperoxidase effect was first observed in milk. *In situ*, the mechanism involves the reaction of lactoperoxidase with hydrogen peroxide (from the presence of existing bacteria) and electron donors like the thiocyanate ion to produce a cascade of antimicrobial metabolites (e.g., hypothiocyanate). Commercially available systems typically use a second component system. The first component consists of the enzymes lactoperoxidase and glucose oxidase. The second component contains the substrates glucose, thiocyanate, and iodide. In combination with oxygen, a reaction is catalyzed, yielding the antimicrobial metabolites hypoiodite and hypothiocyanite (Figure 3.6).

This system has been reported to have both antibacterial and antifungal activity, and when configured in the proper system, can maintain this activity for 18+ months (19). The challenge in employing this system is ensuring that each of the five components in the system is working optimally together and their incorporation is correctly matched to processing conditions. Although the application of the lactoperoxidase system has not reached levels anywhere near those of traditional chemistries, it has been consistently applied by some manufacturers in cosmetic products such as lip balms, toothpastes, and moisturizing creams, with the number of new products having increased in recent years.

Antimicrobial Peptides

Antimicrobial peptides, typically of relatively low molecular weight (2–8 kDA), occur in nature across a variety of life forms, including mammals, insects, and bacteria, and are primarily produced as defense mechanisms. A number of Gram-negative (e.g., *Enterobacter*, *Klebsiella*, *Salmonella*) and Gram-positive bacteria (e.g., *Lactobacillus*, *Clostridium*, *Listeria*) species may produce such molecules, as a mechanism to gain competitive advantage in multiorganism environments. The general name given to these peptides is bacteriocins, although depending on the source organism, they can vary widely in their chemical properties, amino acid sequence, heat stability, and spectrum of activity (20).

The lactic acid bacteria (LAB) are among the most researched organisms for their ability to produce bacteriocins (21). Many bacteriocins have quite a narrow range of inhibitory activity against closely related species and genera, though some may have a broader range of activity.

Nisin, a 34 amino acid bacteriocin shown in Figure 3.7 (22), produced by *Lactococcus lactis* and among the most studied of bacteriocins due to its use in the food industry, is inhibitory to a range of vegetative and spore-forming Gram-positive bacteria, including *Bacillus*, *Clostridium*, and *Listeria*. Some studies suggest that the range of antimicrobial activity can be extended to Gram-negative bacteria via the use of potentiators such as chelants (23) and hurdle technologies.

Some of nisin's properties demonstrate why it has been successfully used in the food industry and why this class of molecules has potential for use as natural preservatives in cosmetics. Nisin has a long history of human consumption since it is a component of many fermented dairy products. It is soluble in aqueous environments and has good stability tolerance in acidic pH. It is relatively heat stable. Nisin has approval as an antimicrobial agent in a variety of food products. In the US, nisin has broad regulatory approval and is generally recognized as safe (GRAS) for use as an antimicrobial in foods. Nisin, and bacteriocins in general, do not impart color and odor, and are thus compatible with product aesthetics.

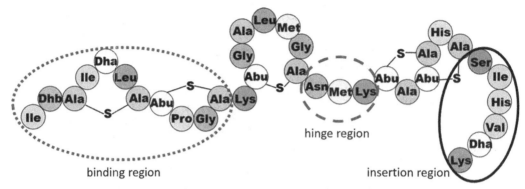

FIGURE 3.7   Structure and relevant regions of nisin (from Han et al. (23) with permission).

One common approach to preservation with bacteriocins is via the use of LAB (lactic acid bacteria) ferments. Although bacteriocins have not been applied broadly in cosmetic preservation, some preservative offerings have been established via the use of ferments of Leuconostoc. While these LAB are known to produce bacteriocins, the broad spectrum activity observed in one study of Leuconostoc ferments of radish root attributed the activity to salicylic acid and didecyldimethylammonium salts rather than bacteriocins (24).

Final Thoughts

Historically, many cosmetic ingredients had some innate hostility to significantly complement preservation approaches. The innate hostility in these formulations was driven by commonly used functional constituents (e.g., perfumes, chelators) and intrinsic parameters (solvents, Aw, pH extremes, etc.). Consumer preference for milder formulations combined with evolving environmental sustainability factors have diminished the overall contribution of innately hostile formula constituents/factors to product preservation. Thus, there is an increased burden on added preservatives to establish sustainable microbial integrity. In recent years, the regulatory and commercial environment surrounding traditional synthetic preservatives has been fluid, with a consistent pressure to recredential, minimize, or eliminate the use of historically mainstream synthetic chemistries. Taken in combination, the development and implementation of innovative and holistic, multi-component preservation strategies will be an ongoing need by the cosmetics industry for the foreseeable future.

As of this writing, there is no obvious new preservative approach or chemistry, synthetic or natural, which stands poised to mitigate current concerns with synthetic chemistries, without introducing many of the technical, regulatory, and commercial challenges discussed in this chapter. Natural preservatives present some interesting options as a means of complementing or potentially replacing traditional synthetic chemistries. One intention of this chapter has been to calibrate the complexities of using natural preservative systems. Compared to synthetic chemistries, natural preservatives—especially extracts and mixtures—will require a more deliberate integration during product development if they are to shoulder the majority of the preservation burden. Even with a highly deliberate intent, natural preservatives may only deliver a portion of the preservation capacity needed and may only be applicable in a portion of cosmetic product categories.

Traditional synthetic preservatives will continue to be under pressure for minimal use or outright removal from formulations. While "preservative-free" labels may broaden product appeal on the shelf, application of this marketing strategy lends itself to further complicating an already murky consumer perception of the benefits of preservation, and the role and implication of certain ingredients as they appear on the label. While assessment, regulation, and customer perspective of preservatives, will continue to be closely watched by the cosmetics industry, consumers will also continue to try to vet the many variants of preservation and establish the "good" from the "bad". Reducing the preservation discussion to these two blunt characterizations does disservice to the nuances of the preservation dynamic. Rather than limiting the discussion to one of these two distinct endpoints, introducing a risk/benefit perspective for preservation would be a more welcomed framework for consideration. Although this is a more nuanced perspective to communicate and understand, it would give a greater depth to the discussion and allow for a more informed decision on the role that preservatives should play in a consumer's product choices.

REFERENCES

1. How FDA evaluates regulated products: cosmetics. (July 07, 2017). Retrieved July 27, 2017, from www.fda.gov.
2. Si, W., Gong, J., Tsao, R., Zhou, T., Yu, H., Poppe, C., Johnson. R., and Du, Z. 2006. Antimicrobial activity of essential oils and structurally related synthetic food additives towards selected pathogenic and beneficial gut bacteria. *J. Appl. Microbiol.* 100:296–305.
3. Browne, B.A., Geis, P., and Rook, T. 2012. Conventional vs. natural preservatives. *Happi.* May: 69–73.
4. Kerdudo, A., Burger, P., Merck, F., Dingas, A., Rolland, Y., Michel, T., and Fernandez, X. 2016. Development of a natural ingredient – natural preservative: a case study. *C.R. Chimie.* 19:1077–1089.
5. Carson, C.F., Hammer, K.A., and Riley, T.V. 2006. *Melaleuca alternifolia* (tea tree) oil: a review of antimicrobial and other medicinal properties. *Clin. Microbiol. Rev.* 19:50–62.
6. Zanettti, M., Ternus, Z.R., Dalcanton, F., de Mello, M.M.J., de Oliveira, D., Araujo, P.H.H., Riella, H.G., and Fiori, M.A. 2015. Microbiological characterization of pure geraniol and comparison with bactericidal activity of the cinnamic acid in gram-positive and gram-negative bacteria. *J. Microb. Biochem.* 7:186–193.
7. Brophy, J.J., Davies, N.W., Southwell, I.A., Stiff, I.A., and Williams, L.R. 1989. Gas chromatographic quality control for oil of Melaleuca terpinen-4-ol type (Australian tea tree). *J. Agric. Food Chem.* 37:1330–1335.
8. International Organization for Standardization. 2004. ISO4730:2004 Oil of *Melaleuca* terpinen-4-ol type (tea tree oil). International Organization for Standardization, Geneva, Switzerland.
9. Prashant, G.M., Chandu, G.N., Murulikrishna, K.S., and Shafiulla, M.D. 2007. The effect of mango and neem extract on four organism causing dental caries: *Streptococcus mutans*, *Streptococcus salivarius*, *Streptococcus mitis*, and *Streptococcus sanguis*: an *in vitro* study. *Indian J. Dent. Res.* 18:148–151.
10. Chia-Jung, L., Li-Wei, C., Lih-Geeng, C., Ting-Lin, C., Chun-Wei, H., Ming-Chuan, H., and Ching-Chiung, W. 2013. Correlations of the components of tea tree oil with its antibacterial effects and skin irritation. *J. Food Drug Anal.* 21:169–176.
11. Subapriva, R. and Nagini, S. 2005. Medicinal properties of neem leaves: a review. *Curr. Med. Chem. Anticancer Agents.* 5:149–156.
13. Raut, R.R., Sawant, A.R., and Jamge, B.B. 2014. Antimicrobial activity of *Azadirachta indica* (neem) against pathogenic microorganisms. *J. Acad. Ind. Res.* 3:327–329.
12. Lakshmi, T., Krishnan, V., Rajendran, R., and Madhusudhanan, N. 2015. *Azadirachta indica*: a herbal panacea in dentistry – an update. *Pharmacognosy Rev.* 9:41–44.
14. Pires, R.H., Lucarini, R., and Mendes-Gianninia, M.J.S. 2012. Effect of usnic acid on *Candida orthopsilosis* and *C. parapsilosis*. *Antimicrob. Agents Chemother.* 56:595–597.
15. Council for Agricultural Science and Technology. 1998. Naturally occurring antimicrobials in food. Task Force Report No. 132.
16. Cowan, M.M. 1999. Plant products as antimicrobial agents. *Clin. Microbiol. Rev.* 12:564–582.
17. Herman, A., Herman, A.P., Domagalska, B.W., and Mlynarczyk, A. 2013. Essential oils and herbal extracts as antimicrobial agents in cosmetic emulsion. *Ind. J. Microbiol.* 53:232–237.
18. Takeoka, G., Dao, L., Wong, R.Y., Lundin, R., and Mahoney, N. 2001. Identification of benzethonium chloride in commercial grapefruit seed extracts. *J. Agric. Food Chem.* 49:3316–3320.
19. Bosch, E.H., Van Doorne, H., and De Vries, S. 2000. The lactoperoxidase system: the influence of iodide and the chemical and antimicrobial stability over the period of about 18 months. *J. Appl. Microbiol.* 89:215–224.

20. Owen Fields, F. 1996. Use of bacteriocins in food: regulatory considerations. *J. Food Protect.* Supplement: 72–77.
21. Klaenhammer, T.R. 1988. Bacteriocins of lactic acid bacteria. *Biochimie.* 70:337–349.
22. Han, D., Sherman, S., Filocamo, S., and Steckl, A.J. 2017. Long-term antimicrobial effect of nisin released from electrospun triaxial fiber membranes. *Acta Biomaterialia.* 53:242–249.
23. Kalchayanand, N., Hanlin, M.B., and Ray B. 1992. Sublethal injury makes Gram negative and resistant Gram positive bacteria sensitive to the bacteriocins, pediocin AcH and nisin. *Lett. in Appl. Microbiol.* 15:239–243.
24. Li, J., Chaytor, J.L., Findlay, B., McMullen, L.M., Smith, D.C., and Vederas, J.C. 2015. Identification of didecyldimethylammonium salts and salicylic acid as antimicrobial compounds in commercial fermented radish kimchi. *J. Agric. Food Chem.* 63:3053–3058.

4

Multifunctional Ingredients

Steven F. Schnittger

Introduction

Every cosmetic manufacturer has a dual responsibility relative to the microbiological quality of its products. The first is to ensure that the product, as purchased, is free from the numbers and types of microorganisms that could affect product quality and consumer health. The second is to ensure that microorganisms formed during normal product use will not adversely affect the quality or safety of the product.

To ensure microbiological quality, all aqueous-based products in multiple use containers—a large percentage of skin care formulations—require preservation and or some form of protection. Product protection can be ensured through a multifaceted approach, and each of these approaches is explained in the section that follows:

a. Protection can be ensured solely based on chemicals whose only function is preservation and are recognized as "conventional preservative systems".
b. Product protection can be confirmed through chemicals whose primary attribute may be humectancy, as an anti-oxidant, emulsifier, chelator but also contribute to the preservative efficacy of a formulation. These chemicals are identified as "multifunctional ingredients or preservative boosters".
c. Protection can also be guaranteed by the physiochemical properties of the product such as pH, reduced water activity, or filling temperatures which creates an environment which is recognized as low risk or hostile to microbial growth. In these types of products the risk of microbiological contamination is very low or non-existent because bacteria cannot survive and grow.

The final method of product protection is through the use of packaging which minimizes the ability of the consumer or the environment to introduce contamination through product contact.

The Microbiological Risk Assessment is the final procedure used by the microbiologist to determine the level of preservation required, the type of testing needed to determine preservative efficacy and product susceptibility, and the risk potential when product/package combination has been determined.

Conventional Preservative Systems

"Preservation is the process by which chemical or physical agents prevent biological deterioration of materials". In this chapter, I discuss preservation of cosmetic products. Cosmetic preservatives are effective against both prokaryotes and eukaryotes cells, and unlike antibiotics they do not act against a defined target cell. Chemical preservation plays the primary role in formula protection whereas pH and reduced water activity are the primary factors in many of the different food groups such as tomato sauce, baked goods, and jellies.

During the manufacturing of a cosmetic product, consumer safety is a major consideration because products are being applied to the body. As a result, careful consideration is given to the choice of preservative(s), inclusion level in a formula, and body surface to which the product is being applied.

Preservation is required in any formulation where there is sufficient free water to support the growth of microorganisms. The antimicrobial effect of a preservative is dependent on the ability to move freely within that water phase but be lipophilic enough to attach and permeate microbial membranes. Traditional preservatives such as the straight-chain parabens, organic acids, and formaldehyde releasers possess sufficient water/lipid solubility to ensure the destruction of target microorganisms.

According to the EC Regulation (EC) No 1223/2009 on cosmetic products (1), "A preservative is a substance which is exclusively or mainly intended to inhibit the development of microorganisms in the cosmetic product". These substances are listed in Annex V of the EC Regulation. Japan also lists preservatives in Annex III of the Japanese "Standard of Cosmetics". In the US, cosmetic ingredients do not require FDA (Food and Drug Administration) approval before they go on to the market. Companies that market cosmetics have the legal responsibility to ensure the safety of their products and so there is no positive list for preservatives there.

Over the past 15 years the global cosmetic industry has seen a significant reduction in the number of conventional preservative systems that are deemed acceptable for use in the marketplace. Even though the European Commission has an extensive list of approved preservatives in Annex V, only a limited number are truly acceptable and presently being used in the Global Market.

Table 4.1 (2) shows the top 23 preservatives used in the US cosmetic industry today. Each of these molecules has some sort of regulatory, environmental, or legal restriction applied to it. Some are being limited for use because of a perceived risk by the consumer and assorted regulatory bodies. The only groups of preservatives which are not restricted are the *organic acids* (sorbic, benzoic, and dehydroacetic acids) and they can be used only in limited applications due to pH restrictions and potential adverse reactions around the eye.

Of the 23 molecules on the list, only phenoxyethanol, Kathon CG, MIT, benzyl alcohol, chlorphenesin, sorbic acid and its salts, and dehydroacetic acid and its salts have shown a significant increase in the past three years. All others have either remained static or showed a decrease. Of these seven, only two are broad spectrum through a wide range of applications with an acceptable regulatory profile (phenoxyethanol, chlorphenesin). Kathon and MIT can be used only in rinse-off products, organic acids are pH dependent, and benzyl alcohol is on the positive allergen list for fragrances.

Eventually because of the lack of acceptability of these and other cosmetic preservatives, the industry has had to look toward other methods to preserve their products and to protect the consumer. One of those avenues has been to investigate the use of ingredients that not only have antimicrobial activity but also other chemical attributes that they could deliver to the formulation. They are identified as *multifunctional ingredients.*

Multifunctional Ingredients

In recent years there has been a growing trend in the cosmetic industry for making "free-from" and "preservative-free" claims. This does not mean that the formula is not preserved or unprotected, but often that the formula may contain ingredients which are generally not recognized as a conventional preservative system.

TABLE 4.1

Frequency of preservative use: number of applications per year, as reported to US FDA

		2007	2010	2013
Methylparaben	Paraben	11609	13434	13423
Propylparaben	Paraben	9329	10421	10423
Phenoxyethanol	Alcohol	5132	8878	11641
Butylparaben	Paraben	2784	5289	5114
Ethylparaben	Paraben	3789	4869	5004
Isobutylparaben	Paraben	1684	2693	2713
Methylisothiazolinone	Isothizolone	1409	2408	3391
MI/CMI	Isothizalone	1392	2235	2774
DMDM Hydantoin	Formaldehyde releaser	1665	2035	2252
Imidazolidinyl urea	Formaldehyde releaser	2266	2007	1822
Benzyl alcohol	Alcohol	1125	1991	3042
Sodium sulfite		2784	1801	1485
Diazolidinyl urea	Formaldehyde releaser	1299	1644	1662
Resorcinol			1447	1423
Chlorphenesin	Halogenated	441	1065	1657
Sorbic acid/K sorbate	Organic acid	1259	1037/1456	1326/2697
Dehydroacetic acid/Na dehydroacetate	Organic acid	866	948	1954
Iodopropynyl butylcarbamate	Halogenated	429	834	972
Salicylic acid			712	951
Benzoic acid/Na benzoate	Organic acid	1153	604/1334	853/2119
Triclosan	Halogenated	565	494	468
Sodium methylparaben	Paraben	272	465	466
Quaternium-15	Formaldehyde releaser	531	389	252

According to the recent requirements by the Annex 7 Recast in the EU, preservative efficacy for every new formulation must be documented. On the basis of this requirement, it can be assumed that these new formulas would pass preservative efficacy testing similar to that of any conventionally preserved system. The increased frequency of use in these types of compounds is directly related to the continued restrictions and perceived risk of conventional systems.

A second reason for the use of multifunctionals and potentiators is the potential reduction in the risk of sensitization due to overuse of those few conventional systems allowed in the marketplace. The combination of a multifunctional with a conventional preservative system can lower the risk of sensitization but increase the efficacy of the preservative system versus used alone.

According to European regulation, the only permitted preservatives are those that are listed in Annex VI of the 7th amendment of the Cosmetic Directive. However, many cosmetic ingredients, such as alcohols, essential oils, chelators, and surfactants have multiple cosmetic functions which can include antimicrobial activity. Some of these materials are used for their beneficial effects and may coincidentally contribute to the preservation of the formulation.

Three of the more commonly used multifunctional ingredients are discussed here:

- **Caprylyl glycol**
  - 1,2-Octanediol or caprylyl glycol is a C8 linear diol with moisturizing properties and exhibits effective viscosity-modulating properties especially in oil in water emulsions. This ingredient can function as emollient, moisturizer, humectant, wetting agent, and co-emulsifier.
  - In certain circumstances the formulation can be adequately preserved by using only caprylyl glycol but in other situations it is used in conjunction with other conventional systems such as phenoxyethanol to lower the overall level of preservatives in a formulation.

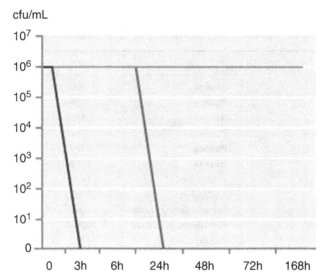

FIGURE 4.1   Ethylhexyl glycerine potentiation of phenoxyethanol (by courtesy of schülke inc., Fairfield, NJ).

- **Ethylhexylglycerin**
  - Has been used for its deodorant, emollient, humectant, and perfume-solubilizing properties.
  - Its mode of action is through reducing the surface tension at the microbial cell membrane and improving exposure of the cell membrane to other antimicrobial substances. It is effective for chemical preservatives. Figure 4.1 shows the potentiation effect of ethylhexylglycerin when used with phenoxyethanol.
- **Monoesters—Glyceryl caprylate**
  - Glyceryl monoesters of caprylic, capric, and lauric acid elicit an antimicrobial activity but also work as emulsifiers, moisturizers, and emollients. Middle-chain fatty acid monoesters of glycerin and diglycerin are frequently used for their deodorant activity, their selective activity against odor-causing *Corynebacterium* species, and other Gram-positive cocci.

Preservative Potentiators

Another activity related to chemical preservation is *potentiation of preservatives*.

Potentiation can be defined as: "The enhancement of an antimicrobial agent through the addition of a microbiologically inactive or only weakly active component that presumably increases the susceptibility of the microbial target to preservative action". On their own, most preservative potentiators would not provide sufficient preservation to ensure consumer safety. Like the multifunctionals they have other benefits when added to a cosmetic emulsion.

Three molecules recognized as a preservative potentiator are discussed here:

- **EDTA**
  - The classic example of a potentiator is ethylene-diamine-tetraacetic acid (EDTA).
  - It has been shown to enhance the activity of a range of preservative agents especially against *Pseudomonas aeruginosa* where its chelating power affects the stability of the protective outer membrane (3).
  - EDTA also stabilizes fragrance components and product color and controls fading.
- **Butylene glycol**
  - Like other humectants, butylene glycol (BG) inhibits the drying out of cosmetics and prevents crystallization of insoluble components in cosmetic vehicles. It also works to retard the loss of

aroma and helps solubilize active ingredients. Since it exhibits mutual solvency in water and oil, it is useful as a coupling agent in emulsions to enhance emulsion stability.
  * It has been shown to enhance the antimicrobial activity of methyl paraben and phenoxyethanol in aqueous solutions and provides more favorable partitioning into the aqueous phase of the emulsion (4).
* **1,2 Propanediol**
  * 1, 2 Propanediol ("Zemea" or PDO) exhibits good skin moisturization effect and boosts moisturization effect when used with glycerin.
  * An added benefit which has been recently documented is its enhanced activity when used with zinc pyrithione against dandruff (5).
  * Up to 75% PDO does not elicit a sensitization reaction as compared to 1.0% Propylene glycol but has equivalent preservative potentiation as compared to propylene glycol (6).

Low-Risk Formulations

According to ISO 29621 (7), a low-risk product is defined as "A product whose composition denies microorganisms the physical and chemical requirements for growth and/or survival".

The risk of microbiological contamination for these types of products is extremely low or non-existent due to product characteristics that create a hostile environment for the growth of microorganisms. Products with certain physio-chemical characteristics do not allow the proliferation of microorganisms of concern to cosmetic products. Any number of physio-chemical factors or combinations thereof in a product can create a hostile environment that will not support microbial growth and/or survival. Combinations of these sub-lethal factors will increase the hostility of the environment and increase the lag phase during the growth of bacteria.

If the environment is hostile enough, the lag phase of the bacteria will be extended to infinity and therefore cause cell death. Combinations of lethal factors can cause rapid cell death. This product category has a very limited product application but does represent a group of formulas where preservation is delivered through physio-chemical characteristics and not through the direct addition of a known chemical preservative.

Those products identified as "low risk" and when produced in compliance with Good Manufacturing Practices (GMPs) pose a very low overall risk to the user. The propensity of a formulation to support the growth of microorganisms or, conversely, to kill microorganisms (self-preserving) is a prime factor in determining the need to add preservatives. A number of factors should be evaluated in order to determine what additional preservative system, if any, is needed for a particular formulation. Listed here are examples of where a hostile formula will not support microbial growth:

* High level of glycols, polyols, or humectants in a cosmetic formulation which limits the amount of available water and, therefore, is not able to support bacterial growth. In this application only an antifungal compound would need to be added.
* Alcohol in a formulation above 25%.
* Formulations where the pH values > 10 and < 3.
* Deodorant and antiperspirants with high levels of aluminum chlorohydrates.

The following characteristics should be considered when determining if a formula requires a preservative, the type of preservative, and the level of preservation. It can also indicate if modifications are required to the test protocol or the pass/fail criteria.

1. Water activity
2. Presence of raw materials recognized as hostile to bacterial growth
3. Emulsifier system
4. pH

5. Physical state
6. Fragrance level and type
7. Alcohol level and type.

It is recommended, when evaluating for preservatives, to run an unpreserved control to determine the susceptibility of the formulation to bacterial and fungal growth.

Manufacturing and Production Conditions

Certain aspects of the manufacturing and filling process (e.g., high temperature) may reduce the microbiological risk of a cosmetic product. As with pH, there is an optimum temperature range for microbial growth. Low temperatures will allow for slow growth and raising temperatures could potentially increase growth. As the temperature rises above optimum, growth is inhibited and microorganisms are killed. Heat is used to control microorganisms either by applying a temperature adequate for rapid kill or by maintaining a temperature above optimum for an extended period of time (8).

Temperature above 65°C can cause thermal inactivation of the microbial bioburden in a product formulation. With a 10-minute hold time at a temperature of above 65°C, most vegetative bacterial cells die due to denaturation and degradation of cellular proteins.

However, it should be noted, from the details given previously, that microbial content testing on product formulations that are filled at a temperature above 65°C is not required. Periodic testing of product or verification of the lethality of process temperature should be considered. It is also recommended that periodic review of manufacturing and filling be performed to ensure there have been no changes to process conditions.

Microbiological Risk Assessment

Microbiological risk assessment is based on a number of factors generally accepted as important in evaluating the adverse effects on product quality and consumer health. It is intended as a guide in determining the level of preservation required for a formulation, the level of testing required, and potential changing of the pass/fail criteria to reflect the product type. The main factors that need to be evaluated are:

- The use of ingredients with antimicrobial or certain physico-chemical properties
- The manufacturing conditions
- The type of packaging
- The conditions for use.

The nature and frequency of testing also vary according to the use of the product. The significance of microorganisms in non-sterile cosmetic products should be evaluated in terms of the use of the product, the nature of the product, and the potential risk to the user.

In ISO 11930—Evaluation of the Antimicrobial Protection of a Cosmetic Product (9), guidelines regarding risk assessment are established as part of the decision process to ensure product safety if it does not comply with the challenge test criteria. In this, other parameters (e.g., protective packaging) are utilized to ensure safety.

Packaging and Product Protection

Packaging can play a major role in product protection. A prime example of where packaging can play a major role is through the use of aerosol sprays, unit-dose packaging, pump type packages, or tubes with one way valves.

Aerosol sprays and pump packages where the neck is crimped around the body of the package ensures complete product protection from the external environment and contact with the consumer. In this case the standard preservative efficacy test is not indicative of evaluating potential risk to the consumer. A consumer use study must be performed to determine product/package risk.

In tube type packages and pump packages the dispensing closure used for containers plays an important role in preventing contamination of cosmetics during use (9). Therefore, even poorly preserved products may withstand consumer use without becoming contaminated if packaged with closures that provide adequate protection from consumer and environmental contact.

Manufacturing concerns, such as raw materials with bio-loads and the need to prevent microbial adaptation to products, usually dictate that preservatives be added to protect products from contamination during manufacturing. Product protection from the addition of preservatives is typically sufficient to prevent consumer contamination in aqueous-based products, but every safeguard should be put in place during product development, manufacturing, and filling to ensure product safety and quality.

Conclusion

Product protection can be ensured from many different directions and approaches. It has been shown in this chapter that it does not always have to be from traditional preservative systems but a multifaceted approach of preservatives, raw materials, and packaging.

Product preservation can be successfully delivered through a combination of molecules that not only deliver functionality to a formulation but also contribute to preservative efficacy. An efficacious preservative system combined with a good closure and packaging design can provide a higher degree of protection to the consumer during product use.

While microbial contamination from manufacturing is controlled by careful attention to good manufacturing practices, contamination from consumer use is controlled by adequate product preservation and by container designs that provide for minimal contact of the product to consumer and the environment.

REFERENCES

1. EC (European Community). Regulation (EC) No. 1223/2009 of the European Parliament and of the Council of 30 November 2009 on Cosmetic Products. *Off J Eur Commun* 2009 (L342).
2. Steinberg, D. 2016. Frequency of Preservative Use Update through 2014. Cosmetic Toiletries. Accessed at: www.cosmeticsandtoiletries.com/regulatory/region/northamerica/Frequency-of-Preservative-Use-Update-Through-2014-367684531.html.
3. Banin, E., Brady, K.M. and Greenberg, E.P., 2006. Chelator-induced dispersal and killing of *Pseudomonas aeruginosa* cells in a biofilm. *Appl. Environ. Microbiol.*, 72(3):2064–2069.
4. Kinnunen, T. and Koskela, M., 1991. Antibacterial and antifungal properties of propylene glycol, hexylene glycol, and 1, 3-butylene glycol in vitro. *Acta dermato-venereologica*, 71(2):148–150.
5. Durham, R.F. and CARE, H., 2014. Improving dandruff shampoo via biobased propanediol. *Personal Care*:77–79.
6. See https://duponttateandlyle.com/zemea.
7. ISO 29621:2017 Cosmetics – Microbiology – Guidelines for the risk assessment and identification of microbiologically low-risk products. Accessed at: www.iso.org/standard/68310.html.
8. ISO 11930:2019 Cosmetics – Microbiology – Evaluation of the antimicrobial protection of a cosmetic product. Accessed at: www.iso.org/standard/75058.html.
9. Brannan, D.K. and Dille, J.C., 1990. Type of closure prevents microbial contamination of cosmetics during consumer use. *Appl. Environ. Microbiol.* 56(5):1476–1479.

5

Preservative Resistance

Donald J. English

Introduction

Preservative resistance is an established phenomenon that occurs when a microorganism becomes largely unaffected and resistant to the antimicrobial activity (e.g., cidal and/or static) of a preservative which will no longer be able to control the survival and proliferation of a microorganism in a product formulation. The development of resistance to the antimicrobial activity of preservatives is not a new problem. It has been a well-known fact for many years in the food and beverage industry that *Saccharomyces cerevisiae* and *Zygosaccharomyces bailii* can become resistant to the antimicrobial activity of organic acid preservatives such as benzoic acid and sorbic acid (1,2). In the cosmetic industry, there are many literature reports of bacteria becoming resistant to the antimicrobial activity to the following types of cosmetic and personal care preservatives: quaternary ammonium compounds (QACs) (3), p-hydroxybenzoic acid esters (4), imidazolidinyl urea (5), methylchloroisothiazolinone (MCIT)/methylisothiazolinone (MIT), dimethylol dimethyl (DMDM) hydantoin, dibromodicyanobutane (DBCB), glutaraldehyde, parabens (6), phenoxyethanol (6), chlorhexidine diacetate (7), and combinations of DMDM hydantoin/ iodopropynyl butylcarbamate (IPBC) and DMDM hydantoin/IBPC/MCIT/MIT (8).

Preservative resistance and accompanying product contamination described in these and other reports is typically attributed to Gram-negative bacterial species including *Alcaligenes faecalis, Enterobacter* species, *Burkholderia cepacia, Pseudomonas aeruginosa, Pseudomonas fluorescens, Pseudomonas putida,* and *Pseudomonas corrugata* (5,8–12).

Mechanisms for the Development of Preservative Resistance

According to A.D. Russell, the mechanism for a microorganism to become resistant to the antimicrobial activity of preservatives is by either intrinsic or acquired means (13). Intrinsic microbial resistance occurs due to the presence of a degrading enzyme or other resistance factors. Acquired resistance to a preservative occurs when a microorganism adapts to the presence of a preservative by either exposure to sub-inhibitory and/or sub-lethal preservative concentrations, mutation, outer membrane changes, or through a capability termed "efflux pump" in the cell membrane.

It should be noted that it is possible for a particular microbial isolate to have various types of mechanisms for the development of preservative resistance. The specific mechanism of preservative resistance by a microorganism is due to the type of selective pressure that is being exerted on a microorganism. However, it is still possible for more than one type of mechanism to exist in a bacterium at the same time to cause preservative resistance. For example, a *Burkholderia cepacia* complex bacterium was found to be resistant to the antimicrobial activity of benzalkonium chloride due to both efflux and metabolic inactivation via biodegradation (14).

Enzymatic Degradation

Enzymatic mechanisms of microorganisms are better understood than any other mechanism of preservative resistance. For example, it was reported in 1985 that five strains of *Pseudomonas* isolated from contaminated cosmetic products were resistant to high concentrations of imidazolidinyl urea (5). In each of these contaminated products, imidazolidinyl urea had been metabolized to formaldehyde which in turn was metabolized to a UV-absorbing lutidine derivative. In addition to imidazolidinyl urea, *Pseudomonas aeruginosa* isolates have also been found to be resistant to the antimicrobial activity of DMDM hydantoin, another formaldehyde-releasing preservative. These resistant isolates were found to have typical patterns of outer membrane proteins (8). It was determined that the development of these *Pseudomonas aeruginosa*-resistant strains was not due to a reduced permeation of DMDM hydantoin or other formaldehyde-releasing preservative across the outer membrane of the bacterial cell, but due to the enzyme formaldehyde dehydrogenase that is able to metabolize formaldehyde to formic acid that is ineffective as a cosmetic/personal care preservative (15,16).

The reported mechanism of antimicrobial mode of action for the parabens is by one of the following: alternating the permeability of the cell membrane (17), inhibiting DNA and RNA synthesis (18), and inhibiting other critical enzyme capabilities such as ATPases and phosphotransferases (19). Resistance to the antimicrobial activity of parabens has been reported in the following types of microbial species: *Acinetobacter* spp. (20), *Pseudomonas aeruginosa* (21), *Cladosporium resinae* (22), *Burkholderia cepacia* (23,24), *Enterobacter cloacae* (25), *Enterobacter gergoviae* (26), and *Escherichia coli* (27). From contaminated, non-sterile solutions of methylparaben and propylparaben, two microorganisms had been found to degrade each of these respective parabens. Using 16S ribosomal ribonucleic acid (rRNA) partial gene sequencing, two paraben-degrading microorganisms were identified as *Pseudomonas beteli* and *Burkholderia latens*. Degradation of various concentrations of methylparaben by *Pseudomonas beteli* followed a logarithmic pattern, but the degradation of propylparaben was found to be linear by *B. latens*. In addition, it was also observed that *Ps. beteli* could not degrade propylparaben, while *B. latens* could degrade both methyl and propylparaben. Absence of High-Performance Liquid Chromatography (HPLC) chromatographic peaks of expected paraben degradation products indicated that these two microbial isolates were able to use the parabens as a carbon source (28). For parabens-resistant *Cladosporium resinae*, *Pseudomonas aeruginosa*, and *Burkholderia cepacia*, Valkova et al speculated that an esterase hydrolyzed parabens to 4-hydroxybenzoic acid. Esterase hydrolysis was confirmed to be the basis for paraben resistance of *Enterobacter cloacae* and *Enterobacter gergoviae* isolates (26,29).

Enterobacter gergoviae is known to cause microbial contamination of cosmetic and personal care product formulations (30,31). In addition to esterase hydrolysis, *E. gergoviae* parabens resistance has also been attributed to overexpression of a 25-kDa peroxiredoxin enzyme that is involved in oxidative detoxification (32). Peroxiredoxins are cysteine-based peroxidases that can act as redox sensors and biomarkers of oxidative stress. Cysteine is oxidized to reduce peroxides by forming an intermolecular disulphide bond with peroxiredoxin. The disulphide-bonded peroxiredoxins are subsequently reduced and reactivated by thiol-containing reductants such as alkyl hydroperoxidase subunit F (AhpF) and thioredoxin (TrxA). It should be noted that the isothiazolinone preservatives are able to inhibit microbial growth and metabolism and to cause the loss of viability due to its interactivity with cysteine (33–36). Excess cysteine is also able to neutralize the antimicrobial activity of (MCIT) (33). Because peroxiredoxins are cysteine-based peroxidases, it is possible that the cysteine component of this enzyme is able to neutralize the antimicrobial activity of MCIT.

Strains of *Pseudomonas putida* and *Alcaligenes xylosoxidans* ssp. *denitrificans* have been reported to exhibit high levels of triclosan resistance due to each of these two bacterial species being able to degrade triclosan by using enzymes (37). Triclosan degradation has also been demonstrated in *Sphingomonas* strain RD1 by the release of 14CO2 from 14C-labeled triclosan (38). Two root fungi, *Trametes versicolor* and *Pycnoporus cinnabarinus*, have been shown to transform triclosan by either glucosylation or xylosylation of the hydroxyl group (39).

It has been reported in the literature that strains of *Pseudomonas putida* and *Acinetobacter calcoaceticus* are able to produce a benzyl alcohol dehydrogenase that oxidizes benzyl alcohol to benzoate (40,41). In the *Pseudomonas putida*-resistant strain, the gene for benzyl alcohol dehydrogenase was encoded on a plasmid that encoded benzyl alcohol dehydrogenase. This *Ps. putida* benzyl alcohol dehydrogenase appears to be remarkably similar to the chromosomally encoded benzyl alcohol dehydrogenase from *Acinetobacter calcoaceticus*. Both of these benzyl alcohol dehydrogenases are soluble, NAD+-dependent enzymes with similar subunit *M* values, pH optima, and substrate specificities. Besides its activity toward benzyl alcohol, benzyl alcohol dehydrogenase has also been shown to degrade phenethyl alcohol which is a fragrance additive that can be used as a non-traditional or alternative preservative in product formulations (42).

By using oxidative degradation, a strain of *Burkholderia cepacia* has also been found to transform benzyl alcohol to salicyl alcohol (43).

Exposure to Sub-Inhibitory and/or Sub-Lethal Preservative Concentrations

Acquired resistance to preservatives by bacteria is a recognized phenomenon propelled by the conditions under which the bacterium is growing (44,45). Exposure of microorganisms to sub-inhibitory or sub-lethal preservative concentrations during manufacturing is an acquired mechanism that can cause the development of antimicrobial resistance to preservatives. Antimicrobial resistance to chlorhexidine and quaternary ammonium compounds (QACs) has been previously described, but this resistance is often unstable. When chlorhexidine and QAC preservative–resistant cells are transferred to a preservative-free growth conditions, eliminating the selective pressure, the cells become re-sensitized to the antimicrobial activity of both chlorhexidine and QAC (46).

In experiments performed by Orth and Lutes, laboratory strains of *Pseudomonas* a*eruginosa*, *Escherichia coli*, and *Staphylococcus aureus* were adapted to preservatives by exposing them in sub-inhibitory and sub-lethal concentrations of the following preservatives: methylparaben, imidazolidinyl urea, Quaternium-15, a 3:1 blend of MCIT/MIT, phenoxyethanol, DMDM hydantoin, and formaldehyde (9). In this study, *E. coli* and *S. aureus* isolates did not adapt to the presence of methylparaben whereas *Ps. aeruginosa* isolate was capable of this adaption to methylparaben. Although each laboratory test microorganism tested was capable of adaption and resistance to imidazolidinyl urea, Quaternium-15, DMDM hydantoin, a 3:1 blend of methylchloroisothiazolinone/methylisothiazolinone and formaldehyde. However, none of the laboratory test microorganisms were found to adapt to the presence of phenoxyethanol.

During the 1990s, bacterial isolates with reduced antimicrobial susceptibility to triclosan were produced in laboratory experiments by repeated exposure to sub-lethal concentrations (47).

Outer Membrane Changes

Outer membrane changes of the bacterial cell have been implicated to cause the development of preservative resistance. For example, Favet determined that adapted bacteria could survive in low concentrations of Kathon CG (a blend of 3:1 MCIT/MIT) and imidazolidinyl urea (45). It was postulated that this preservative adaptation could be due to changes in the outer membrane of the cell by its implanted proteins because they play an important role in excluding harmful compounds into the cell (46). For an antimicrobial agent to have a detrimental effect, it must enter the interior of the cell and attain a sufficient concentration at the target site by passing through these outer membrane proteins (48). Therefore, the development of resistance to some antimicrobial agents is effected by a change in the permeability of the outer membrane by either the overexpression or loss of certain outer membrane proteins (48,49). An isolate of *Pseudomonas aeruginosa* exposed to increasing concentrations of Kathon CG demonstrated a surge in resistance to the preservative (12). It was noted that there was also the disappearance of a 35-kDa outer membrane protein (Protein T) in this adapted *Ps. aeruginosa* Kathon CG resistant strain. By using the pure forms of MCIT and MIT, sub-minimum inhibitory concentrations had been found to cause *Ps. aeruginosa* cultures to become resistant to each component of Kathon CG (50). With the development of antimicrobial resistance to each component of Kathon CG, there was also the disappearance of this 35-kDa outer membrane protein. When the resistant *Ps. aeruginosa* culture was subsequently cultured in the absence of MCIT or MIT, this 35-kDa outer membrane protein had reappeared.

Resistant *Pseudomonas aeruginosa* isolates had also been found to adapt to benzalkonium chloride by serially cultivating in increasing concentrations of this preservative. Characteristics accompanying the development of antimicrobial resistance to benzalkonium chloride included alterations in outer membrane proteins, cell surface charge and hydrophobicity, and fatty acid content of the cytoplasmic membrane all apparently effecting reduced benzalkonium chloride uptake and transport (51). In a different study, two-dimensional polyacrylamide gel electrophoresis analysis was conducted on the outer membrane of a benzalkonium-resistant *Pseudomonas aeruginosa* strain. In a benzalkonium chloride–resistant *Ps. aeruginosa* strain, the authors found a significant increase in the level of a 26-kDa outer membrane protein (named OprR) (52). Although the function of the OprR protein in the outer cell membrane is not yet clear, there was a correlation between the levels of expression of the OprR protein and the antimicrobial resistance of a *Ps. aeruginosa* strain to benzalkonium chloride. These results suggested that the OprR protein plays a significant role in the adaptation of *Ps. aeruginosa* strains to benzalkonium chloride.

Overexpression of flagellin components has been reported in triclosan-resistant *E. coli* isolates (53,54). Flagellin is a globular protein that forms a filament in the bacterial flagellum. By having a modification in the flagellin expression, there was a decrease in the levels of intracellular ethylenediaminetetraacetic acid (EDTA) and sodium deoxycholate uptake which indicates the involvement of the outer membrane of the cell as a permeability barrier to preservatives as mentioned for *Pseudomonas aeruginosa* (55). It has been previously speculated that changes to the outer membrane of the cell can cause antimicrobial resistance by changing the permeability of the cell to the entry of compounds (56). In a separate study, it was found that high concentrations of sodium benzoate did not limit proliferation and control adaptability of *Enterobacter gergoviae* in cosmetic product formulations (57). It was speculated that outer membrane changes in *Enterobacter gergoviae* could be responsible for this sodium benzoate resistance.

Efflux Pump

The presence of the efflux pump within the cytoplasmic membrane of the bacteria cell has also been implicated in microbial adaption and resistance to preservatives. Efflux pumps are transport proteins that can cause the extrusion of toxic substrates such as antibiotics and preservatives from within the interior of microbial cells and move them back into the external environment. In *Escherichia coli* and *Enterobacter gergoviae* isolates, the presence of an efflux pump had been found to establish the antimicrobial resistance to parabens (27,31). In a different study, Minimum Inhibitory Concentration (MIC) and Minimum Lethal Concentration (MLC) testing conducted on 83 selected *Burkholderia cepacia* complex industrial strains found increased resistance to DMDM hydantoin, benzisothiazolinone, MIT, a blend of 3:1 MCIT/MIT, methylparaben, phenoxyethanol, benzethonium chloride, and sodium benzoate (58). Since *Burkholderia lata* was found to be the most common industrial *Burkholderia cepacia* complex species of this study, the type strain—383T (LMG 22485T)—was used to study preservative tolerance because it had developed a stable preservative resistance to benzisothiazolinone, MIT, a 3:1 blend of MCIT/MIT, and benzethonium chloride. Several subcultures of the *Burkholderia lata* strain had been carried out in the presence of sub-lethal preservative concentrations of a 3:1 blend of MCIT/MIT. Transcriptomic analysis was used to determine the molecular basis for this *Burkholderia lata* strain adaptive resistance and it demonstrated that an efflux pump had played a major role in the development of resistance to a 3:1 blend of MCIT/MIT. By using the inhibitor L-Phe-Arg-β-napthylamide, the role of an efflux pump had been confirmed in the resistant *Burkholderia lata* 383-M-MCIT strain.

Efflux pumps have also been implicated in the development of triclosan resistance in bacteria. In general, these efflux pumps belong to the resistance nodulation cell division (RND) family. In clinical and laboratory strains of *Escherichia coli*, triclosan is a substrate of the AcrABTolC multidrug efflux pump (59). It has also been shown that clinical and environmental *Pseudomonas aeruginosa* isolates are also intrinsically resistant to the antimicrobial activity of triclosan by virtue of constitutive expression of the MexAB-OprM efflux pump. In addition, the MexCD-OprJ efflux pump has also been implicated in causing *Pseudomonas aeruginosa* to become resistant to triclosan (60).

Mutation

Mutation of the DNA in bacterial cells has also been speculated as a mechanism to cause preservative resistance because a formaldehyde-resistant gene had been located to be present on the cell chromosome of *Pseudomonas* (61–63). Isolates of the *Enterobacteriaceae* have been found to be resistant to the antimicrobial activity of formaldehyde-releasing preservatives, and the source of this resistance has been determined to be located on a cellular DNA plasmid and is self-transmissible (62,63).

Oxidative stress induced by triclosan is the selective mechanism that can cause genetic bacterial mutations (64). In Gram-negative and Gram-positive bacteria as well as Mycobacteria, triclosan has been shown to have a specific target of antimicrobial action against an enzyme in the bacterial fatty acid biosynthetic pathway, NADH-dependent enoyl-[acyl carrier protein] reductase (FabI) and its homolog InhA (65). Exposing *Escherichia coli* and *Staphylococcus aureus* to triclosan resulted in FabI mutations in the fatty acid biosynthetic pathway that caused each of these organisms to become resistant to triclosan (66,67). Studies have shown that some mutations affecting InhA will also lead to the development of triclosan resistance in *Mycobacterium smegmatis* and *Mycobacterium tuberculosis* (68,69).

The nfxB gene is a regulatory gene that controls the MexCD-OprJ efflux system in *Pseudomonas aeruginosa* (70). Exposing a susceptible *Pseudomonas aeruginosa (mexAB-oprM)* strain to triclosan caused triclosan resistance by the hyperexpression of the MexCD-OprJ efflux system following mutations in the nfxB regulatory gene (60).

Inhibiting the Development of Preservative Resistant Strains

Preservatives too can accommodate the development of antimicrobial-resistant microbial strains as do antibiotics. However, it is highly unlikely that antimicrobial resistance to preservatives originates during consumer product usage because preservative concentrations in finished cosmetic and personal care product formulations are generally high enough to prevent the development of adapted or mutated resistant strains of microorganisms. However, antimicrobial resistance to preservatives by a microorganism could easily develop in a manufacturing plant if it has one of the following conditions: a low standard of plant hygiene (poor cleaning and sanitization procedures), finished product formulations having a poorly designed preservative system, and using chemical disinfectants that use the same active ingredient as the preservative in a product formulation.

If manufacturing equipment surfaces are not properly cleaned and sanitized, finished product residuals and/or remains of process water rinses from cleaning and sanitization procedures can dilute the preservative system of a newly manufactured finished product formulation. Diluting a newly manufactured batch of finished product results in sub-inhibitory and/or sub-lethal concentrations of the preservative system components that could now act as a selective pressure that could generate a preservative-resistant isolate.

Subsequent development of a relevant biofilm of the resistant isolate becomes possible somewhere in the manufacturing equipment.

The presence of an equipment microbial biofilm consisting of preservative-resistant microorganisms will result in intermittent and erratic contaminations of product formulations. I personally observed a newly manufactured finished product contaminated due to microbiological compromise of product residuals improperly removed during the cleaning process of the manufacturing equipment. Similarly, water remains that had been improperly drained from manufacturing equipment following cleaning and sanitization procedures can support microbial growth. What results from both scenarios is the proliferation and potential development of resistance typically involving Pseudomonads and *Enterobacteriaceae*, which are preservative-resistant strains in which the diluted preservative system of the newly manufactured product batch had fallen to be below the sub-inhibitory levels driving both greater resistance and the development of a microbial biofilm harboring these resistant strains.

An improperly designed preservative system in a finished product formulation is also a risk that could cause the development of preservative-resistant strains especially in manufacturing facilities as well as microbial contamination that is introduced during consumer usage. For example, a recalled eye makeup remover that included a relatively weak preservative system consisting of only 0.2% methylparaben and 0.15% propylparaben was contaminated with paraben-resistant isolates of *Enterobacter cloacae, Klebsiella pneumoniae,* and *Klebsiella oxytoca.* Generally, parabens are used as preservatives in product formulations to establish antifungal activity, but have weak antimicrobial activity against bacteria. In the absence of a strong bactericidal preservative, selective pressure allowed parabens resistance in these incidental microbial contaminants. If a strong or potent bactericidal preservative such as phenoxyethanol, DMDM hydantoin, or imidazolidinyl urea with a chelator had been included, the product would have been more robustly preserved and the risk for the development of preservative resistance would have been greatly reduced. In the absence of such robust preservative efficacy to migrate risks of inadequate current Good Manufacturing Practices (cGMPs) and compromised manufacturing hygiene issues, a poorly designed product preservative system can allow the accidental generation of preservative-resistant strains even in a manufacturing system that is under appropriate cGMPs and controls. Similarly, inadequate preservation of a product formulation during consumer usage could pose a risk to preservative resistance and cause contamination of the finished product.

If a microorganism is resistant to the antimicrobial activity of a chemical disinfectant, it is possible that it is also resistant to a preservative in a product formulation if the active ingredient is in both the disinfectant and preservative. For example, a strain of *Pseudomonas aeruginosa* has been found to be resistant to N-dodecylpyridinium iodide (P-12), whose structure is similar to that of a common disinfectant, cetylpyridinium chloride (71). *Pseudomonas aeruginosa* has been well known to survive and proliferate in solutions of benzalkonium chloride (72). Benzalkonium chloride and cetylpyridinium chloride are QACs. It is well known that Gram-negative bacteria are less susceptible to QACs than Gram-positive bacteria, and *Pseudomonas* spp. have generally high intrinsic resistance compared to other Gram-negative bacteria (44). In addition, *Pseudomonas* spp. may adapt to survive against higher concentrations of QACs (73). In addition to being active ingredients in disinfectants, benzalkonium chloride and cetylpyridinium chloride can be used as preservatives in product formulations. If a microbial isolate in the manufacturing equipment is resistant to the antimicrobial activity of a benzalkonium chloride or cetylpyridinium chloride disinfectant, they could contaminate a finished product. If a finished product contains either benzalkonium chloride or cetylpyridinium chloride as the preservative, the resistant isolate may survive and eventually proliferate in that formulation.

Because the mechanism for the development of antimicrobial resistance is not fully understood for all of the different types of preservatives that are commonly used by the cosmetic and personal care industry, there are several steps that need to be in place in order to prevent their generation. One prevention step is to ensure that all of the cleaning and sanitization procedures of manufacturing equipment are validated and followed correctly at all times to prevent product residuals and rinse water remains in manufacturing equipment before a new finished product batch is compounded.

A second prevention step is that the use of sub-lethal or sub-inhibitory concentrations of preservatives be avoided for usage in a product formulation in order to prevent either preservative adaptation or mutation by a contaminating microorganism. The concentration of a preservative in a product formulation must be above the MIC and/or MLC in which there would be either static or cidal activity against contaminating microorganisms (74). The third prevention step is the use of other hurdle technology factors to prevent the growth of microorganisms. Included are product formulation factors such as a low or high pH, hostile manufacturing temperatures, low water activity, and modified finished product packaging that could prevent the introduction of microorganisms during consumer usage. The fourth prevention step involves the design of a preservative system for a susceptible product formulation to include the several different preservative system components to prevent the generation of a selective pressure and preservative- resistant strains to a single preservative system component of limited efficacy. The fifth prevention step is to use physical disinfectant methods such as heat in place of chemical sanitizers that may generate resistant isolates in which the active ingredient of the disinfectant is the same as the preservative in a product formulation. If a chemical disinfectant has to be used for sanitizing manufacturing equipment surfaces, it is recommended that a stronger disinfectant be used that has an active ingredient such as chlorine, peracetic acid, or glutaraldehyde to prevent the survivability and proliferation of resistant microorganism in a product formulation.

Confirming the Presence of a Preservative-Resistant Microorganism in a Product Formulation

In the context of several consecutive production batches of a cosmetic/personal care product formulation that are not in compliance with the Quality Control microbial release test specifications, it is highly possible that the contaminating microorganism could be preservative resistant. As part of the microbial root cause investigation to determine the source of the microbial contamination in the rejected finished product batches, it is recommended that qualitative and quantitative analytical chemical analysis be conducted to verify whether each of the preservative system components is indeed present at the indicated levels. If one or more of the preservative system components in a product formulation are either not present or at a low concentration in the rejected product formulations, it is highly likely that the formulation preservative system has been compromised by a contaminating microorganism. If all of the components of product preservative system are still present in the affected rejected product formulations, it may still be likely that a contaminating microorganism has a resistance mechanism consisting of either an efflux pump or there have been permeability changes to the outer cell membrane.

To confirm preservative resistance of a contaminating microorganism, it is recommended that MIC and MLC testing (75) be conducted on the contaminating genotypic or phenotypic identified microbial isolate(s) and its corresponding American Type Culture Collection (ATCC) type strain(s). If there is more than a two-fold resistance difference in the MIC/MLC values for the contaminating isolate in comparison to the corresponding ATCC type strain, the isolate can be considered to be resistant to the antimicrobial activity of the preservative.

As further confirmation that the recovered microbial contaminant is preservative-resistant, it is recommended that a microbial challenge test such as the United States Pharmacopeia Antimicrobial Effectiveness Test (AET) be conducted using the recovered microbial contaminant and its corresponding ATCC type strain as separate inoculums in an uncontaminated laboratory-prepared batch of the rejected finished product formulation. If the recovered microbial contaminant is able to survive at high levels (e.g., less than 1 logarithmic reduction from the calculated inoculum count [5–6 logarithmic count]) and the corresponding ATCC type strain had been reduced by 3 or more logarithmic counts in the finished product by seven days after inoculation, the recovered microbial contaminant is in all probability a preservative-resistant strain.

Elimination of Preservative-Resistant Isolates from a Manufacturing Facility

It is highly unlikely for preservative-resistant microbial isolates to be isolated from process or purified water and compressed air systems since a selective pressure is not present in these areas to cause the development of preservative resistance because isolated microorganisms are not exposed to preservatives. However, these systems can serve as a microbial contamination source where microorganisms can become preservative resistant if a corresponding selective pressure is present in the manufacturing equipment for a finished product.

A four-step process needs to be conducted to remove this preservative-resistant isolate from finished product manufacturing equipment. The first step is to determine sources of contamination in the finished product by conducting microbial monitoring of manufacturing equipment surfaces using swabs, contact plates, and rinse water samples. The purpose of this microbial monitoring is to detect the location of the preservative-resistant isolate in the manufacturing equipment. The second step is to ensure that all manufacturing equipment surfaces do not have finished product remains from previous manufactured batches. The effectiveness of cleaning manufacturing equipment procedures can be ensured by conducting either total organic carbon (TOC) analysis or conductivity readings on the final deionized water equipment rinse of the cleaning process. The third step is to ensure that there is no residual water in the manufacturing equipment after the completion of the cleaning process. The fourth and most difficult step is to sanitize equipment surfaces that have a preservative-resistant isolate. It is highly likely that this preservative-resistant isolate exists in a biofilm somewhere in the manufacturing equipment. Because preservative-resistant cells in a biofilm are embedded in a slimy extracellular matrix that is difficult to remove, the preservative-resistant isolate is protected against chemical disinfectants. The most effective sanitization means to remove a manufacturing equipment biofilm containing a preservative-resistant isolate is to use purified hot water as a physical disinfectant at a temperature between 60.0°C with 30-minute exposure and 80.0°C with 10-minute exposure. Heat from the hot water will pass through the extracellular matrix and kill the embedded preservative-resistant isolate. If a chemical disinfectant is used as a sanitizer, it may take several attempts to remove several layers of the microbial biofilm from the surface of the manufacturing equipment. A second source of microbial contaminants in non-sterile cosmetic and personal care products is raw ingredients. The most likely raw ingredient types to be contaminated with microorganisms are those either susceptible to microbial contamination such as botanical ingredients, starches, sugars, proteins, natural gums, etc., or those preserved such as with surfactants, natural extracts, and botanical solutions. For those raw ingredients that can support the growth of microorganisms, it is highly unlikely that they would contain preservative-resistant isolates due to the lack of a preservative that is part of the raw ingredient composition. However, there is potential for preserved raw ingredient to be contaminated with preservative-resistant isolates due to supplier problems in the cleaning and sanitization of raw ingredient manufacturing equipment. If a preserved raw ingredient is contaminated with a preservative-resistant isolate, it likely will contain a high number of microorganisms. To prevent the entry of preservative-resistant isolates from those raw ingredients that had been preserved, appropriate Quality Control microbial release testing will need to be performed to ensure compliance with the microbial test specifications.

Antibiotics Resistance to Preservative Resistance

In November 2011, the United States Food and Drug Administration (FDA) held a public meeting entitled "Cosmetic Microbiological Safety Issues" (Fed. Reg. 76.67461). During a discussion on preservative challenge testing of finished products, a question was asked regarding antibiotic-resistant bacteria in finished products posing a specific health risk to users of cosmetics. One aspect of cosmetic microbiology that has not been adequately addressed is the susceptibility of cosmetic/personal care product formulation contaminants to preservatives and antibiotics. During consumer in-use testing of prototype product formulations during development, it is not unusual to isolate microbial contaminants that are antibiotic resistant due to the widespread presence of these organisms in the general population. For example, Flores et al. had isolated several bacterial species from contaminated cosmetics and found that many of these isolates exhibited resistance to more than one preservative category, but found correlation between preservatives and antibiotic resistance (6). However, Osungunna et al. reported that bacterial contaminants of cosmetics were resistant to many antibiotics, but again this resistance did not correlate to that of the respective preservatives (76).

Preservatives are effective against a wide spectrum of bacteria and function through a variety of mechanisms that can differ from those mechanisms of action for antibiotics (44,77). *Pseudomonas aeruginosa* cells adapted to benzalkonium chloride, did show resistance to other membrane-active agents but not to clinically relevant antibiotics (78). In a different study, the adaptive mechanisms of *Enterobacter gergoviae, Pseudomonas putida,* and *Burkholderia cepacia* against several different formaldehyde-releasing preservatives (i.e., DMDM hydantoin, Quaternium 15, imidazolidinyl urea, diazolidinyl urea, sodium hydroxymethylglycinate) were studied to determine if these resistant bacterial species were able to generate cross-resistance to other preservatives as well as cross-resistance to antibiotics (79). MIC testing of formaldehyde-releasing preservative-resistant strains showed a diminished susceptibility to the formaldehyde-releasing preservatives, but not to other commonly used cosmetic preservatives (i.e., methylparaben, propylparaben, MCIT/MIT, phenoxyethanol, chlorphenesin, etc.). However, MIC testing of these formaldehyde-releasing resistant strains showed an increasing antimicrobial resistance to several types of antibiotics (e.g., β-lactams, quinolones, rifampicin, and tetracycline) when compared to the results of strains that are susceptible to formaldehyde-releasing preservatives. However, it should be noted in this study that some of the formaldehyde-releasing resistant isolates had MIC levels for certain of the antibiotics 2–8-fold higher from the susceptible strains, but these increased MIC levels for antibiotic resistance were found to be insufficient to cause the development of clinical antibiotic resistance. The increase in the antibiotic MIC levels for the tested formaldehyde-releasing resistant strains may have been due to the presence of an efflux mechanism effecting removal of antibiotics rather than due to the presence of a formaldehyde dehydrogenase enzyme.

Confirmation of the effectiveness of several preservative systems against antibiotic-resistant staphylococci in cosmetic formulations has been reported based on MIC/MLC and microbial challenge testing (80). In one study, a total of 21 different ATCC *Staphylococcus* strains compromising 12 antibiotic susceptible and 9 resistant isolates were employed. For each *Staphylococcus* isolate, MIC/MLC testing was conducted on 12 commonly used cosmetic preservatives and preservative blends and no significant differences were observed in MIC and MLC values between the antibiotic susceptible and resistant isolates. In addition, microbial challenge testing was conducted on 27 different marketed skin care, hair care, and color cosmetic product formulations with each of the antibiotic susceptible and resistant of *Staphylococcus* strains. At 4 hours, 2, 5, 7, 14, 21 and 28 days post-inoculation, the recovery for each isolate was determined in each of the inoculated product formulations. None of the *Staphylococcus* isolates was recovered from 24/26 of the aqueous formulations after the 2-day sampling point. In contrast, post-inoculation recovery of several strains of both antibiotic susceptible and resistant *Staphylococcus* isolates were observed in the oil-based anhydrous formulation and 2 of the aqueous formulations, although recovery decreased between the time of inoculation and 5–14 days post-inoculation. There was no recovery of antibiotic-resistant or susceptible strains at or beyond the 14-day sampling point for any of the 3 formulations; thus each was considered adequately preserved according to the criteria (≥ 2 log reduction at 14 and 28 days) in the USP AET. On the basis of these observations, it was concluded that adequately preserved cosmetic formulations are no less effective against antibiotic-resistant staphylococci compared to those which are not.

Using a similar approach, the effectiveness of several preservative systems that are commonly used in cosmetic formulations were evaluated against several antibiotic susceptible and resistant Gram-negative bacilli (81). A total of 23 ATCC strains (*Acinetobacter baumannii, Enterobacter. cloacae, Escherichia coli, Pseudomonas aeruginosa, Klebsiella pneumoniae,* and *Stenotrophomonas maltophilia*) comprising 6 susceptible and 17 resistant isolates had been employed. MIC/MLC values of 15 preservatives and preservative blends were determined for each of the tested Gram-negative bacilli isolates, and the results showed no significant differences between the antibiotic susceptible and resistant isolates. In addition, 15 different marketed aqueous skin care, hair care, personal care, and color cosmetic product formulations containing one or more of the preservative systems were used to conduct microbial challenge testing based on inoculation with each of the 23 isolates. At 4 hours, 2, 5, 7, 14, 21 and 28 days post-inoculation, sample aliquots were removed to determine the plate count recovery of each isolate. At the 2-day sampling point, isolates of both antibiotic susceptible and resistant strains of *Enterobacter, Escherichia, and Klebsiella* were recovered (at 10^1–10^4 CFU/gram) from 6 of the 15 formulations. After 5 days, isolates of antibiotic-resistant (but not antibiotic-susceptible) strains of *Escherichia coli* were recovered at levels of 620 and 630 CFU/gram, respectively, in 2 of the 15 cosmetic formulations. However, there was no recovery of either antibiotic-resistant or susceptible Gram-negative bacilli at or beyond the 7-day sampling point from any of the 6 formulations, and thus each was considered adequately preserved according to the criteria ($\geq$ 2 log reduction at 14 and 28 days) of the United States Pharmacopeia Antimicrobial Effectiveness Test. These observations indicate that adequately preserved cosmetic formulations are no less effective against antibiotic-resistant Gram-negative bacilli compared to those which are antibiotic susceptible. Besides these two studies, there have been several additional studies that failed to demonstrate a correlation between resistance to preservatives and antibiotics (76,82,83).

At this time, there are no data showing that a microorganism resistant to the antimicrobial activity of preservatives demonstrates cross-resistance to antibiotics or antibiotic resistant microorganisms showing resistance to preservatives. In general, the mode of action of antibiotics include inhibition of nucleic acid, cell-wall, or protein synthesis (84). However, bacterial resistance to antibiotics involves a single mechanism such as antibiotic inactivation, changes in the outer membrane permeability, target site alternation, and efflux pump mechanisms (85). A possible reason for the absence of cross resistance between antibiotics and preservatives may be due to the fact that preservatives have several different reported mechanisms of action involving multiple targets such as bacterial cell wall disruption, inhibition of protein biosynthesis, and inhibition of biosynthetic pathways (44,77). In addition, the absence of such cross-resistance be related to the relatively high preservative concentrations used in cosmetic/personal care product formulations (e.g., a single paraben ester is used at a concentration between 10 to 40 grams/kilogram in a product formulation) when compared that of antibiotic applications (e.g., amoxicillin standard dosage is between 20 to 40 milligrams/kilogram of body weight) (86,87). Because preservatives are used at a far higher concentration in a product formulation, it is highly unlikely that an antibiotic-resistant strain will develop resistance to the antimicrobial activity of a preservative.

Summary

In conclusion, the potential development of antimicrobial resistance to cosmetic/personal care preservatives in microorganisms is documented risk. There are several different intrinsic and acquired mechanisms in how microorganisms can become resistant to the antimicrobial activity of preservatives. However, steps can be taken to prevent the development of these preservative-resistant strains. If a microbial contaminant from a product formulation is suspected to be preservative resistant, MIC and MLC tests can be performed to verify its resistance. In addition, there is no evidence that antibiotic-resistant isolates are able to generate resistance to the antimicrobial activity of preservatives and vice versa due to preservatives having multiple sites of antimicrobial action in comparison to antibiotics.

REFERENCES

1. Warth, A.D. Resistance of yeast species to benzoic and sorbic acids and to sulfur dioxide. *J. Food Protec.* 1985, 48 (7): 564–569.
2. Piper, P., Ortiz-Caleron, C., Hatzixanthis, K., Mollapour, M. Weak acid adaptation: the stress response that confers yeasts with resistance to organic acid food preservatives. *Microbiol.* 2001, 147 (10): 2635–2642.

3. Adair, F.W., Geftic, S.G., Gelzer, J. Resistance of *Pseudomonas* to quaternary ammonium compounds. *Appl. Microbiol.* 1971, 21 (3): 1058–1063.

4. Close, J., Nielson, P.A. Resistance of a strain of *Pseudomonas cepacia* to esters of p-hydroxybenzoic acid. *Appl. Envir. Microbiol.* 1976, 31 (5): 718–722.

5. Bowman, P.I., Lindstrom, S.M. Resistance of *Pseudomonas* strains to imidazolidinylurea. *J. Soc. Cosmet. Chem.* 1985, 36: 413–423.

6. Flores, M., Mirillo, M., Crespo, M.L. Deterioration of raw materials and cosmetic products by preservative resistant microorganisms. *Int. Biodeter. Biodegrad.* 1997, 40 (2–4): 157–160.

7. Thomas, L., Maillard, J.–Y., Lambert, R.J.W., Russell, A.D. Development of resistance to chlorhexidine diacetate in *Pseudomonas aeruginosa* and the effect of a residual concentration. *J. of Hosp. Infec.* 2000, 46 (4): 297–303.

8. Chapman, J.S., Diehl, M.A., Fearnside, K.B. Preservative tolerance and resistance. *Int. J. Cosm. Sci.* 1998, 20: 31–39.

9. Orth, D.S., Lutes, C.M. Adaptation of bacteria to cosmetic preservatives. *Cosm. & Toiletr.* 1985, 100 (2): 57–64.

10. Borovian, G.E. *Pseudomonas cepacia*: growth in and adaptability to increased preservative concentrations. *J. Soc. Cosmet. Chem.* 1983, 34: 197–203.

11. Brozel, V.S., Cloete, T.E. Resistance of *Pseudomonas aeruginosa* to isothiazolone. *J. Appl. Bacteriol.* 1994, 76 (6): 576–582.

12. Chapman, J.S. Characterizing bacterial resistance to preservatives and disinfectants. *Int. Biodeter. & Biodegrad.* 1998, 41 (3–4): 241–245.

13. Russell, A.D. A review: mechanisms of bacterial resistance to non-antibiotics: food additives and food and pharmaceutical preservatives. *J. Appl. Bacteriol.* 1991, 71 (3): 191–201.

14. Ahn, Y., Kim, J.M., Kweon, O., Kim, S.J., Jones, R.C., Woodling, K., Gamboa da Costa, G., LiPuma, J.J., Hussong, D., Marasa, B.S., Cerniglia, C.E. Intrinsic resistance of *Burkholderia cepacia* complex to benzalkonium chloride. *mBio*. 2016, 7 (6): e01716-16.

15. Sondossi, M., Rossmoore, H.W., Wireman, J.W. The effect of fifteen biocides on formaldehyde resistant strains of *Pseudomonas aeruginosa*. *J. Indus. Microbiol.* 1986, 1 (2): 87–96.

16. Kummerele, N., Feucht, H.H., Kaulfers, P.M. Plasmid-mediated formaldehyde resistance in *Escherichia coli*: characterization of resistance gene. *Antimicrob. Agents Chemother.* 1996, 40 (10): 2276–2279.

17. Freese, E., Sheu, C.W., Galliens, D.E. Function of lipophilic acids as antimicrobial food actives. *Nature*. 1973, 2341: 321–328.

18. Nes, I.F., Eklund, I. The effect of parabens on DNA, RNA, and protein synthesis in *Escherichia coli* and *Bacillus subtilis*. *J. Appl. Bacteriol.* 1983, 54 (2): 237–242.

19. Ma, Y., Marquis, R.E. Irreversible paraben inhibition of glycolysis by *Streptococcus mutans* GS-5. *Lett. Appl. Microbiol.* 1996, 23 (5): 329–333.

20. Kok, R.G., D'Argenio, D.A., Ornston, L.N. Mutation analysis of PobR and PcaU, closely related transcription activation in *Acinetobacter*. *J. Bacteriol.* 1998, 180 (19): 5058–5069.

21. Zedan, H.H., Serry, F.M. Metabolism of esters of p-hydroxybenzoic acid by a strain of *Pseudomonas aeruginosa*. *Egypt. J. Microbiol.* 1984, 19: 41–54.

22. Sokolski, W.T., Chiderster, C.G., Honeywell, G.E. The hydrolysis of methyl p-hydroxybenzoate by *Cladosporium resinae*. *Dex. Ind. Microbiol.* 1962, 3: 179–187.

23. Close, J.-A., Nielsen, P.A. Resistance of a strain of *Pseudomonas cepacia* to esters of p-hydroxy benzoic acid. *Appl. Environ. Microbiol.* 1976, 31 (5): 718–722.

24. Suemitsu, R., Horiuchi, K.S., Yanagawase, S., Okamatsu, T. Biotransformation activity of *Pseudomonas cepacia* on p-hydroxybenzoates and benzalkonium chloride. *J. Antibact. Antifung. Agents*. 1990, 18: 579–582.

25. Valkova, N., Lepine, F., Valeanu, L., Dupont, M., Labrie, L., Bisaillon, J.-G., Beaudet, R., Shareck, F., Villemur, R. Hydrolysis of 4-hydroxybenzoic acid esters (parabens) and their aerobic transformation into phenol by the resistant *Enterobacter cloacae* strain EM. *Appl. Envir. Microbiol.* 2001, 67 (6): 2404–2409.

26. Valkova, N., Lepine, F., Bollet, C., Dupond, M., Villemur, R. *prbA*, a gene coding for an esterase hydrolyzing parabens in *Enterbacter cloacae* and *Enterobacter gergoviae* strains. *J. Bac.* 2002, 184 (18): 5011–5017.

27. Bredin J., Davin-Regli, A., Pages, J-M. Propyl paraben induces potassium efflux in *Escherichia coli*. *J. Antimicrob. Chemother.* 2005, 55 (6): 1013–1015.
28. Amin, A., Chauhan, S., Dare, M., Ansal, A.K. Degradation of parabens by *Pseudomonas betali* and *Burkholderia latens*. *Eur. J. Pharm. Biopharm.* 2010, 75 (2): 206–212.
29. Valkova, N., Lepine, F., Labrie, L., Dupond, M., Beaudet, R. Purification and characterization of PrbA, a new esterase from *Enterobacter cloacae* hydrolyzing the esters of 4-hydroxybenzoic acid (parabens). *J. Biol. Chem.* 2003, 278 (15): 12779–12785.
30. Anelich, L.E., Korston, L. Survey of microorganisms associated with spoilage of cosmetic creams manufactured in South Africa. *Int. J. Cosmet. Sci.* 1996, 18 (1): 25–40.
31. Davin-Regli, A., Chollet, R., Bredin, J., Chevalier, J., Lepine, F., Pages, J.M. *Enterobacter gergoviae* and the prevalence of efflux in paraben resistance. *J. Antimicrob. Chem.* 2006, 57 (4): 757–760.
32. Periame, M., Pages, J-M., Devin-Regi, A. *Enterobacter gergoviae* membrane modification are involved in the adaptive response to preservatives used in the cosmetic industry. *J. Appl. Microbiol.* 2015, 118 (1): 49–61.
33. Collier, P.J., Ramsey, A.J., Austin, P., Gilbert, P. Growth inhibitory and biocidal activity of some isothiazolone biocides. *J. Appl. Bacteriol.* 1990a, 69 (4): 569–577.
34. Collier, P.J., Ramsey, A.J., Waigh, R.D., Douglas, K.T., Austin, P., Gilbert, P. Chemical reactivity of some isothiazolone biocides. *J. Appl. Bacteriol.* 1990b, 69 (4): 578–584.
35. Collier, P.J., Austin, P., Gilbert, P. Isothiazolone biocides: enzyme-inhibiting pro-drugs. *Int. J. Pharm.* 1991, 74 (2-3): 195–201.
36. Williams, T.M. The mechanism of action of isothiazolone biocide. *Power Plant Chem.* 2007, 9: 14–22.
37. Meade, M.J., Waddell, R.L., Callahan, J.M., Soil bacteria *Pseudomonas putida* and *Alcaligenes xylosoxidans subsp. denitrificans* inactivate triclosan in liquid and solid substrates. *FEMS Microbiol. Lett.* 2001, 204 (1): 45–48.
38. Hay, A.G., Dees, P.M., Sayler, G.S. Growth of a bacterial consortium on triclosan. *FEMS Microbiol. Ecol.* 2001, 36 (2–3): 105–112.
39. Hundt, K., Martin, D., Hammer, E., Jonas, U., Kindermann, M.K., Schauer, F. Transformation of triclosan by *Trametes versicolor* and *Pycnoporus cinnabarinus*. *Appl. Environ. Microbiol.* 2000, 66 (9): 4157–4160.
40. Fewson, C.A. The growth and metabolic versatility of the Gram-negative bacterium NCIB 8250 ("Vibrio 01"). *J. Gen. Microbiol.* 1967, 46 (2): 255–266.
41. Chalmers, R.M., Scott, A.J., Fewson, C.A. Purification of the benzyl alcohol dehydrogenase and benzaldehyde dehydrogenase encoded by the TOL plasmid pWW53 of *Pseudomonas putida* MT53 and their preliminary comparison with benzyl alcohol dehydrogenase and benzaldehyde dehydrogenases I and II from *Acinetobacter calcoaceticus*. *J. Gen. Microbiol.* 1990, 136(4): 637–643.
42. Landete, J.M., Rodríguez, H., de Las Rivas, B., Muñoz, R. Characterization of a benzyl alcohol dehydrogenase from *Lactobacillus plantarum*. WCFS1. *J. Agric. Food Chem.* 2008, 56 (12): 4497–4503.
43. Horiuchi, K., Morimoto, K., Ohta T, Suemitus, R. Biotransformation of benzyl alcohol by *Pseudomonas cepacia. Biosci. Biotech. Biochem.* 1993, 57(8): 1346–1347.
44. Russell, A.D., Chopra, I. *Understanding Antibacterial Action and Resistance.* 2nd ed. Chichester, UK: Ellis Horwood. 1996.
45. Favet, J., Fehr, A., Griffiths, W., Amacker, P.A., Schorer, E. Adaptation of *Escherichia coli*, *Pseudomonas aeruginosa*, and *Staphylococcus aureus* to Kathon CG and Germall II in an O/W Cream. *Cosm. & Toiletr.* 1982, 2 (12): 75–85.
46. Nikaido, N., Vaara, M. Outer membrane. In:. *"Escherichia coli"* and *"Salmonella typhimurium"; Cellular and Molecular Biology.* (Neidhardt, F.C., Curtiss, R., eds.) Washington, DC: ASM, 1987, 7–22.
47. Yazdankhah, S.P., Scheie, A.A, Arne Høiby, E.A., Lunestad, B-T, Heir, E., Fotland, T.O., Naterstad, K., Kruse, H. Microbial drug resistance. 2006, 12 (2): 83-90.
48. Nikaido, N. Non-specific and specific permeation channels of the *Pseudomonas* outer membrane. In: *"Pseudomonas"; Molecular Biology and Biotechnology.* (Galli, E., Silver, S., Witholt, B., eds.). Washington, DC: ASM, 1992, 146–155.
49. Hancock, R.E.W, Siehnel, R., Martin, N. Outer membrane proteins of *Pseudomonas. Mol. Microbiol.* 1990, 4: 1069–1075.

50. Winder, C.L., Al-Adham, I.S., Abdel Malek, S.M., Buultjens, T.E., Horrocks, A.J., Collier, P.J. Outer membrane protein shifts in biocide-resistant *Pseudomonas aeruginosa* PAO1. *J. Appl. Microbiol.* 2000, 89 (2): 289–295.

51. Loughlin, M.F., Jones, M.V., Lambert, P.A. *Pseudomonas aeruginosa* cells adapted to benzalkonium chloride show resistance to other membrane-active agents but not to clinically relevant antibiotics. *J. Antimicrob. Chemother.* 2002, 49 (4): 631–639.

52. Tabata, A., Nagamune, H., Maeda, T., Murakami, K., Miyake, Y, Kourai, H. Correlation between resistance of *Pseudomonas aeruginosa* to quaternary ammonium compounds and expression of outer membrane protein OprR. *Antimicrob. Agents Chemother.* 2003, 47 (7): 2093–2099.

53. Bailey, A.M., Constantinidou, C., Ivens, A., Garvey, M.I., Webber, M.A., Coldham, N., Hobman, J.L., Wain, J., Woodward, M.J., Piddock, L.J. Exposure of *Escherichia coli* and *Salmonella enterica serovar Typhimurium* to triclosan induces a species specific response, including drug detoxification. *J. Antimicrob. Chemother.* 2009, 64 (5): 973–985.

54. Sheridan, A., Lenahan, M., Condell, O., Bonilla-Santiago, R., Sergeant, K., Renaut, J., Duffy, G., Fanning, S., Nally, J.E., Burgess, C.M. Proteomic and phenotypic analysis of triclosan tolerant verocytotoxigenic *Escherichia coli* O157:H19. *J. Proteomics.* 2013, 80: 78–90.

55. Zhou, G., Shi, Q.S., Ouyang, Y.S., Chen, Y.B. Involvement of outer membrane proteins and peroxidesensor genes in *Burkholderia cepacia* resistance to isothiazolone. *World J. Microbiol. Biotechnol.* 2014, 30 (4): 1251–1260.

56. Cloete, T.E. Resistance mechanisms of bacteria to antimicrobial compounds. *Int Biodeterior. Biodegrad.* 2003, 51 (4): 277–282.

57. Périamé, M., Pagès, J.M., Davin-Regli, A. *Enterobacter gergoviae* adaptation to preservatives commonly used in cosmetic industry. *Int. J. Cosmet. Sci.* 2014, 36 (4): 386–395.

58. Rushton, L., Sass, A., Baldwin, A., Dowson, C.G., Donoghue, D., Mahenthiralingam, E. A key role for efflux in the preservative susceptibility and adaptive resistance of *Burkholderia cepacia* complex bacteria. *Antimicrob. Agents Chemother.* 2013, 57 (7): 2972–2980.

59. McMurry, L.M., Oethinger, M., Levy, S.B. Overexpression of marA, soxS, or acrAB produces resistance to triclosan in laboratory and clinical strains of *Escherichia coli*. *FEMS Microbiol. Lett.* 1998. 166 (2); 305–309.

60. Chuanchuen, R., Beinlich, K., Hoang, T.T., Becher, A., Karkhoff-Schweizer, R.R., Schweizer, H.P. Cross-resistance between triclosan and antibiotics in *Pseudomonas aeruginosa* is mediated by multidrug efflux pumps: exposure of a susceptible mutant strain to triclosan selects nfxB mutants overexpressing MexCD-OprJ. *Antimicrob. Agents Chemother.* 2001, 45 (2): 428–432.

61. Kaulfers, P-M., Brandt, D. Isolation of a conjugative plasmid in *Escherichia coli* determining formaldehyde resistance. *FEMS Microbiol. Lett.* 1987, 43 (2): 161–163.

62. Kaulfers, P-M., Wollmann, A. Cloning and expression of formaldehyde resistance from *Escherichia coli*. *FEMS Microbiol. Lett.* 1988, 55 (3): 299–302.

63. Wollmann, A., Kaulfers, P-M. Formaldehyde resistance in *Enteriobacteriaceae* and *Pseudomonas aeruginosa*: identification of resistance genes by DNA – hybridization. *Zentrabl. Bakteriol. Parasitenkd. Infecktion- SKR. Hyg.* Abst 1 Orig. 1991, 191 (5-6): 449–456.

64. Lu, J., Jin, M., Nguyen, S.H., Mao, L., Li, J., Coin, L.J.M., Yuan, Z., Guo, J. Non-antibiotic antimicrobial triclosan induces multiple antibiotic resistance through genetic mutation. *Environ Int.* 2018, 118 (September 2018): 257–265.

65. Schweizer, H.P. Triclosan: a widely used biocide and its link to antibiotics. *FEMS Microbiology Letters.* 2001, 202 (1): 1–7.

66. Heath, R.J., Yu, Y.T., Sharpiro, M.A., Olson, E., Rock, C.O. Broad spectrum antimicrobial biocides target the FabI component of fatty acid synthesis. *J. Biolog. Chemother.* 1998, 273 (46): 30316–30320.

67. Heath, R.J., Li, J., Roland, G.E., Rock, C.O. Inhibition of the *Staphylococcus aureus* NADPH-dependent enoyl-acyl carrier protein reductase by triclosan and hexachlorophene. *J. Biolog. Chemother.* 2000, 275 (7): 4654–4659.

68. McMurry, L.M., McDermott, P.F., Levy, S.B. Genetic evidence that InhA of *Mycobacterium smegmatis* is a target for triclosan. *Antimicrob. Agents Chemother.* 1999. 43 (3): 711–713.

69. Mdluli, K., Sherman, D.R., Hickey, M.J., Kreiswirth, B.N., Morris, S., Stover, C.K., Barry. C.E. Biochemical and genetic data suggest that InhA is not the primary target for activated isoniazid in *Mycobacterium tuberculosis*. *J. Infect. Dis.* 1996, 174 (5): 1085–1090.

70. Gotoh, N., Tsujimoto, H., Tsuda, M., Okamoto, K., Nomura, A., Wada, T., Nakahashi, M., Nishino, T. Characterization of the MexC-MexD-OprJ multidrug efflux system in Δ*mexA-mexB-oprM* mutants of *Pseudomonas aeruginosa*. *Antimicrob. Agents Chemother*. 1998; 42 (8): 1938–1943.

71. Tabata, A., Maeda,T., Nagamune, H., Koura, H. 2002. Characterization of *Pseudomonas aeruginosa* resistant to a quaternary ammonium compound. *Biocontrol Sci*. 2002, 7 (3): 147–153.

72. Adair, F.W., Geftic, S.G., Gelzer, J. Resistance of *Pseudomonas* to quaternary ammonium compounds. I. Growth in benzalkonium chloride solution. *Appl. Microbiol*. 1969, 18 (3): 299–302.

73. Langsrud, S., Sundheim, G., Borgmann-Strahsen, R. Intrinsic and acquired resistance to quaternary ammonium compounds in food-related *Pseudomonas* spp. *J Appl. Microbiol*. 2003, 95: 874–882.

74. DGK MAHEG, Microbiology – Do microorganisms develop resistance to antimicrobial biocides? *IFSCC Magazine*. 2000, 3 (2): 35–37.

75. National Committee for Clinical Laboratory Standards. 2000. Methods for dilution antimicrobial susceptibility tests for bacteria that grow aerobically: Approved standard M7-A5 National Committee for Clinical Laboratory Standards, Wayne, PA.

76. Osungunna, M.O., Oluremi, B.B., Adetuyi, A. Bacteriological and antibiotic sensitivity patterns of bacterial isolates from creams and lotions hawked in Sagamu. *Ogun State. Pakistan J. Nutri*. 2010, 9 (8): 773–775.

77. Poole, K. Mechanisms of bacterial biocide and antibiotic resistance. *J. Appl. Microbiol. Sympos. Suppl*. 2002, 92: 55S–64S.

78. Loughlin, M.F., Jones, M.V., Lambert, P.A. *Pseudomonas aeruginosa* cells adapted to benzalkonium chloride show resistance to other membrane-active agents but not to clinically relevant antibiotics. *J. Antimicrob. Chemother*. 2002, 49 (4): 631–639.

79. Orús, P., Gomez-Perez, L., Leranoz, S., Berlanga, M. Increasing antibiotic resistance in preservative-tolerant bacterial strains isolated from cosmetic products. *Int. Microbiol*. 2015, 18 (1): 51–59.

80. English, D.J., Yang, Y., Tran-Osowski, L., Pungitore, S., Lapointe, K., Chu, V., Scotti, M., Gettings, S.D. Evaluation of commonly used preservatives in cosmetic formulations against antibiotic susceptible and resistant *Staphylococcus* isolates. American Society for Microbiology 113th General Microbiology Meeting Poster, Denver, Colorado. 2013.

81. English, D.J., Yang, Y., Tran-Osowski, L., Lapointe, K., Ceccarelli, C., Kowal, L., Rivas, M., Gettings, S.D. Evaluation of commonly used preservatives in personal care formulations against antibiotic-susceptible and antibiotic-resistant Gram-negative isolates. American Society of Microbiology 114th Meeting Poster, Boston, Mass. 2014.

82. Shaqra, Q.M.A., Al-Momani, W., Al-Groom, R.M. Susceptibility of some bacterial contaminants recovered from commercial cosmetics in Jordan to preservatives and antibiotics. *Trop. J. Pharm. Res*. 2014, 13 (2): 255–259.

83. Martins, R.X., Viana, A.A.G., Ferreiral, G.F., Cavalcanti, T.C., Amaral, I., Travassos, R., Vasconcelos, U. Preservative and antimicrobial susceptibility of non-fermenting bacilli recovered from solid waste of beauty salons in Brazil. *J. Appl. Pharm. Sci*. 2018, 8 (6): 169–174.

84. Kapoor, G., Saigal, S., Elongavan, A. Action and resistance mechanisms of antibiotics: a guide for clinicians. *J. Anaesthesiol. Clin. Pharmacol*. 2017. 33 (3): 300–305.

85. Wise, R. A review of the mechanisms of action and resistance of antimicrobial agents. *Can. Respir. J*. 1999 Jan–Feb, 6 Suppl. A: 20A-2A.

86. Wallhausser, K.H. Appendix B Antimicrobial Preservatives Used by the Cosmetic Industry. In: *Cosmetic and Drug and Drug Preservation, Principles and Practice*. (Kabara, J.J. ed.) New York: Marcel Dekker. 1984: 605–745.

87. www.mayoclinic.org/drugs-supplements/amoxicillin-oral-route/proper-use/drg-20075356.

6

Antimicrobial Preservative Efficacy and Microbial Content Testing*

Scott V.W. Sutton with Philip A. Geis

Introduction

Cosmetics do not need to be sterile, but they must be adequately preserved or protected from microbial contamination and spoilage. When consumers use cosmetic products, they repeatedly challenge the cosmetics with microorganisms in saliva, on dirty hands, and in tap water. Microbial growth may occur in cosmetics and toiletry articles kept in a bathroom and subjected to heat and humidity (1). These products include mascaras, eye shadows, shampoos, facial powders, and facial lotions (foundations and moisturizers).

Microbes in cosmetic products can lead to infection, discoloration, production of gas, and odor formation. Typical contaminants of cosmetics include *Enterobacter* spp., *Klebsiella* spp., *Serratia* spp., *Burkholderia* and *Pseudomonas* spp (2–4). Contaminated cosmetics intended for use in the eye area are of particular concern. The cornea especially, if compromised, can be extremely vulnerable to serious infection potentially resulting in blindness. Several cases of such infection due to mascara contamination from *Pseudomonas aeruginosa* (5) have occurred (1,6,7).

Although cosmetics occasionally are contaminated with spoilage microorganisms, the biggest threat of contamination is the presence of pathogens that may potentially pose health threats (8). Even nonpathogenic spoilage microbes in a cosmetic may cause disease under appropriate conditions. For example, a microbe contaminating a cosmetic product may be invasive if one applies the cosmetic to cover a blemish or break in the skin (9). Tragically, as reviewed in Chapter 2 fatal infections have even been traced to contaminated shampoos. People most at risk to serious infection from contaminated cosmetics are those whose immunities have been temporarily or permanently compromised by conditions such as broken skin, chronic diseases such as AIDs and diabetes, chemotherapy, and antirejection treatment for organ transplant, age, and the very old and very young (10).

---

* This chapter is an update to Dr. Sutton's 2006 chapter.

The microbiologist uses a variety of chemical preservatives to prevent contamination by pathogens or spoilage microorganisms. This extends the shelf life of products. The preservatives include benzyl alcohol, boric acid, sorbic acid, chlorhexidine, formaldehyde and formaldehyde releasers, parabens, quaternary ammonium compounds (QACs), phenol, imidazolidinyl compounds, isothiazolinones and others as reviewed in Chapter 2. Extant literature is available on these preservatives (1,11–13).

The survival and growth of microorganisms in cosmetic products is well known. The purpose of this chapter is to review the technologies of two methodologies central to cosmetic microbiology: preservative efficacy determination and microbial content testing.

Preservative Efficacy Methods

Current Preservative Efficacy Test Methods

Three organizations serve as primary sources for guidelines and methods covering testing of preservative efficacy in cosmetics and toiletry products in the United States. These sources are the Personal Care Product Council (PCPC) via its "CTFA" guidelines and methods, the American Society for Testing Materials (ASTM), and the United States Pharmacopeia (USP). The International Standards Organization (ISO) has established methods (14,15) largely derived from those of the above organizations and will not be addressed here. All three involve challenging cosmetic formulations with microorganisms. However, there are differences among the procedures that address the specific intention of the parent organizations (16–21). For example, the U.S. Food and Drug Administration (FDA) microbiological methods for cosmetics; Chapter 23 of its *Bacteriological Analytical Manual* (9) refers to validation of the CTFA method.

Preservation Efficacy Testing: General Procedure

The PCPC, ASTM, and USP have developed their own specific recommendations for organisms, media, growth and storage conditions, and test methods (Tables 6.1, 6.2, and 6.3). Standardization of all the requirements of a challenge must be achieved in order to obtain reproducible data.

The preparation of the challenge organisms is of special importance. The growth and preparation of a challenge organism determines the physiological state of cells that exert a direct influence on the results of any assay of disinfection efficacy (22,23). It is essential to maintain cultures of microorganisms that are subcultured on appropriate media to assure viability and resistance. Standard conditions for organism preparation and storage are essential for reproducible results.

It is important to remember that these tests use populations of cells—not individual cells. The data generated from these tests will be less variable if the cell population assayed is homogeneous. Liquid cultures or confluent growths on solid media are adequate for the reproducible growth of inocula, but reports about which mode provides the most reproducible results are conflicting (23). Whenever growth is slowed due to stress (including exposure to biocides) or because of some nutrient limitation, microbes have the potential to change their responses to a biocide (24).

Bacteria used as an inoculum are usually at a concentration of 1.0×10^8 colony-forming units per milliliter (CFU/mL). This allows for a 1:100 ratio of inoculum to product dilution, giving a final recommended concentration of bacterial challenge of 1.0×10^6 CFU/mL or gram. The high initial concentration of the challenge organism reduces the dilution of product upon inoculation. It is typical to use molds and yeasts at a final concentration of 1.0×10^4 mold spores or yeast/mL or gram (PCPC). The ASTM recommends 1.0×10^5 mold spores or yeast/mL or gram. The USP calls for standardization of the yeast or mold inoculum to 1.0×10^8 yeast/spores per mL. This translates to an initial inoculation of 1.0×10^6 microorganisms per milliliter or gram of product (see Table 6.2). Note that the dilution of the test product should not exceed 1%.

The challenge inoculum for the test consists of inoculating a known amount of test sample with the test organism. The technician then removes aliquots from the test sample and dilutes them in a neutralizing broth. Neutralization of the preservative must occur in the broth to avoid inflated estimates of efficacy. In

TABLE 6.1

Suggested organisms for testing. Consult individual method for isolate choice and inoculum composition

Organism	ATCC	USP	PCPC	ASTM
Bacteria				
Gram negative				
Klebsiella pneumoniae	10031		+	
Enterobacter cloacae	13047		+	
Escherichia coli	8739	+	+	+
Enterobacter gergoviae	33028		+	+
Pseudomonas aeruginosa	9027	+	+	
Burkholderia cepacia	25416		+	+
Pseudomonas fluorescens	13525		+	+
Pseudomonas putida	31483		+	
Gram positive				
Bacillus subtilis	6051		+	
Staphylococcus aureus	6538		+	+
Staphylococcus epidermidis	12228		+	
Fungi				
Candid albicans	10231	+	+	+
Aspergillus brasiliensis	16404	+	+	+
Penicillium sp.	Not specified		+	
Eupenicillium leviticum	10464			+
Other				
Isolate relevant to product			+	+

these procedures, some residual preservative will carry over into the recovery medium, and a neutralizer should be used to inactivate this residual and permit the organisms to grow. The CTFA and the ASTM both address the neutralization of the preserved test solution.

One determines the number of surviving CFUs by plating the broth dilutions on the proper agar. Table 6.3 lists several of these media and their uses. Thereafter, the plates are inoculated at the optimal temperatures until the colonies grow large enough to be countable. The number of surviving CFUs is then calculated from the dilution, yielding countable plate growth (traditionally 30–300 CFU/plate).

Criteria for passage of these tests vary. Surviving organisms are evaluated either as *percent survivors* (i.e., no more than 0.1% of inoculum surviving) or as *log_{10} unit reductions*. In practice, these are not different measures since the log reduction is calculated by subtracting the log_{10} unit of the survivors at a time point from the log_{10} unit of the inoculum concentration.

PCPC Method

These guidelines (25) were first issued in 1974 by CTFA's (Cosmetic Toiletry and Fragrance Association was the former name of the PCPC) Preservation Subcommittee.

Challenge Organism Inoculum

The challenge organisms suggested for testing cosmetics are listed in Table 6.1. In addition, it is often useful to include organisms that may be acquired from indigenous microflora around the eye, clinical isolates, or isolates from contaminated products.

One should culture the organisms on suitable media. Generally recommended media for bacteria include nutrient agar (26), tryptic soy agar (27), or Eugonagar (28). Culture media for fungi include Sabouraud dextrose agar (29), potato dextrose agar (30,31), or mycophil agar (32–34).

TABLE 6.2

Comparison of compendial challenge protocols

Parameter Specified	PCPC	ASTM	USP
Detailed passage information	yes	no	yes
Harvesting solution	3 identified	sterile saline	sterile saline
Use of actual contaminants	yes	yes	no
Specifics of mold harvesting	yes	yes	yes
Standardization procedures	no	yes	yes
Mixed culture inoculum	yes	yes	no
Pure culture inoculum	yes	yes	yes
Standardized inoculum			
Bacteria	no	$1X10^8$/mL	$1X10^8$/mL
Fungi	no	$1X10^7$/mL	$1X10^8$/mL
Challenge CFU/product volume			
Bacteria	$1X10^6$/mL	$1X10^6$/mL	10^5–10^6/mL
Fungi	$1X10^5$/mL	$1X10^5$/mL	10^5–10^6/mL
Inoculum amount	<1%	0.2mL	0.5–1%
Product sample size	no	20 g	no
Specified sample intervals (days)	weekly to 28	0,7,14,28	7,14,28
Rechallenge	no	yes	no
Neutralizers	yes	yes	yes
Neutralizer validation	yes	no	yes
Control products	no	yes	no

The storage of the working cultures is another concern. Once growth occurs, it is possible to maintain bacteria and yeast at 5°C on slants for a period dependent on the cell type. For example, most bacteria and *Candida* spp. remain viable for up to one month in refrigerated conditions, while *Pseudomonas aeruginosa* may not be useful after two weeks (depending on specific conditions).

One effective means of maintaining mold spores is to store them at room temperature in culture on slants. Weekly or periodic subculturing can be done to assure the viability of the microorganisms, but this practice raises the risk of loss of resistance. Cultures may also be frozen or lyophilized as an alternative to maintain the stability of the microorganism and end frequent subculturing. The main advantage to these latter storage means is that they prevent loss of genetic resistance factors. These factors, as well as those requiring phenotypic expression, are sometimes lost with frequent subculturing in media without the selective pressure of a biocide to maintain resistance due to genotypic and phenotypic characteristics. One may also maintain contaminating microorganisms in the same marginally preserved products from which they were isolated. This practice sustains continued resistance to the preservatives.

Conducting Test

The microorganism challenge is usually done in at least 20 g or mL of product. A recommended challenge level is 1.0×10^6 bacteria or 1.0×10^5 molds and yeast per gram of product. The PCPC prefers use of single cultures for the challenge or pooling of similar organisms to provide specific data for each organism or category of organism (35). Inoculum volume should be less than 1% of the final volume.

These challenge levels represent a larger microbial challenge of the product than might be expected from normal consumer use. Therefore, most challenge tests are far more stringent than they need to be in order to ensure that a product withstands contamination during consumer use. This is especially true when we consider that many products also have protective mechanisms for delivering the product without

TABLE 6.3

Media used in preservative efficacy testing

Agar	Microorganisms	Purpose	Ref.
Tryptic soy agar	Bacteria	General	27
Nutrient agar	Bacteria	General	26
Eugonagar	Variety	General	28
Sabouraud dextrose agar	Yeasts and molds	General	29
Potato dextrose agar	Yeasts and molds	General	30, 31
Mycological (mycophil) agar	Fungi	General	32, 33, 34, 43, 44
Mycophil agar, pH 4.7	Molds	General	32, 33, 34, 43, 44
	Acidic Bacteria		
	Yeast (saprophytic)		
Letheen agar	Bacteria	Neutralization/general	25, 35, 37, 38, 39
	Yeast, molds, anaerobic microorganisms		
Tryptic digest of casein and soy agar	Bacteria	General	40
	Yeasts and molds		
Infusion agar	Bacteria	General	25
Thioglycollate agar	Bacteria	Neutralization/general	25
Tryptone–glucose–yeast extract agar	Bacteria	General	30, 31
Dey–Engley agar	Bacteria	Neutralization/general	41, 63
Trypticase soy agar with lecithin and Polysorbate 80	Bacteria	Neutralization/general	29, 40
Soybean–casein digest agar	Bacteria, yeasts, and molds	General	29, 40
Letheen broth with lecithin	Bacteria	Neutralization/dilution	25, 37
Letheen broth with lecithin and Triton X-100	Bacteria	Neutralization/dilution	25
Thioglycollate broth	Bacteria	Neutralization/dilution	25, 37
	Yeast/mold		
Williamson-buffered suspending fluid (modified)	Bacteria, yeasts, and molds	Neutralization/dilution	25, 37

contact with the consumer; such protective mechanisms would be metered dosages or a closure system that encourages separation of the consumer from the product. Challenge tests do not measure the protection afforded by these delivery mechanisms (36).

Once the sample is inoculated, the technician mixes the contents thoroughly. A sample is taken and diluted in the proper neutralization broth to inactivate the preservative. If the neutralizer's effectiveness cannot be established, then physical dilution or membrane filtration may aid in inactivating the preservatives (see the section that follows).

Most procedures require pour plating of 1 g or 1 mL of the inoculated product. Some laboratories use an alternate streaking method to estimate the number of microorganisms present. Spread plating also can be used, especially when the organisms are sensitive to temperatures required for tempering agar (45–47°C). The inoculated samples are incubated at room temperature or at a temperature that encourages proliferation of the test organisms used in the challenge. The incubation temperature for the plates is typically 32–37°C for bacteria and 25–30°C for fungi.

Most test method development organizations such as PCPC, USP, and ASTM recommend sampling on the following days after each challenge: 0, 1, 2, 3 (eye cosmetics only), 7, 14, and 28 (other products). Some tests may need more than 28 days, depending on a product's intended usage. Rechallenges (multiple, sequential inoculations) are often conducted to estimate preservative adequacy in certain products.

Repeatedly challenging the product with a particular organism will show the number of challenges needed to inactivate the preservative system (25).

Neutralization and Recovery

The PCPC recommends diluting the inoculated sample with the neutralizers including: Letheen broth, Letheen broth with lecithin Tryptic soy broth and Eugon broth (25,37). Lecithin or Polysorbate 80 added to a medium is usually enough to neutralize most preservative carry-over and disperse the product when using the pour plate method (25). Letheen agar is a standard recommendation for bacteria, yeasts, and molds (35). This medium was originally intended as an anaerobic growth medium (38), but it is also effective for neutralizing QACs (39). Other media recommended by the PCPC (25,35) include tryptic digest of casein and soy agar (40), nutrient agar (26), thioglycollate agar (38), infusion agar (brain, heart, veal, or combinations), Eugonagar (28), tryptone–glucose–yeast or trypticase–glucose–yeast extract agars (30,31), Dey Engley (D–E) medium (41,42) and trypticase soy agar with lecithin and Polysorbate 80. Other media that may produce more luxuriant growths of fungi include Sabouraud dextrose agar (29), mycophil agar, mycological agar (32–34,43,44), and Eugonagar (28).

A neutralizer should be incorporated in the plated agar when recovering bacteria by plating (39,45–47). Most of these methods recommend Letheen agar (25,37). However, an agar with sodium thioglycollate should be used with a preservative containing mercury or other heavy metals. Alternatively, recovery of microorganisms can be facilitated by the dilution of a preservative, if appropriate for that preservative (48). The critical concern is the removal of residual antimicrobial activity to allow quantitative recovery of surviving microorganisms.

ASTM Method

Challenge Organism Inoculum

This method (49) is used to test preserved samples compared to nonpreserved samples. The ASTM provides a list of challenge organisms (Table 6.1). The method recommends maintaining the microorganisms per ATCC criteria. Relevant methods use nutrient agar (20) for bacteria and on mycophil agar at pH 4.7 for molds, yeasts, and acidophilic bacteria (32–34,43,44). Transfers should be performed monthly, with bacteria incubated at 32°C and fungi at 25°C.

One prepares fresh cultures for the inoculum. This is done by growing them on the proper solid medium for 25–37 hours at 35°C (bacteria) or 48–72 hours at 25°C (yeasts). Mold cultures should grow for 5–7 days (until full sporulation) at 25°C on proper media.

The method provides for harvesting the organisms with a sterile inoculating loop and transferring them to sterile distilled water. The optical density measured a McFarland Standard 32 to yield 1.0×10^8 bacteria/mL. Mold spores are dislodged from mycelial cultures by rubbing gently with a sterile inoculating loop or removal with a sterile glass hockey stick. Then the spores are filtered with sterile nonabsorbent cotton to remove the hyphae and break up any clumps. One may use a hemocytometer count to adjust the spore level to 1.0×10^7/mL.

Conducting Test

ASTM allows two types of challenges: a mixed culture or single culture method. The mixed culture challenge permits three separate inocula preparations. These preparations usually include equal portions of (1) Gram-positive bacteria, (2) Gram-negative bacteria, and (3) yeast and mold suspensions. To determine the number of CFUs, the method uses serial dilution. Plating is done in duplicate using Letheen agar (25,37). Incubation is carried out at 35°C for 48–72 hours for bacteria and at 25°C for 3–5 days for fungi.

ASTM suggests preparing three 120-g samples in glass containers with lids and inoculating each sample with 1 mL of each microorganism suspension (final concentration of 1×10^6 bacteria/mL or 1×10^5 yeasts or spores/mL). The inoculated samples are then mixed and stored at ambient temperature. At the proper times (0, 7, 14, 21, and 28 days), one part test sample is mixed with nine parts Letheen broth. Additional 10-fold dilutions are done, and duplicate plating of each dilution is performed with Letheen agar. Incubations of bacteria are done at 35°C (fungi at 25°C) for at least 48 hours (3–5 days for fungi). The CFU number per plate is then counted to determine the number of surviving microorganisms per gram of the test product.

Some cosmetics are subjected to repeated exposure or contamination. If that is the case, ASTM allows a rechallenge with the microorganisms at 21 or 28 days. ASTM, however, does not specify an inoculum level. The test would then continue for an additional 28 days.

Neutralization and Recovery

The ASTM does not directly address a protocol for neutralome haveization. Some have used a method that checks the neutralization of the preservative if no growth is seen on any plates. This is done by streaking plates from the 10^{-1} and 10^2 plates with a 10^{-3} dilution of nutrient broth culture of mixed inoculum. This mixed inoculum may be Gram-negative bacteria, Gram-positive bacteria and yeast, or a mixed culture of mold incubated 18–24 hours. Lack of growth after incubation at 32 and 25°C for 72 hours suggests that neutralization of the biocide did not take place. Unfortunately, this procedure does not prove that neutralization occurred at the time of plating.

The original plates used for the test have already been incubated at least 3 days. Therefore, the preservative is not in the condition it was in at the time of sampling. Growth in this system cannot be taken as evidence of effective biocide neutralization at the time of the sampling. Another far more appropriate method offered by ASTM is detailed in the section that follows.

Criteria for Passing

ASTM crtieria require at least 99.9% reduction for bacteria and yeast within 7 days and no increase thereafter. Within 7 days, fungi should show a 90% decrease and again show no increase within the remaining test period. Unpreserved controls should fail both these criteria.

USP Method

The USP method (27) has undergone a great number of changes in an attempt to harmonize with the European Pharmacopeia and the Japanese Pharmacopeia. In addition, many changes have been introduced in an effort to minimize variability between tests and between laboratories (50).

Challenge Organism Inoculum

Table 6.1 lists the recommended test organisms. One may also include any other organisms that are likely contaminants. A medium such as soybean–casein digest agar supports vigorous growth and is recommended for initial cultivation of such organisms (27,40).

Freshly grown stocks of a particular culture are prepared by inoculating a solid agar medium. Incubate bacterial cultures at 30–35°C for 18–24 hours. Incubate yeasts at 20–25°C for 44–52 hours, and molds at 20–25°C for 6–10 days. Then harvest the bacteria and yeast using sterile saline (0.9% NaCl) and dilute the suspended cells to 1×10^8 CFU/mL. The mold is harvested with sterile saline containing 0.05% Polysorbate 80, adjusting the spore count to 1×10^8 CFU/mL. The number of colony forming units per milliliter determines the amount of inoculum to use in the test. The viability of the suspension should be monitored, especially if not used promptly.

Conducting Test

A 20-mL sample of the product is transferred to a sterile, capped bacteriological tube if it is not possible to inoculate the product container and sample it aseptically. Inoculation of the test sample with the suspension is done using a 0.5 to 1% mL inoculum to 20 mL test sample. The concentration of microorganisms in solution should be between 1×10^5 and 1×10^6 CFU/mL. Numbers of viable microorganisms in the inoculum suspension are determined by the plate count method. This value is used to calculate the initial concentration of CFU/mL in the test product.

The inoculated containers are incubated at 20–25°C and examined 7, 14, 21, and 28 days after inoculation. Microbial numbers (CFU/mL) are determined by the plate count method at each of these intervals, and percentage change is estimated by comparison to initial viability.

Criteria for Passage

According to this method, an effectively preserved system will reduce the viable bacteria 1 log by day 7 and 3 logs by day 14. For yeasts and molds, the viable level must decrease or remain the same. The concentration for all microorganisms must remain at or below these designated levels for the remainder of the test.

Comparison of Methods

Of the three methods discussed, the ASTM includes the most detail. The CFTA procedure leaves more room for customizing a test for a specific target. The USP recognizes that many drugs are not subjected to the same rigors of consumer use and abuse as are cosmetics. Table 6.1 provides an overview of the three methods along with American Type Culture Collection (ATCC) data.

Challenge Microorganisms

Challenging a product with appropriate organisms is a major concern in determining how effective a preservative must be. Organisms representing possible contaminants obtained following consumer use or manufacture failures are ideal for challenge testing. Because organisms can develop resistance to preservatives and cause opportunistic infections (1,8), we must always be looking for new sources of challenge organisms.

Staphylococcus aureus (ATCC 6538) is a common skin organism (25). Most preservative challenge test methods use it to challenge frequently used cosmetic products because it is a common contaminant that may pose threats to consumers (8). It represents Gram-positive cocci in many tests. Since its nutrient needs are comparatively demanding, it does not always seem to be a logical choice as a challenge inoculum.

Pseudomonas aeruginosa is a non-fermentative Gram-negative rod suggested by all three testing groups. The ASTM and USP recommend ATCC strains 9027 and the PCPC recommends strains 15442 and 13388. *P. aeruginosa* is a well known, highly ubiquitous pathogen. It also shows high resistance to many preservatives (35). Burkholderia cepacia, another nonfermantative Gram negative is often used as it with P. aeruginosa is a very common contaminant of cosmetics.

Both the PCPC and the USP methods recommend *Escherichia coli*, ATCC 8739, a fermentative Gram-negative rod. It is a member of one of the largest bacterial families, the *Enterobacteriaceae*, and is considered an indicator of fecal contamination (35). Like most of the coliform bacteria, it can easily develop biocide resistance. *Enterobacter,* and *Klebsiella* are sometimes used for or with *E. coli*.

All three institutions recommend *Candida albicans* as naturally occurring representative yeast. It can be pathogenic (35) and also represent the resistance of yeasts to preserved systems. The PCPC, ASTM and USP recommend ATCC isolate 10231.

A major cause of product decomposition is contamination by filamentous fungi such as *Penicillium* or *Aspergillus* spp (35). All three methods recommend the use of *Aspergillus brasiliensis*. The PCPC, ASTM, and USP use the ATCC strain 16404, while PCPC also suggests the use of a Penicillium sp. isolate but offered no specific strain.

Microorganisms indigenous to the normal eye, clinically significant isolates, and product isolates are recommended by CTFA for challenging eye cosmetics. These include the organisms detailed in Table 6.1. Gram-positive spore formers are represented by *Bacillus subtilis*. Eye cosmetics and inadequately preserved systems may allow Gram-positive spore formers to survive, germinate, and actively proliferate. Using spore formers such as *B. subtilis* for a challenge inoculum should be done carefully in order to evaluate susceptibility of the vegetative forms (versus spores) to the preservative. If the inoculum preparation procedure promotes sporulation, then the challenge may be too rigorous for a product to pass until it is over-preserved and toxicologically unsafe for use.

Maintenance and Harvesting of Organisms

PCPC and ASTM specifically refer to ATCC culture maintenance recommendations for maintenance of cultures. PCPC also observes to option of storage of isolates in product to maintain unique characteristics, especially in evaluation of similar materials. USP does not address culture maintenance as it anticipates cultures from ATCC and specifies treatment. This is an important consideration as standardization of culture preparation is a critical concern for achieving reproducible results. Considerable work has been done by Peter Gilbert and his colleagues to show that a great deal of phenotypic variance occurs simply due to growing organisms under nutrient-limited conditions such as the one that occurs when grown to late log or early stationary phase (23,24). USP specifies that viable organisms used in the test be no more than five passages from the original ATCC culture. The ASTM and USP methods also cover harvesting and standardizing conditions that may involve filtration of mold spores (49).

Harvesting methodology differs for the ASTM and USP methods and this factor may influence the viability of organisms (50). Neither method specifies buffering the solutions to the pH or ionic range of the culture medium. Suspension of the cells in a solution that is at an incorrect pH or osmolarity compared with the culture medium may produce inhibitory toxic effects (51). Orth found that broth inocula decreased the rate of inactivation of the test organisms compared to the use of saline inocula prepared from surface growth on agar media (52). Although not specifically mentioned by Orth, this result was likely due to the broth medium serving as a preservative inactivating agent.

Preparation and Standardization of Inoculum

Dilution of the cell suspension should not occur in an unfavorable environment. Diluted cells are more susceptible to harm than denser cell concentrations. A buffered solution will protect against a pH change after the cells have been suspended (51). The ASTM uses sterile water while the USP uses sterile saline when washing the organisms from the transferred stock culture. The CTFA does not specify any recommendations for harvesting.

The ASTM is specific about the standardization of bacteria, yeasts, and molds. It recommends a certain spectrophotometer, spectrophotometric tube, and a specific absorbance wavelength. Neither the USP nor CFTA is are as specific. They require only a final inoculum level. The inoculum level is different for each of the three methods. Before inoculation, the ASTM recommends that the concentration of a microbial suspension be 1×10^8 CFU/mL for bacteria and 1×10^7 CFU/mL for yeasts and molds. The USP recommends adjusting the microbial or spore count to 1×10^8 CFU/mL while the PCPC does not address standardization of the suspension.

The resulting challenge level of the product is more similar between the methods than the inoculum levels. All three methods recommend a level of 1×10^6 CFU/mL or gram of product for bacteria. The USP actually gives a range between 10^5 and 10^6. For yeasts and molds, the CFU levels per milliliter or gram are slightly different. The ASTM recommends 1×10^5, the CTFA 1×10^4, and the USP again gives a range of 1×10^5–1×10^6 CFU/mL. The CTFA challenge level is comparatively low. As a result, it limits the measurable reduction to less than four $\log_{10}$ units.

Pure versus Mixed Cultures

The PCPC and ASTM recommends using a pure or mixed culture inoculum, while the USP method anticipate pure cultures. Mixed cultures may more accurately reflect the normal contamination profile of a product used by a consumer. However, pure cultures may exhibit more resistance to a preservative than a mixed culture (8,21). One recommendation is that mixed or pooled isolates used as inocula should be composed of related microorganisms (8). For example, one would combine Gram-positive or Gram-negative species.

Incubation Conditions, Interpretation, Rechallenge

Although all methods specify a ratio of inoculum to product, only ASTM identifies a specific product volume—20g. All three methods require sampling after inoculation at 0, 7, 14, and 28 days. In a separate protocol, PCPC also specifies sampling at days 1 through 3 for eye area cosmetics. By 7 days, according to the PCPC and ASTM, the vegetative bacterial counts should reach a 3 log or 99.9% reduction. The USP allows 14 days for this reduction of bacteria. The yeast and mold counts must be reduced by 90.0% at day 7 for the CTFA method and 28 days per ASTM. USP specifies that by 7, 14 and 28 days the levels of yeasts and molds remain the same or below the initial concentrations within a certain tolerance level (e.g., 0.5 log).

In discussing these criteria, it is interesting to note that an apparent increase in the number of microorganisms recovered may be noted under conditions where no increase is expected. This can happen even with well-characterized formulations in tests performed by experienced technicians. Orth characterized this as the "Phoenix Phenomenon" and argued that it is to be expected in tests of this type (53).

PCPC and ASTM recommend consideration of a rechallenge with microorganisms at 28 days. Repeat challenges may provide better indications of potential problems of product contamination while in consumer use (1). For example, rechallenge may be important for assessing hand and body lotion contamination or testing mascaras that are repeatedly used. Rechallenging or repeating the inoculations may indicate how the preservative system of a particular product will withstand insult before failure (36).

Other Published Methods

D-Value Methods

Orth proposed a rapid method for estimating preservative efficacy (52,54). This method uses short sample times and estimates the final response at 28 days by linear regression as a D-value. Orth claimed that each organism has a characteristic rate of death. When this rate is multiplied by the log of the inoculum challenge, it can predict the time required to inactivate the entire challenge (55).

This method is not a new one, but an adaptation from heat destruction D-values of food microbiology. One weakness inherent in this method is the extrapolation of kill beyond the measured data. This extrapolation has not been validated for linear regression analysis (56).

A second weakness of the method is that it assumes a linear relationship between the time of exposure to the biocide and the number of surviving microorganisms. One can usually analyze the logarithmic nature of biocide killing by log transforms. However, even this relationship does not exist for a variety of microorganisms and biocides (57).

If one performs all the D-value assays in precisely the same manner, it may be possible to show reproducible results. This would allow a rapid preliminary screening of preservatives, but should not be relied upon as the sole method of testing.

Capacity Tests

The capacity test assesses the efficacy of concentration and the antimicrobial spectrum of a preserved cream, suspension, or solution. Mixed bacterial cultures are grown in nutrient broth for 48 hours. Yeasts and molds are grown in 2% v/v malt extract in distilled water (58). The test method permits storage of mixed mold spore suspensions in distilled water at 4°C. These suspensions are from cultures grown on malt extract agar plates.

In a capacity study by Barnes and Denton (58), the mixed cultures consisted of: (1) Gram-negative bacteria (*Escherichia coli, Proteus vulgaris, Pseudomonas aeruginosa, P. fluorescens*), (2) Gram-positive bacteria (*Staphylococcus aureus, S. albus, Micrococcus flavus, M. luteus*), (3) aerobic spore formers (*Bacillus subtilis, Bacillus cereus, Bacillus megaterium*), (4) mold spores (*Mucor plumbeus, Aspergillus brasiliensis, Cladosporium herbarum, Penicillium spinulosum, Trichoderma* spp.), and (5) yeasts (*Saccharomyces cerevisiae, Sporobolomyces* spp., *Schizosaccharomyces pombe, Candida albicans*). The preservatives tested included benzalkonium chloride, Bronopol, chlorhexidine gluconate, chlorocresol, Dowicil 200, methyl parabens, Phenonip, propyl parabens, thimerosal, and "Preservative C". Barnes and Denton incorporated the preservatives into creams, suspensions, or solutions at recommended use levels and also tested two lower concentrations.

The test protocol required a thorough mixing of 1 mL inoculum into 20 g of the cream, suspension, or test formula. They stored the formulae at room temperature for 48 hours, then sampled the creams and suspensions with a sterile loop; 1 mL was removed from each of the solutions. Barnes and Denton dispersed the samples into either 5 mL (for creams and suspensions) or 9 mL (for solutions) of nutrient broth containing Lubrol® and lecithin as neutralizers for all preservatives except thimerosal, which required sodium thioglycollate as the neutralizer.

A sample of this dispersion was then plated on nutrient agar (bacteria) or malt extract (molds and yeasts) containing neutralizers. The authors incubated the plates at 37°C for 24 hours (bacteria) or for 25°C for 48 hours (molds and yeasts). They repeatedly cycled through the reinoculation and sampling 15 times or until 3 consecutive positive results occurred.

A preservative must reduce the number of viable organisms in an inoculated formulation by 10^3 within 48 hours for creams and suspensions to produce a single negative result according to Barnes and Denton (58). This ability diminishes gradually due to dilution and biocide absorption by the added organisms.

Bean (12) cited the need for a performance test rather than a typical preservative efficacy test. He felt that a performance test would measure "the ability of the contaminating organisms to destroy the product". Such a test may be more rapid than a typical preservative efficacy test and more quantitative in assessing the ability of a product to handle contamination.

Tests Predictive of Consumer Contamination

Brannan et al. (59) conducted a study designed to validate corporate preservative efficacy test as a predictive model of consumer contamination. This is a critical concern. One can control the microbial insults from the manufacturer by sanitary processing, but a product must also provide consumer protection from pathogens during use.

In a later study, Brannan evaluated two cosmetic formulations—a lotion and a shampoo—at three different preservative levels using a modified preservative efficacy test method. They first challenged products diluted to four concentrations (30, 50, 70, and 100%) with mixed cultures of bacteria known to contaminate cosmetics. After 28 days, they used these results to classify the formulations as (1) poorly preserved, (2) marginally preserved, or (3) well preserved. The formulae were then used by consumers and evaluated after use for contamination.

For the consumer contamination part of the study, the products were packaged in containers to allow direct contact with consumers. This assured that package design was not a significant factor in preventing exposure to microbial contaminants from the consumer or the environment. Brannan's group defined contamination as recovery of >100 CFU/g or the presence of Gram-negative bacteria at initial receipt and 4–7 days post-receipt.

No samples of the well-preserved products were contaminated after consumer use, while 46–90% of the poorly preserved products were contaminated after consumer use; 0–21% of the marginally preserved products were contaminated. Thus, the method accurately predicted the potential for consumer contamination. It did not, however, account for the significant role that containers play in preventing consumer contamination.

Farrington et al. (60) evaluated the abilities of nine antimicrobial systems to preserve an experimental water-based cosmetic formulation in a round-robin format among several manufacturers. Six microbiological challenge tests were evaluated: the USP, the British Pharmacopeia (BP), the CTFA, an experimental rapid screen test, a test that incorporated a rechallenge after 14 days, and a simulated use/post-use test (product was challenged with 10^7 CFU/g *P. aeruginosa* following simulated use). The simulated products used in these assays were several combinations of varying amounts of two parabens and a quaternary compound.

The products were then also used to evaluate the maintenance of product purity in an 8-week-simulated in-use study. The level of contamination in the simulated in-use study was then determined to be the accurate measure and all laboratory tests were compared to it. The experimental rapid screen test was determined to be the best for predicting differences at intermediate levels of preservation, although the authors determined that:

> Statistically, all of the tests were equivalent predictors of preservation efficacy in the in-use test ($P = 0.05$). At the $P = 0.10$ level, only the U.S. Pharmacopeia, British Pharmacopeia, rapid screen, and Cosmetic, Toiletry, and Fragrance Association tests were significantly predictive. The results of prediction by a test, based on the preservative levels used, agreed well with the in-use test results ($P = 0.01$).
>
> Farrington et al. (60)

Susan Lindstrom presented a different design in an attempt to model contamination occurring through consumer use (61). While Brannan and the CTFA Round Robin Study both attempted to correlate laboratory tests to consumer use, Lindstrom focused on designing repeatable consumer panels to use in product testing. Four parameters are essential to the consumer use test: (1) consumer panel selection, (2) product selection, (3) test design, and (4) product evaluation. The panel selection is designed to be representative of the target consumer and the product selection to evaluate products of interest. The test design is important in that Lindstrom recommends a double-blind cross-over design, with the duration of use dependent on the product under test (mascaras tested for up to 8 weeks, for example) and the use conditions reflecting actual use. The evaluation phase is determined by the desired level of antimicrobial efficacy, but testing should be done within 24 hours of last use to prevent loss of viable microorganisms.

The pharmaceutical industry has also been concerned about in-use testing, particularly in Europe. In this regard, Urban et al. (62) presented a laboratory test utilizing multiple low-level challenges. The Committee for Proprietary Medicinal Products (CPMP)[*] has published standards on testing methodologies (63,64), and the entire subject has been recently reviewed (65). Fundamentally, the approach resembles that recommended by Lindstrom (61).

Tests for Factors Affecting Preservative Efficacy

A number of factors can influence the results of assays of preservation efficacy. Russell provides a review of some of these factors (66,67), correctly noting that the condition of the challenge microorganism and the conditions of the assays can play large roles in the measured activity of an antimicrobial. While directing their discussion to antibiotic test methodologies, Gilbert et al. presented an excellent discussion of preservation issues in 1991 (68). The central theme of their discussion is that the treatment received by an inoculum will affect a microorganism's susceptibility to antimicrobial agents, particularly the manner in which it was harvested and the medium in which it was suspended.

Inoculum Preparation and Handling

A recent review of the role inocula play in the apparent activities of disinfectants was prepared by Bloomfield et al. (69) They argue that much of the lab-to-lab and day-to-day variability seen in disinfectancy testing is due to poor control over the challenge microorganism cultures and inocula preparation and they offer

---

[*] The reference standards from the CPMP are available through the European Medicines Evaluation Agency (EMEA) Web site: www.emea.eu.int/index/indexh1.htm

specific suggestions to address these sources of variability. Many of their suggestions have found their way into the current USP chapter (57) on antimicrobial effectiveness testing (27).

The USP recommends the use of freshly prepared inoculum, a recommendation in line with the Pharmacopeia Europaea (50,70). However, Muth and Casey present data suggesting that there is no difference in response to three different antimicrobial agents (sodium hypochlorite, benzalkonium chloride, and propyl paraben) if the challenge inoculum is freshly prepared or a frozen preparation recently thawed (71). It should be noted, however, that the activities of the agents were not measured in the standard antimicrobial efficacy test. Rather than measuring surviving CFUs after exposure, Muth and Casey measured the length of time required for challenge microorganisms to grow in trypticase soy broth (TSB) containing different concentrations of the antimicrobial agent. Although this study sounds interesting, it is not clear whether it is relevant to questions of bactericidal activity or relates only to inhibition of growth.

Orth recommended standardized conditions of inoculum preparation in 1989 (72). Using the linear regression model for data analysis, he reported on two different methods for inoculum preparation: growth in broth and growth on solid agar with a saline wash. Upon addition of 0.2% broth inocula (0.1 mL in 50 mL of sample), he saw a decrease in the antimicrobial activity compared to that seen with a saline rinse of cells grown on agar. Not investigated were the effects of media constituents on antimicrobial activity and it would be of interest to see whether similar effects would be seen with broth-grown microorganisms that had been centrifuged and then resuspended in saline, eliminating the potential inhibition of the organic load introduced by medium carry-over.

The size of the inoculum can also have an effect on the apparent activity of the antimicrobial as reported by Van Doorne and Vringer (73) in 1994 after a study conducted with *Candida albicans* and *Aspergillus niger* and by Steels et al. in 2000 (74). When conducting a laboratory preservative efficacy test, it is necessary to have a large inoculum so that the microbiologist can measure the required reduction. It is difficult to measure a 3-$\log_{10}$ reduction if an inoculum is smaller than 100,000 (10^5) CFU/mL. However, these authors showed microbial growth in a cream formulation when the inoculum was relatively small, a growth not observed with greater inocula. They note that these results are not consistent with earlier work that employed prokaryotic challenge organisms.

Other authors have argued that the laboratory tests are so far removed from the real world situation that they are all but meaningless (75). Factors seen as critical in this regard are the prevalence of biofilm as a contaminating agent, the extremely slow growth (and subsequent physiological changes) of naturally occurring microorganisms, and the extraordinary post-growth treatments to which inocula are subjected (including putative damage from centrifugation).

In a somewhat opinionated article, Gilbert et al. describe several aspects of inocula preparation of concern for reducing variability in antimicrobial tests through tight control of the inocula (76). Of particular interest in this article are the discussions on the growth on solid agar and the difficulties in generating reproducible inocula due to differences in growth rates. Liquid growth is recommended, however, in another article (77). Gilbert et al. describe injury to the challenge organism *Pseudomonas aeruginosa* by centrifugation. One is left with a dilemma: how to grow organisms in liquid media (and so enhance reproducibility) while avoiding problems of media carry-over into the product tested. The pharmacopeias have elected to allow centrifugation.

Recovery Conditions

Media used for the recovery of microbial survivors will have direct effects on the estimates of antimicrobial activity. It is well established that some media, while capable of supporting the growth of healthy microbial cells, are unable to support the growth of sub-lethally injured microorganisms (78,79). In addition to the nutritive properties of the media, the temperature and duration of incubation are of particular concern in providing opportunity for cell recovery and proliferation (80).

Plating Concerns

It must be stressed that a significant amount of variation occurs strictly as a result of the methods used to count microorganisms. Standard practice utilizes duplicate plating to provide an estimate of the number of viable CFUs present in the suspension. This is acknowledged to be a different measure from the number of viable cells present as a colony could arise from 100 cells in a cluster or chain as easily as from a single cell. However, this consideration is not the only element of the variability introduced by the plating technique.

Wilson and Kullman looked at the advisability of increasing the number of replicate plates (81). Using *Rhizobium trifolii*, they evaluated the errors of estimates in cell density taking three or four parallel plates to derive an estimate of plating error. On the basis of this study, the authors recommended the use of at least three plates and preferably more to decrease the inherent variability and allow elimination (without bias) of plates containing markedly different colony numbers. Jennison and Wadsworth described two components to variability in plating: sampling error and dilution error (82). While Wilson and Kullman assumed that dilution error was a small contributor to variability, Jennison and Wadsworth argued that errors in the volume of dilution blanks, variability in pipettes, and the number of dilutions made were large contributors to variability in the derived microbial counts. These errors were examined in greater detail by Hedges (83) who recommended larger numbers of replicate plates as well as the preparation of tables estimating the errors particular to the pipettes used in each laboratory and the method employed for enumeration.

The other source of plating variability comes, of course, from the actual number of colonies on a plate. If too few colonies are present, random sampling error becomes too great to allow accurate estimates. Too many colonies on a plate will mask each other and compete for nutrients, thus depressing the observed numbers (84,85). Breed and Dotterer determined the most accurate counting range for milk-borne bacteria to be between 30 and 400 colonies/plate (86). The FDA's *Bacteriological Analytical Manual* notes a specific range of 25–250 colonies per plate, citing Tomasiewicz et al (87).

Neutralizer Evaluation

Functions of Neutralizers

A neutralizer should inactivate a preservative or biocide and allow for unrestrained microbial growth (88). If a biocide is not inactivated, the antimicrobial activity of the biocidal agent will be overestimated because killing will continue in the recovery medium (42). Included in the evaluation of a neutralizer should be controls to measure neutralizer toxicity toward the microorganisms (89).

Types of Neutralization

Chemical Neutralization

Lecithin, Polysorbate 80, and sodium thiosulfate are examples of chemical inactivators for QACs, phenolics, and halogens, respectively. The type of neutralizer and the effective concentration must be determined for each biocide and microorganism permutation (see Table 6.4) (52). Disinfectants and preserved products are typically tested by inoculating either directly or via contaminated carriers. When sampling an inoculated disinfectant or preserved product, one must stop the killing activity of the biocide immediately.

Some biocides are difficult to inactivate. For example, sodium bisulfite is the neutralizer for formaldehyde and glutaraldehyde. Unfortunately, sodium bisulfite also inhibits the growth of bacteria and the germination of spores (22). Thus, in addition to efficacy, it is equally important that a neutralizer be nontoxic to the microorganisms.

Neutralizer toxicity can be determined by comparing growth in the neutralizing medium alone to growth in a typical medium such as tryptic soy agar or Sabouraud dextrose agar (45). Most test procedures require the chemical neutralizers to be included as part of the dilution broths into which the samples are placed. One may also include the chemical neutralizer in the plating agar.

One effective general neutralizing medium is Dey–Engley. It contains sodium thioglycollate, sodium thiosulfate, sodium bisulfite, lecithin, and Polysorbate neutralizing agents (41,42,45) and is available in broth and agar preparations. Some common diluting fluids are in the *USP XXII*: diluting fluid A with 0.1% meat peptone, diluting fluid D with meat peptone plus Polysorbate 80, and diluting fluid K with meat peptone, Polysorbate 80, and beef extract. Another variant on this broth has been described for use in membrane filtration testing (88).

Dilution and Membrane Filtration

Some preservatives are sensitive to concentration and are effectively neutralized by dilution (see Table 6.4). Several excellent papers discuss this subject (22,42,48). One method of neutralizing a preservative is membrane filtration. Bacteria are isolated on a filter and then rinsed free of preservative. The surviving bacteria are then transferred to a growth medium. Bloomfield (22) suggests washing the membrane with nutrient broth and transferring it to the surface of an agar plate to count the surviving colonies. The nutrients from the agar diffuse through the membrane to support the microorganism's ability to grow into visible colonies.

Another test for the neutralization of a biocide on a membrane filter involves placing a known number of microorganisms on the membrane without the biocide and placing the same number of microorganisms again on another membrane that has been exposed to a disinfectant. The disinfectant is rinsed through (and thus off) the membrane filter by placing neutralizing agent onto the filter and allowing the neutralizer to go through the filter using vacuum or pressure. If the two membranes show equal counts, then the disinfectant has been neutralized. If the disinfectant is bound to the membrane, then counts will be significantly lower than the counts on the membrane not exposed to the biocide (22).

TABLE 6.4

Neutralizing agents in disinfectant testing

Substance or Group	Neutralizing Agent or Dilution
Aldehydes	Glycine
	Sodium sulfite
	Dimedone-morpholine?
Phenolics	Dilution
	Polysorbate 80
Mercury compounds	Sodium thioglycollate
	Cysteine
Hydrogen peroxide	Catalase
Alcohols	Dilution
Organic acids and esters	Dilution
	Polysorbate 20 or 80
Acridines	Nucleic acids
Quaternary ammonium compounds (QACs), biguanides	Lecithin + Lubrol W
	Lecithin + Polysorbate 80
Tego compounds	Polysorbate 80
EDTA and related chelating agents	Dilution
	Mg^{2+}
Hypochlorites	Sodium thiosulfate
	Nutrient broth
Iodine	Polysorbate 80
	Sodium thiosulfate

Methods for Testing Biocide Neutralizers

The ASTM methods (90) actually comprise a series of experiments to show whether a neutralizer is non-toxic and effective. Testing is first done to determine the maximum tolerated concentration (MTC) of the inactivator using the correct liquid test medium. Often, the medium will be buffered peptone water. After adding the target organism, one determines the microbial counts at 0 and 30 minutes. The peptone water should not cause a significant decrease in microbial survival over the 30 minutes.

One can add several concentrations of the neutralizer to the peptone water system and compare the number of microbial survivors of the 30-min exposure in the neutralizer–peptone solution to the number of 30-min peptone control survivors. This comparison yields the MTC of neutralizer that does not decrease the microbial survivors of the targeted microorganism.

The next procedure determines the effect of the MTC on the antimicrobial. It involves adding specific concentrations of the antimicrobial to the MTC of the neutralizer and comparing the numbers of microbial survivors at the 30-min point. The number of survivors of the neutralizer–antimicrobial system should not differ significantly from the counts of the peptone–neutralizer controls.

The ASTM method uses square root transforms of the plate count data for the different treatment groups and controls. It assumes that the plate count data are Poisson-distributed. The method then uses the T test to determine significant mean differences.

The USP dedicated an entire guidance chapter (91) for the demonstration of neutralizer efficacy and toxicity. The chapter clearly distinguishes methods useful for demonstrating recovery on agar and in liquid. It also provides a method for determining the maximum number of colonies allowable on a plate, which is especially useful information if you encounter an unusual microorganism with odd colonies. Finally, the chapter highlights concerns about the accuracy of very low numbers of colonies on a plate.

Rapid Methods Used in Preservative Testing

Two approaches noted in the literature make the preservative test less labor-intensive and time-consuming. The first is to design a screening test that will allow predictions of the activity of the test formulation when tested by the official method. An example of this is Orth's linear regression method discussed previously. Mulberry et al. discuss other options in an excellent review (92) in which they reinforce the point that these methods must be validated against the accepted method and should not be relied upon without evaluation.

A second approach is to utilize an alternative technology (avoiding the use of plate counts). Relatively little has been published on this topic, perhaps as the need for a 28-day sampling period lessens the impact of a rapid enumeration of survivors. However, studies of several technologies have been reported in the literature. Impedance techniques are the most commonly reported for this application (93,94). Connolly et al. compared impedance, direct epifluorescence (DEFT-MEM), and ATP bioluminescence for applicability to preservative testing and found that only impedance yielded results similar to the traditional method (95). Another approach that shows promise, at least for *E. coli*, is the use of green fluorescent protein to monitor viability. Casey and Nguyen (96) utilized a genetically engineered strain of *E. coli* that contained the green fluorescent protein, which provided an easily distinguished marker for viable cells. When this strain is used, less than 2 minutes per sample is required for the determination of viable cells.

A third, empirical approach used by some establishes risk assessment based upon complete elimination of challenge viability at an early (e.g., 7 or 14 days) sampling point. Especially if no recovery at enrichment level of detection, such observations in context of familiarity with formulations and preservatives allows such consideration to speed decision-making and facilitating speed to market.

General Considerations for Formulating Preserved Products

Interactions of Preservatives

The chemical and biological activities of a preservative may be influenced by the overall formulation of the product. For example, a minor alteration of pH may change the ionic character of a preservative, change the chemical groupings on the bacterial surface, or increase the partitioning of the preservative between the product and microbial cells (12).

Some preservatives can bind to surfactants. Nonionic surfactants in particular can impair the antimicrobial activities of some preservatives such as the parabens. Some preservatives might be inactivated by proteins and exhibit reduced antimicrobial activity as a result (97). In oil-based emulsions, most of the emulgen disperses throughout the water phase as emulgent micelles. This redistributes the preservative and changes the concentration level in the aqueous phase (12).

In addition, the buffer system may affect the activity of the preservative. For example, borate-buffered formulations are more easily preserved than phosphate-buffered formulations, presumably because the boric acid also acts as an inhibitor of the membrane potential. It is mandatory to understand all factors of the formulation, not simply the ingredients recognized as preservatives.

The level of solids present in a formulation can also impact the effectiveness of a preservative. Inorganic solids (carbonates, silicates, and oxides) and organic solids (cellulose and starch) absorb preservatives such that they require higher concentrations. Talc, for example, decreases the antimicrobial activity of methyl parabens by as much as 90% (97). Preservation strategies are reviewed in more detail by Philip A. Geis in Chapter 2.

Water Activity

As reviewed in detail by Peter King in Chapter 1, microorganisms require available water for metabolism. Water activity (A_w) is the measure of available water, expressed as the ratio of the vapor pressure of a sample to the pressure of pure water at a constant temperature. An A_w value of 1.0 (100% relative humidity) can be obtained only with pure water. Restriction of this necessary component for life is an effective means of preserving a formulation (98–100). The consideration of water activity in product formulation may well allow for a decrease or total elimination of conventional preservatives (101). Water activity considerations are proposed in compendia as justification for reduced finished product testing and as basis for projecting low risk for contamination (102,103).

Container Considerations

The type of container used for packaging a cosmetic will influence the concentration and activity of a preservative (36). Generally, the more lipid-soluble preservatives are associated with greater risk of absorption by containers and their closures (12). Containers must be tested in order to determine the actual preservative effectiveness under real storage conditions. Adsorption, complexation, and volatility can erode antimicrobial activity. Certain containers are not compatible with certain preservatives, such as nylon and parabens or polyethylene with certain phenolics, mercurials, and benzoates (97).

Dispensing closures can also be important considerations in preventing microbial contamination during consumer use. A study by Brannan and Dille (104) showed that, during consumer use, unpreserved shampoo in bottles with flip-type caps exhibited the greatest degree of protection from contamination (0%). For an unpreserved skin lotion, a pump-top dispenser afforded the best protection from contamination (10%). Other types of closures tested included the standard screw cap and slit cap. The screw cap closure provided the least amount of protection, while the slit cap provided moderate protection from contamination. This study underscores the need for considering preservation as an attribute of an entire product, not simply a characteristic of an active preservative. It also points out the fallacy of the argument that a preservative test in a laboratory can predict final product performance. A preservative test cannot fulfill this broad function. Its intended purpose is to provide an indication of the ability of a formulation to withstand microbial challenge.

Packaging development has substantially diminished the risk of contamination in use. Though the use of bacteriologic filters that remove potential contaminants in air drawn into package replacing product dispensed via pump, in-use exposure is effectively eliminated and protocol have been proposed for validation of this package efficacy (105).

Alternative Tests

Methods discussed in the chapter presume product forms that allow relatively even distribution of challenge microorganisms are fluid products or gel products. Derived from these protocols and adapted to unique product forms, methods have been developed to test preservative efficacy of wipes (106), powders (107,108) as well as integrity of barrier packaging (105). In addition, protocols that address preservative efficacy of "atypical" products have been established. These attempt to provide guidance to project contamination risks of novel product forms—those that may present unique susceptibilities (109).

Risk Assessment

Performance of a preserved formulation in efficacy testing discussed earlier is a necessary but insufficient data base for the completion of a microbial risk assessment. Whereas the primary purpose of preservation is the prevention of in-use contamination, some level of efficacy is needed to address low-level microbial exposure during manufacture in nonsterile systems, and addition of Gram-negative bacteria in the CTFA protocol anticipates that risk. Manufacturing hygiene and controls that limit such exposure assume a role in risk assessment. Similarly, preservation versus in-use contamination is a function of formulation efficacy and exposure making packaging and dispensing elements essential considerations in the risk assessment. These are discussed in more depth in Chapter 2.

Microbial Content Testing

The survival and growth of microorganisms in cosmetic products are known facts (110–113). Some incidents of microorganism growth involve health risks, as in the case of eye infections caused by mascara contaminated with microorganisms (5,114,115). Some incidents have led to product spoilage (112,116–118). Whatever the outcome, the knowledge that microbes can grow in cosmetics means the manufacturer is responsible for detecting them.

For microbial content testing, the currently used methods include traditional plate counting and enrichment testing (9,119,120). These methods share the limitations of plate counts as estimates of viable cells discussed earlier in this chapter. An additional limitation is that counts at very low CFU/plate numbers rapidly approach errors of 100% relative to the mean as the number of colonies per plate drops below 10 CFU (91).

The plate count is a pragmatic and practical method that has survived because of its simplicity and long acceptance, not because of its scientific validity. Thus, we must continue using it until new methods supersede it. A variety of new methods are currently used for microbial content testing, and there are chances for more to be developed (121,122). This will be interesting because virtually all raw material and product specifications are currently stated as CFUs per unit of measure.

Two concerns surround the current use of CFU measurements in our specifications as the alternative methods grow in prominence. The first is that the number of CFUs per milliliter in a suspension is at best an estimate of the number of cells in the suspension because many bacteria clump or grow in chains, and thus confound counts—a single colony may arise from a single cell or hundreds of cells in a clump. The second issue is that many of the new technologies do not require bacterial growth, and may allow us to "see" organisms in ways not achievable with present methods (123).

As discussed for the Antimicrobial Effectiveness Test (AET), care must be taken to ensure that any residual preservative or antimicrobial property of the material tested should be completely neutralized. This "method suitability" study should be done prior to the establishment of the material test method and specifications.

General Product and Raw Materials Tests

The aim of these tests is to obtain an estimate of the aerobic population of potential contaminants in a product. The product is sampled aseptically (usually in 1 g amounts) into a diluent meant both to neutralize the product's antimicrobial nature and to dilute the organisms present to countable values. The diluted and neutralized product is then plated onto a medium that promotes growth and recovery of injured organisms.

In order to conduct any of the content tests, a well-supplied microbiology laboratory is needed. The lists of the needed equipment and supplies are available and will not be enumerated here. Each laboratory should document in its SOPs how the equipment should be used, how the materials and reagents (media, dyes, biochemical test solutions) should be prepared, and how the tests should be conducted (e.g., aseptic technique, room features, air circulation, and handling) (124).

Most products and raw materials received are packed for consumer use or delivered in sterile containers. Typically, if a product or raw material is in aqueous form, 10 g of product or raw material is placed into 90 mL of a dilution blank with appropriate neutralizing media. The bottle is then capped and shaken thoroughly. Anywhere from 0.5 to 1.0 mL of this dilution is pour-plated or 0.1 mL is spread-plated on the recovery medium.

The plates are incubated at 33–37°C for anywhere from a few days to a week and at lower temperatures for detection of yeasts and molds. Some microbiologists prefer using a specific medium for recovery of yeasts and molds (e.g., potato extract agar or Sabouraud). The colonies on the plate are counted and the value is multiplied by the dilution factors required.

If a product is a powder or a solid, then it should be dissolved or resuspended into the diluent using a solubilizing agent such as Polysorbate 80. If the material cannot be made into a solution, an alternative for conducting the test is the most probable number (MPN) method that utilizes a dilution series approach with the sample suspended in growth media. This approach allows the testing of samples that cannot be plated and samples that are so full of particulate matter that plate counts cannot be determined. Interested readers are referred to several excellent treatments of the subject (9,125–128).

USP Tests

The USP microbial tests (Chapters 61–62) have been harmonized globally with the Pharmacopeia Europaea and the Japanese Pharmacopoeia and reproduced in recent method development by the International Standards Organization. This process and the work of the USP for the past 10 years have been summarized in the literature (129,130). As part of the harmonization, three new chapters were established:

61—Microbiological Examination of Nonsterile Products: Microbial Enumeration Tests.
62—Microbiological Examination of Nonsterile Products: Tests for Specified Microorganisms.
1111—Microbial Contamination Limits for Nonsterile Products.

Chapter 61—Microbial Enumeration Tests

The harmonization of the microbial limits tests that began in the 1995–2000 revision cycle was completed in 2009 (131). The chapter provides elaborate details on the generation of the inocula, growth promotion testing of microorganisms, and controls.

Chapter 62—Tests for Specified Microorganisms

The 2001 publication of the Stage 4 harmonized Chapter 62 (132) placed a good deal of emphasis on the absence of "objectionable" microorganisms. After years of debate, three major pharmacopeia organizations decided that this objective was too vague and indeed outside the scope of the pharmacopeia. A revised Stage 4 document was published (133) with renewed emphasis on the absence of "specified" microorganisms, simplification of the identification scheme, and more detailed information about controls, growth promotion, and incubation conditions. This is now the basis for the harmonized protocol.

1111—Microbiological Contamination Limits for Nonsterile Products

This chapter is intended to provide some guidance covering nonsterile pharmaceutical products, but it can also be used as general guidance related to certain cosmetics. The chapter is very brief, consisting mainly of several tables providing recommended target values for bioburdens and absence of specified microorganisms.

Package Tests

These tests are usually conducted on empty packages received from suppliers that are not expected to be free of microorganisms. Typically, the first step is pouring a specific amount of sterile diluent into a bottle (or other container) which is then capped with the type of cap used in ordinary production. The bottle is then shaken thoroughly and the diluent is plated or diluted further with sterile diluent and then plated. Frequently, the number of CFUs in containers, particularly molded plastic containers, is very low and the entire volume of the rinse is filtered through a 0.45μm (nominal) pore size filter, laid on a plate, and incubated for growth (134,135).

The plates are incubated and counted as described previously. The CFUs per sample are determined by multiplying the count by the appropriate dilution factors employed in the test.

Environmental Tests and Monitoring

A variety of environmental tests may be conducted to determine bioburden in the air or on equipment. A good review of the topic can be found in Chapter 9 and another was published for the pharmaceutical industry (136) in response to the industry's great concern about maintenance of total clean room environments for aseptic processing (136). However, environmental monitoring is also a consideration for nonsterile facilities (137). The primary concern in cosmetic manufacture is the number of organisms present on product contact surfaces inside a plant.

A simple way to test this issue is to moisten a swab with Letheen broth (or any other neutralizing diluent that would support growth) and swab the equipment. The portion of the swab that is not contaminated by technician handling is broken off into the medium and incubated. If turbidity occurs after incubation, then sterility has not been achieved on the product contact areas. Alternatively, the diluent may be immediately plated or diluted further and plated to determine the actual numbers of contaminants per surface area.

Another way to these tests is through the use of RODAC (replicate organism detection and counting) plates. A RODAC plate is slightly overfilled so that the medium projects above the lip of the plate (138,139). The medium is then pressed on the surface to be sampled, removed, and the cover is returned to its position for incubation. A replica of the viable counts that were on the flat surface can then grow on the surface of the agar.

Whichever way the test is conducted, the operator must be aware of the sampling efficiency of the method used in that facility. Even the best technician will succeed in sampling only a relatively small proportion of the microorganisms present in any location, and studies should be conducted in the facility to estimate this efficiency (140–142). Such testing and its interpretation is addressed in more depth in the manufacturing controls discussed elsewhere in this text.

Identification of Microbes

Considerable space in the literature is typically devoted to the identification of the microbes isolated from the above tests. A thorough resource for the identification of microorganisms is the *Manual for Clinical*

Microbiology of the American Society for Microbiology (ASM). Use of rapid identification techniques is replacing many of the traditional culture methods. Although the techniques can be adapted from their clinical uses to cosmetic microbiology, it must be kept in mind that most of the organisms encountered in cosmetic microbiology are environmental isolates. Thus, rapid ID systems geared for environmental isolates should be preferred over those developed primarily for clinical use.

There are two major categories of commercially available microbial identification systems: those that rely on phenotypic characteristics for identification and those that rely on genotypic characteristics. Phenotypic identification systems are more commonly found in industrial microbiology labs. The archetype is the collection of test tubes we dealt with as undergraduates trying for example to determine whether an unknown was urease positive or negative or able to ferment different sugars. The first improvement on those was the API strip, followed by the Vitek, and now the Vitek 2 Compact. A different approach to phenotypic identification is incorporated in the Biolog systems that rely on a pattern of carbohydrate utilization among a standard set of carbohydrates to identify microorganisms. A final approach is the Sherlock fatty acid analysis system that uses gas chromatographs of cellular fatty acids to identify microorganisms.

Genotypic methods are fundamentally different in that they look directly at nucleic acids to achieve identification. DuPont Qualicon markets the Riboprinter that uses the restriction endonuclease fragment patterns of sequences homologous to 16S rDNA as the identifying characteristics. Diversilab markets the Bacterial Barcode system that utilizes re-PCR (polymerase chain reaction) technology in a similar fashion. The other general identification system in this category is the MicroSeq that sequences the first 500 base pairs of the unknown organism's 16S rDNA to identify it. Of course, if you are looking for a specific microorganism, several choices of PCR technologies are directed to organisms of interest.

All of these systems are completely dependent on the adequacies of their databases to make correct identifications. Genotypic methodology is a fascinating and rapidly changing field, and the reader is referred to several recent review articles on the identification of environmental isolates and the different methodologies currently available (143–146).

Summary

This chapter has attempted to provide an overview of preservative efficacy and microbial content tests used by the pharmaceutical and personnel care industries. Several points should have been made clear to readers:

1. The classical antimicrobial efficacy test is a control test of a formulation. By itself, it is insufficient to predict contamination during use because it neither includes the effects of the container in preventing contamination nor does it utilize all possible microbial contaminants that might be introduced into the product. Additional test designs that mimic consumer use conditions to varying degrees are described in the literature.
2. No single test design meets all needs. Each user must determine his or her company's needs (regulatory compliance, rapid answer, etc.) and use a design or a group of designs that addresses those needs.
3. The goal of antimicrobial efficacy tests is to provide reproducible results to assist in the determination of product quality. Therefore, unrealistically high inocula are used to assist the technician in determining kill over time, and a limited range microorganism species is used under tightly controlled conditions to minimize variability of test results.
4. Estimates of preservative efficacy are dependent upon the accurate counting of surviving microorganisms over time. Therefore, complete neutralization of the preservative system during plating to avoid residual inhibition of growth is essential to obtaining accurate results.

REFERENCES

1. Durant, C., and Higdon, P., Methods for assessing antimicrobial activity, in *Society for Applied Bacteriology Technical Series 27: Mechanisms of Action of Chemical Biocides*, Denyer, S.P., and Hugo, W.B., Eds., Blackwell Scientific, Bedford, UK, 1991.

2. Geis, P.A. Preservation strategies, in *Cosmetic Microbiology: A Practical Handbook*, 2nd Ed., Geis, P.A., Ed., New York; Taylor & Francis, 2006, pp.163–180.

3. Fainstein, V., Andres, N., Umphrey, J., and Hopfer, R., 1988. Hair clipping: another hazard for granulocytopenic patients? *J. Infect Dis.*, 158 (3), 655, 1988.

4. Madani, T.A., Alsaedi, S., James, L., Eldeek, B.S., Jiman-Fatani, A.A., Alawi, M.M., Marwan, D., Cudal, M., Macapagal, M., Bahlas, R., and Farouq, M., Serratia marcescens-contaminated baby shampoo causing an outbreak among newborns at King Abdulaziz University Hospital, Jeddah, Saudi Arabia. *J. Hosp. Infect.*, 78 (1), 16, 2011.

5. Wilson, L.A., and Ahearn, D.G., *Pseudomonas*-induced corneal ulcers associated with contaminated eye mascaras, *Am. J. Ophthalmol.*, 84, (1) 112, 1997.

6. Block, S.S., *Disinfection, Sterilization, and Preservation,* 4th ed., Lea & Febiger, Philadelphia, 1992, pp. 18, 887, 1009.

7. Tenenbaum, S., Pseudomonads in cosmetics, *J. Soc. Cosmet. Chem.*, 18, 797, 1967.

8. Cowen, R.A., and Steiger, B., Antimicrobial activity: a critical review of test methods of preservative efficacy, *J. Soc. Cosmet. Chem.*, 27, 467(10), 1976.

9. U.S. Food and Drug Administration, *Bacteriological Analytical Manual*, 8th ed., 2001. www.cfsan. fda.gov/~ebam/bam-23.html.

10. Gerba, C.P., Rose, J.B., and Haas, C.N. Sensitive populations: who is at the greatest risk? *Int. J. Food Microbiol.*, 30 (1–2), 113–123, 1996.

11. Kabara, J.J., *Cosmetics and Drug Preservation, Principles and Practices.* Marcel Dekker, New York, 1984.

12. Bean, H.S., Preservatives for pharmaceuticals, *J. Soc. Cosmet. Chem.*, 23 (2), 703, 1972.

13. Chapman, D.G., Preservatives available for use, in *Society for Applied Bacteriology Technical Series 22, Preservatives in the Food, Pharmaceutical and Environmental Industries*, Board, R.G., Allwood, M.C., and Banks, J.G., Eds., Bedford, UK, 1987.

14. International Standards Organization. ISO 17516:2014. Cosmetics — Microbiology — Microbiological limits.

15. International Standards Organization. ISO 11930:2019. Cosmetics — Microbiology — Evaluation of the antimicrobial protection of a cosmetic product.

16. Brannan, D.K., Cosmetic preservation, *J. Soc. Cosmet. Chem.*, 46, 199, 1995.

17. Orth, D.S., *Handbook of Cosmetic Microbiology,* Marcel Dekker, New York, 1993.

18. Ray, B., Injured Index and Pathogenic Bacteria, CRC Press, Boca Raton, FL, 1989.

19. Madden, J.M., Microbiological methods for cosmetics, in *Cosmetic and Drug Preservation: Principles and Practices*, Kabara, J.J., Ed., Marcel Dekker, New York, 1984, p. 573.

20. Orth, D.S., Principles of preservative efficacy testing, *Cosmet. Toilet.*, 96 (1), 43, 1981.

21. Cosmetic, Toiletry, and Fragrance Association Preservation Subcommittee, Evaluation of methods for determining preservative efficacy, *Cosmet. Toilet. Frag. Assoc. J.*, 5, 1, 1973.

22. Bloomfield, S., Methods for assessing antimicrobial activity, in *Society for Applied Bacteriology Technical Series 27, Mechanisms of Action of Chemical Biocides*, Denyer, S.P., and Hugo, W.B., Eds., Blackwell Scientific, Oxford, UK, 1991, p. 1.

23. Gilbert, P., Brown, M.R.W., and Costerton, J.W., Inocula for antimicrobial sensitivity testing: a critical review, *J. Antimicrob. Chemother.*, 20, 147 (2), 1987.

24. Gilbert, P., Collier, P.J., and Brown, M.R.W., Influence of growth rate on susceptibility to antimicrobial agents: biofilms, cell cycle, dormancy, and stringent response, *Antimicrob. Agents Chemother.*, 34 (10), 1865, 1990.

25. Personal Care Products Council. M-4 Method for Preservation Efficacy Testing of Eye Area Personal Care Products *PCPC Microbiology Guidelines*. p. 217. 2018.

26. American Public Health Association, *Standard Methods for the Examination of Water and Wastewater*, Washington, DC, 2017.

27. U.S. Pharmacopeia Convention, Antimicrobial preservatives: effectiveness, in *U.S. Pharmacopeia 2005,* Rockville, MD, 2004, chap. 51.

28. Bacto® Eugon agar, in *DIFCO Manual*, 11th ed., DIFCO Laboratories, Detroit, MI, 1986, p. 190.

29. Odds, F.C., Sabouraud['s] agar, *J. Med. Vet. Mycol.*, 29, 355, 1991.

30. American Public Health Association, *Standard Methods for the Examination of Dairy Products*, 14th ed., Washington, DC, 1978.

31. American Public Health Association, *Compendium of Methods for the Microbiological Examination of Foods*, Washington, DC, 1976.

32. Von Reisen, V.L., and Jensen, T., Acid mycophil agar for the selective isolation of yeasts, *Am. J. Med. Technol.*, 24 (2), 123, 1958.

33. Beneke, E.S., and Rogers, A.L., *Medical Mycology Manual*, 3rd ed., Burgess, Minneapolis, 1971, p. 23.

34. Mycological media, in *DIFCO Manual*, 10th ed., DIFCO Laboratories, Detroit, 1985, p. 589.

35. Personal Care Products Council. M-3 Method for Preservation Efficacy Testing of Water_Miscible Personal Care Products. *PCPC microbiology Guidelines*. p. 217. 2018.

36. Brannan, D.K., The role of packaging in product preservation, in *Preservation-Free and Self-Preserving Cosmetics and Drugs*, Kabara, J.J., and Orth, D.S., Eds., Marcel Dekker, New York, 1996, Chap. 10, pp. 227–242.

37. el-Falaha, B.M., Furr, J.R., and Russell, A.D., Quenching of the antibacterial activity of chlorhexidine and benzalkonium by Letheen broth and Letheen agar in relation to wild-type and envelope mutant strains of Gram-negative bacteria, *Microbios.*, 49 (198), 31, 1987.

38. Brewer, J.H., A clear liquid medium for the "aerobic" cultivation of anaerobes, *JAMA*, 155 (8), 598, 940.

39. Quisro, R.A., Gibby, I.W., and Foster, M.J., A neutralizing medium for evaluating the germicidal potency of the quaternary ammonium salts, *Am. J. Pharm.*, 118 (9), 320, 1946.

40. U.S. Pharmacopeia Convention, Microbial limit tests, in *U.S. Pharmacopeia 2005*, Rockville, MD, 2004, Chap. 61. www.pharmacopeia.cn/v29240/usp29nf24s0_c61.html.

41. Engley, F.B., Jr., and Dey, B.P., A universal neutralizing medium for antimicrobial chemicals, in *Proceedings of the 56th Mid-Year Meeting of the Chemical Specialties Manufacturers Association*, New York, 1970, p. 100.

42. Dey, B.P., and Engley, F.B., Jr., Methodology for recovery of chemically treated *Staphylococcus aureus* with neutralizing medium, *Appl. Environ. Microbiol.*, 45 (5), 1533, 1983.

43. Martinelli, S.D., Media, *Prog. Ind. Microbiol.*, 29, 829, 1994.

44. Microbial limit test for cosmetics. EU/ASEAN Document TH-02, 2004.

45. Sutton, S.W.V., Wrzosek, T., and Proud, D.W., Neutralization efficacy of Dey–Engley medium in testing of contact lens disinfecting solutions, *J. Appl. Bacteriol.*, 70 (4), 351, 1991.

46. MacKinnon, I.H., Use of inactivators in evaluation of disinfectants, *J. Hyg. Cambr.*, 73 (2), 189, 1974.

47. Singer, S., The use of preservative neutralizers in diluents and plating media, *Cosmet. Toilet.*, 102 (12), 55, 1987.

48. Hugo, W.B., and Denyer, S.P., Concentration exponent of disinfectants and preservatives (biocides), in *Preservatives in the Food, Pharmaceutical and Environmental Industries*, Board, R.G., Allwood, M.C., and Banks, J.G., Eds., Blackwell Scientific, Boston, 1987, p. 281.

49. American Society for Testing and Materials. E640-06. Standard method for preservatives in water containing cosmetics. 019.

50. Sutton, S.V.W., and Porter, D. Development of the antimicrobial effectiveness test as USP Chapter 51, *PDA J. Pharm. Sci. Tech.*, 56 (6), 300, 2002.

51. Gerhardt, P., Murray, R.G.E., Costilow, N., Nester, R., Eugene, W., Wood, W.A., Krieg, N.R., and Phillips, G.B., *Manual for Methods for General Bacteriology*, American Society for Microbiology, Washington, DC, 1981, pp. 67, 174, 504.

52. Orth, D.S., Lutes, C.M., and Smith, D.K., Effect of culture conditions and method for inoculum preparation on the kinetics of bacterial death during preservative efficacy testing, *J. Soc. Cosmet. Chem.*, 40 (2), 193, 1989.

53. Orth, D.S., Putting the phoenix phenomenon into perspective, *Cosmet. Toilet.*, 114 (4), 61, 1999.

54. Orth, D.S., Linear regression method for rapid determination of cosmetic preservative efficacy, *J. Soc. Cosmet. Chem.*, 30 (5), 321, 1979.

55. Orth, D.S., Preservative efficacy testing of cosmetic products: rechallenge testing and reliability of the linear regression method, *Cosmet. Toilet.*, 97 (5), 61, 1982.

56. Zar, J.H., Simple linear regression, in *Bio-Statistical Analysis*, Prentice-Hall, Englewood Cliffs, NJ, 1984, p. 261.

57. Sutton, S.V.W., Franco, R.G., Mowrey-McKee, M.F., Busschaert, S.C., Hamberger, J., and Proud, D.W., D-value determinations are an inappropriate measure of disinfecting activity of common contact lens disinfecting solution, *Appl. Environ. Microbiol.*, 57 (7), 2021, 1991.

58. Barnes, M., and Denton, G.W., Capacity tests for the evaluation of preservatives in formulations, *Soap Perf. Cosmet.*, October, 729, 1969.

59. Brannan, D.K., Dille, J.C., and Kaufman, D.J., Correlation of *in vitro* challenge testing with consumer use testing for cosmetic products, *Appl. Environ. Microbiol.*, 53 (8), 1827, 1987.

60. Farrington, J.K., Martz, E.L., Wells, S.J., Ennis, C.C., Holder, J., Levchuk, J.W., Avis, K.E., Hossman, P.S., Hitchins, A.D., and Madden, J.W., Ability of lab methods to predict in-use efficacy of antimicrobial preservatives in an experimental cosmetic, *Appl. Environ. Microbiol.*, 60 (6), 4553, 1994.

61. Lindstrom, S.M., and Hawthorne, J.D., Validating the microbiological integrity of cosmetic products through consumer-use testing, *J. Soc. Cosm. Chem.*, 37 (5), 481, 1986.

62. Urban, S., Hecker, W., and Shiller, I., Low-level challenge test for the examination of the microbiological susceptibility, during the period of use, of liquid and semi-solid dosage forms in multiple-dose containers [in German], *Zbl. Bakt. Hyg. I. Abt. Orig. B.*, 172 (6), 478, 1981.

63. European Union, EMEA/CVMP/127/95, Note for guidance: in-use stability testing of veterinary medicinal products, Brussels, 1995.

64. European Union, EMEA/QWP/2934/99, Note for guidance: in-use stability testing of human medicinal products, Brussels, 2001.

65. Sutton, S.V.W., In-use stability testing: what data are required and when? *Reg Affairs J.*, 9 (Oct), 728, 1998.

66. Russell, A.D., Factors influencing the activity of antimicrobial agents: an appraisal, *Microbios.*, 10 (38), 151, 1974.

67. Russell, A.D., Neutralization procedure in the evaluation of bactericidal activity, in *Society for Applied Bacteriology Technical Series 16, Disinfectants: Their Use and Evaluation of Effectiveness*, Collins, C.H., Allwood, M.C., Bloomfield, S.F., and Fox, A., Eds., Academic Press, London, 1981, p. 45.

68. Gilbert, P., and Brown, M.R.W., Out of the test tube into the frying pan: post-growth, pre-test variables, *J. Antimicrob. Chemother.*, 27 (6), 859, 1991.

69. Bloomfield, S., Development of reproducible test inocula for disinfectant testing, *Int Biodet. Biodegrad.*, 38 (3-4, 311, 1996.

70. Matthews, B.R., Preservation and preservative efficacy testing: European perspectives, *Eur. J. Parenteral Pharm. Sci.*, 8 (3), 99, 2003.

71. Muth, H., The effects of antimicrobial preservatives on organisms derived from fresh versus frozen cultures, *Pharmacop. For.*, 26 (2), 51, 2000.

72. Orth, D.S., Effect of culture conditions and method of inoculum preparation on the kinetics of bacterial death during preservation efficacy testing, *J. Soc. Cosmet. Chem.*, 40, 193 (2), 1989.

73. Van Doorne, H., Effect of inoculum size on survival rate of *Candida albicans* and *Aspergillus niger* in topical preparations, *Lett. Appl. Microbiol.*, 18 (50, 289, 1994.

74. Steels, H., James, S.A., Roberts, I.N., and Stratford, M., Sorbic acid resistance: the inoculum effect, *Yeast,* 16, 1173 (13), 2002.

75. Gilbert, P., Some perspectives on preservation and disinfection in the present day, *Int. Biodeter. Biodegrad.*, 36 (3-4), 219, 1995.

76. Gilbert, P., Brown, M.R., and Costerton, J.W., Inocula for antimicrobial sensitivity testing: a critical review, *J. Antimicrob. Chemo.*, 20 (2), 147, 1987.

77. Gilbert, P., Coplan, F., and Brown, M.R., Centrifugation injury of Gram-negative bacteria, *J. Antimicrob. Chemo.*, 27 (4), 550, 1991.

78. Mossel, D.A., and Van Nette, P., Harmful effects of selective media on stressed microorganisms: nature and remedies, in *The Revival of Injured Microbes*, Academic Press, New York, 1984, p. 328.

79. Gilbert, P., The revival of microorganisms sublethally injured by chemical inhibitors, in *The Revival of Injured Microbes*, Academic Press, New York, 1984, p. 175.

80. Harris, N.D., The influence of the recovery medium and the incubation temperature on the survival of damaged bacteria, *J. Appl. Bact.*, 26 (3), 387, 1963.
81. Wilson, P.W., and Kullman, E., Statistical inquiry into methods for estimating numbers of Rhizobia, *J. Bacteriol.*, 22 (1), 71, 1931.
82. Jennison, M., and Wadsworth, G., Evaluation of the errors involved in estimating bacterial numbers by the plating method, *J. Bacteriol.*, 39 (4), 389, 1940.
83. Hedges, A.J., Estimating the precision of serial dilutions and viable bacterial counts, *Intl. J. Food Microbiol.*, 76 (3), 207, 2002.
84. Jennison, M.W., Relations between plate counts and direct microscopic counts of *Escherichia coli* during the logarithmic growth period, *J. Bacteriol.*, 33 (5), 462, 1937.
85. Jennison, M.W. and Wadsworth, G.P., Evaluation of the errors involved in estimating bacterial numbers by the plating method, *J. Bacteriol.*, 39 (4), 389, 1940.
86. Breed, R., and Dotterrer, D.W., The number of colonies allowable on satisfactory agar plates, *J. Bacteriol.*, 1 (3), 321, 1916.
87. Tomasiewicz, D.M., Hotchkiss, D.K., Reinbold, G.W., Read, R.B., Jr., and Hartman, P.A., The most suitable number of colonies on plates for counting, *J. Food Prot.*, 43 (4), 282, 1980.
88. Proud, D.W., and Sutton, S.V.M., Development of a universal diluting fluid for membrane sterility testing, *Appl. Environ. Microbiol.*, 58 (3), 1035, 1992.
89. Sutton, S.V.M., Proud, D.W., Rachui, S., and Brannan, D.K., Validation of microbial recovery from disinfectants, *PDA J. Sci. Technol.*, 56 (5), 255, 2002.
90. American Society for Testing and Materials, Evaluating Inactivators of Antimicrobial Agents in Disinfectant, Sanitizer, and Antiseptic Products, Philadelphia, 1991, p. 1054.
91. U.S. Pharmacopeia Convention, Validation of microbial recovery from pharmacopeial articles, in *U.S. Pharmacopeia 2005*, Rockville, MD, 2004, Chapter 1227.
92. Mulberry, G., Entrup, M.R., and Agin, J.R., Rapid screening methods for preservative efficacy evaluations, *Cosmet. Toilet.*, 102 12), 47, 1987.
93. Basa, E., Preservative efficacy testing for stability using impedance, *Cosmet. Toilet.*, 115 (4), 61, 2000.
94. Zhou, X., and King, V.M., An impedimetric method for rapid screening of cosmetic preservatives, *J. Indust. Microbiol.*, 15 (2), 103, 1995.
95. Connolly, P., Study of the use of rapid methods for preservative efficacy testing of pharmaceuticals and cosmetics, *J. Appl. Bacteriol.*, 75 (5), 456, 1993.
96. Casey, W.M., and Nguyen, N.T., Use of the green fluorescent protein to rapidly assess viability of *E. coli* in preserved solutions, *PDA J. Sci. Pharm. Tech.*, 50 (6), 352, 1996.
97. Sabourin, J.R., Evaluation of preservatives for cosmetic products, *Drug Cosmet. Ind.*, 146 (2) 24, 1990.
98. Friedel, R.R., and Cundell, A.M., The application of water activity measurement to the microbiological attributes testing of nonsterile over-the-counter drug products, *Pharmacop. For.*, 24 (2), 6087, 1998.
99. Curry, J., Manipulation of water activity for developing products intrinsically hostile to microbial growth, *Cosmet. Toilet. Manuf.*, 107, 53, 1993.
100. Curry, J., Water activity and preservation, *Cosmet. Toilet.*, 100 (2), 53, 1985.
101. Cowen, R., Why a preservative system must be tailored to a specific product, *Cosmet. Toilet.*, 92 (3), 15, 1977.
102. USP 47 2018. ⟨1112⟩ Application of water activity determination to nonsterile pharmaceutical products.
103. International Standards Organization. 29621. Cosmetics – Microbiology – Guidelines for the risk assessment and identification of microbiologically low-risk products, 2017.
104. Brannan, D.K., and Dille, J.C., Type of closure prevents microbial contamination of cosmetics during consumer use, *Appl. Environ. Microbiol.*, 56 (5), 1476, 1990.
105. Devlieghere, F., De Loy-Hendrickx, A., Rademaker, M., Pipelers, P., Crozier, A., De Baets, B., Joly, L., and Keromen, S. A new protocol for evaluating the efficacy of some dispensing systems of a packaging in the microbial protection of water-based preservative-free cosmetic products. *Int. J. Cosm. Sci.*, 37 (6), 627, 2015.
106. Cremieux, A., Cupferman, S., and Lens, C. Method for evaluation of the efficacy of antimicrobial preservatives in cosmetic wet wipes. *Int. J. Cosm. Sci.*, 27 (4), 223, 2005.

107. Tran, T.T, Hitchins, A.D., and Collier A.W. Direct contact membrane method for evaluating preservative efficacy in solid cosmetics, *Int. J. Cosmet. Sci.*, 12 (4), 175, 1990.

108. Souza, M.R., and Ohara, M.T. The preservative efficacy testing method for powdered eye shadows. *J. Cosm. Sci.*, 54 (4), 411, 2003.

109. Yablonski, J.I., and Mancuso, S.E. Preservation of atypical cosmetic product systems. *Cosm. Toiletr.*, 117 (4), 31, 2002.

110. Baird, R.M., Microbial contamination of cosmetic products, *J. Soc. Cosmet. Chem.*, 28 (1), 17, 1977.

111. Baird, R.M., Bacteriological contamination of products used for skin care in babies, *Int. J. Cosmet. Sci.*, 6 (2), 85, 1984.

112. Ashour, M.S., Hefnai, H., Tayeb, O., Abdelaziz, A.A., Microbial contamination of cosmetics and personal care items in Egypt, *Cosmet. Toilet.*, 102 (1), 61, 1987.

113. Goldman, C.L., Microorganisms isolated from cosmetics, *Drug Cosmet. Ind.*, 117, 40, 1979.

114. Wilson, L.A., Julian, A.J., and Ahearn, D.G., Survival and growth of microorganisms in mascara during use, *Am. J. Ophthalmol.*, 79 (4), 596, 1975.

115. Gabriel, H., Gable, E.M., Sauser, K., and Rice, J., Testing the inhibitory effects of mascara life on bacterial growth in mascara, *Optometry*, 72 (4), 251, 2001.

116. Wolven, A., and Levenstein, I., Cosmetics: contaminated or not? *Soap Cosme.t Chem. Spec.*, 45 (1), 60, 1969.

117. O'May, G.A., Allison, D.G., and Gilbert, P., Rapid method for the evaluation of both extrinsic and intrinsic contamination and resulting spoilage of water-in-oil emulsions, *J. Appl. Microbiol.*, 96 (5), 1124, 2004.

118. Smart, R., and Spooner, D.F., Microbiological spoilage in pharmaceuticals and cosmetics, *J. Soc. Cosmet. Chem.*, 23 (11), 721, 1972.

119. Tran, T.T., Hurley F.J., Shurbaji, M., Koopman F.B., Adequacy of cosmetic preservation: chemical analysis, microbial challenge and in-use testing, *Int. J. Cosmet. Sci.*, 16 (2), 61, 1994.

120. Yablonski, J., and Mancuso, S.E., Personal care wipes: manufacturing practices and microbiological control, *Cosmet. Toilet.*, 119 (8), 53, 2004.

121. Jimenez, L., Molecular diagnosis of microbial contamination in cosmetic and pharmaceutical products: a review, *J. AOAC Intl.*, 84 (3), 671, 2001.

122. Swaminathan, B., Rapid detection of foodborne pathogenic bacteria, *Ann. Rev. Microbiol.*, 48, 401, 1994.

123. Rappe, M., and Giovannoni, S.J., The uncultured microbial majority, *Ann. Rev. Microbiol.*, 57 (1), 69, 2003.

124. U.S. Pharmacopeia Convention, Microbiological best laboratory practices, Chapter 1117, *Pharmaco. For.*, 30, 1713, 2004.

125. Garthright, W.E., and Blodgett, R.J., FDA's preferred MPN methods for standard, large, or unusual tests with a spreadsheet, *Food Microbiol.*, 20 (4), 439, 2003.

126. Roser, D.J., Bavor, H.E., and McKersie, S.A., Application of most-probable-number statistics to direct enumeration of microorganisms, *Appl. Env. Microbiol.*, 53 (6), 1327, 1987.

127. Loyer, M., and Hamilton, M.A., Interval estimation of the density of organisms using a serial dilution experiment, *Biometrics,* 40 (4), 907, 1984.

128. Aspinall, L.J., and Kilsby, D.C., Microbiological quality control procedure based on tube counts, *J. Appl. Bacteriol.*, 46 (2), 325, 1979.

129. Sutton, S.V.W., Knapp, J.E., and Dabbah, R., Activities of the USP microbiology subcommittee of revision during the 1995–2000 revision cycle, *PDA J. Pharm. Sci Tech.*, 55 (1), 33, 2001.

130. Sutton, S.V.W. Activities of the USP microbiology subcommittee of revision during the 2000–2005 revision cycle, *PDA J. Pharm. Sci. Tech.*, 59, 157, 2005.

131. U.S. Pharmacopeia Convention, Microbial limits tests, Chapter 61, *Pharmaco. For.*, 29, 1714, 2003.

132. U.S. Pharmacopeia Convention, Microbiological examination of nonsterile products: microbial enumeration tests, Chapter 61, *Pharmaco. For.*, 27, 2299, 2001.

133. U.S. Pharmacopeia Convention, Microbiological examination of nonsterile products: tests for specified microorganism harmonization, Chapter 62, *Pharmaco. For.*, 29, 1722, 2003.

134. U.S. Pharmacopeia Convention, Microbiological quality of nonsterile pharmaceutical products, Chapter 1111, *Pharmaco. For.*, 29, 1733, 2003.

135. Means, E.G., Hanami, L., Rdgeway, H,F., and Olsen, B.H., Evaluating mediums and plating techniques for enumerating bacteria in water distribution systems, *J. Amer. Water Works Assn.*, 72 (11), 585, 1981.

136. Parenteral Drug Association, Fundamentals of an environmental monitoring program, Technical Report 13 (Revised), 55, 19.,2001.

137. U.S. Food and Drug Administration, Guidance for industry: sterile drug products produced by aseptic processing – current good manufacturing practice, 2004.

138. One, J., An approach to developing a microbial environmental control program for non-sterile pharmaceutical manufacturing, *Amer. Pharm. Rev.*, 8, 32, 2005.

139. Rohde, P.A., A new culture plate: its applications, *PDA Bull. Parent. Drug Assn.*, 17, 1, 1963.

140. Bruch, M., Improved method for pouring RODAC plate, *Appl. Microbiol.*, 16 (9), 1427, 1968.

141. Whyte, W., Methods for calculating the efficiency of bacterial surface sampling techniques, *J. Hosp. Infect.*, 13 (1), 33, 1989.

142. Poletti, L., Comparative efficiency of nitrocellulose membranes versus RODAC plates in microbial sampling on surfaces, *J. Hosp. Infect.*, 41 (3), 195, 1999.

143. Salo, S. Laine, A., Alanko, T., Sioberg, A-M., and Writanen, G., Validation of microbiological methods: hygicult dipslide, contact plate, and swabbing in surface hygiene control: a Nordic collaborative study, *J. AOAC Intl.*, 83 (6), 1357, 2000.

144. Sutton, S.V.W., and Cundell, A.M., Microbial identification in the pharmaceutical industry, *Pharm. Forum,* 30 (5), 1884, 2004.

145. Meays, C.L., Source tracking fecal bacteria in water: a critical review of current methods, *J. Environ. Mgt.*, 73 (1), 71, 2004.

146. O'Hara, C.M., Manual and automated instrumentation for identification of Enterobacteriaceae and other aerobic Gram-negative bacilli, *Clin. Microbiol. Rev.*, 18, (1) 147, 2005.

7

Rapid Methods in Cosmetic Microbiology

Michael J. Miller

Introduction

Most modern laboratories use liquid or agar media to evaluate samples for the presence of microorganisms. The media is incubated for a period of time at some specified temperature to encourage the growth and recovery of microorganisms that may be present in the test sample. This standard practice is universal across a wide range of industries, including cosmetics, personal care, pharmaceutical, environmental, municipal water and clinical/healthcare sectors.

For microbiologists who support the development and manufacture of cosmetics, microbiological quality and long-term stability is a significant concern. Quality control laboratories must demonstrate product batches are within acceptable microbial specifications prior to release, and this is related to the ability of the manufacturing site to control adventitious contamination in raw materials, containers, operational equipment and processes, as well as the manufacturing environment. Moreover, cosmetics must be adequately preserved to prevent the growth of organisms that gain entry into product containers during routine use. To demonstrate this, antimicrobial effective testing (AET) in combination with re-challenge studies will normally predict the ability of a formulation to kill or prevent the proliferation of organisms during the shelf life of the product. Of course, this assumes the product will not be adulterated or otherwise misused by the consumer.

Microbiology testing conducted by the cosmetic quality control laboratory (as well as the product development sector) most often mirror the same methods developed by our founding microbiology subject matter experts from the 19th century, such as Louis Pasteur, Robert Koch, Walther and Angelina Hesse, Hans Christian Joachim Gram and Julius Richard Petri. For instance, growth-based and enrichment methods specified in the United States Pharmacopeia (USP) Chapters 61 and 62 are used to enumerate the number of microorganisms present in a test sample and to determine the presence (or absence) of specified or objectionable microbial species. Unfortunately, these methods are hampered by a variety of scientific limitations.

First, the time to recover microorganisms is relatively long. Days or weeks may elapse before microorganisms are visually observed, and confluent growth on an agar plate may prevent individual microbial colonies from being isolated, necessitating sub-culturing onto additional media, delaying the time to result even further. And the longer it takes to confirm the presence of microorganisms, the longer it takes to confirm the microbiological safety of a product. This is especially true for the cosmetic industry, in which the concentration and specific type of microorganisms must be assessed before a product batch can be released for distribution to consumers.

Next, in many cases the test sample will need to be diluted before plating; for example, when the sample is antimicrobial in nature and/or when it contains preservatives. Dilutions will help neutralize the antimicrobial effect during testing; however, assay sensitivity may be reduced, such as the limit of detection or quantification.

Furthermore, microorganisms that are stressed due to nutrient deprivation or exposure to antimicrobial agents may not replicate when cultured on artificial media, because the incubation environment is not optimal for the resuscitation and subsequent growth of the organisms. This may result in an underestimation of the number or types of microorganisms present, which may include organisms considered objectionable for a particular formulation and/or indication for use.

Finally, when the same assays are utilized in support of a product contamination issue, the same technical limitations will be realized, often delaying the time to find a root cause and close out microbial out-of-specification investigations.

For these and other technical and business reasons, the modern laboratory should look toward developing innovative approaches to the detection, quantification and identification of microorganisms. These include the implementation of rapid microbiological methods.

Rapid Microbiological Methods

Rapid microbiological method (RMM) technologies are designed to offer a greater level of sensitivity, accuracy, precision and robustness when compared with conventional or traditional growth-based methods (e.g., those that are described in most pharmacopeia microbiology chapters). Furthermore, RMMs may provide increased sample throughput, operate in a continuous data-collecting mode, afford significantly reduced time-to-result (e.g., from days or weeks to hours or minutes). They may also promise increased automation capabilities and for some technologies that do not rely on microbial growth, results in real-time.

Commercially available rapid methods can detect the presence of specific microbial species, quantify the concentration of microorganisms in a sample and identify recovered organisms to the genus, species and sub-species level. The manner in which microorganisms are detected, enumerated or identified will be dependent on the specific technology and instrumentation employed.

For example, growth-based RMM technologies are the closest to traditional microbiology methods because they rely on the measurement of biochemical or physiological parameters that reflect the growth of microorganisms. These types of systems require organisms to divide and multiply, either on solid or in liquid media, so as to be detected and/or quantified. Viability-based systems utilize viability stains that will indicate the presence of living microorganisms without the need for microbial growth. For this reason, viability-based RMMs have been shown to detect slow growing, fastidious, dormant and viable but non-cultural (VBNC) microorganisms as compared with standard methods. Cellular component-based technologies rely on the analysis of specific cellular targets, such as proteins, surface macromolecules or adenosine triphosphate (ATP), or the use of probes that are specific for microbial sites of interest. Nucleic acid amplification technologies utilize polymerase chain reaction (PCR) with DNA as a starting material, RNA-based transcription-mediated amplification, 16S ribosomal RNA (rRNA) typing, gene sequencing techniques or other novel applications for the detection of target microorganisms and in some cases, an estimation of viable cell counts. Spectroscopic methods make use of light scattering and other optical techniques, such as Raman spectroscopy for the detection, quantification and identification of viable organisms. And because these systems do not require microbial growth for detection, results may be realized in real-time. Finally, micro-electro-mechanical systems (MEMS), such as microarrays, biosensors and lab-on-a-chip or microfluidic systems provide significantly scaled-down versions of much larger bench-top instrumentation. A number of rapid method technologies are discussed in greater detail later in this chapter.

Many growth-based rapid methods or other technologies which require an enrichment incubation period (e.g., to generate sufficient cellular targets of interest, such as ATP) can still be faster than conventional methods. Depending on the amount of microbial growth required for detection and/or quantification, the time to result could be as little as a few days. However, non-growth-based methods can attain results in real-time or close to real-time (e.g., minutes or hours). Eliminating the need for microbial growth while obtaining microbiology data in real-time can help facilitate a cultural shift from operating the microbiology laboratory in a reactive mode (i.e., when contamination occurs) to a proactive one (i.e., preventing contamination and maintaining a state of microbial control). Real-time rapid methods can also allow immediate technical and business decisions to be made on in-process material and finished product batches during the normal course of manufacturing operations.

The use of rapid methods may also provide additional benefits including releasing finished product faster to meet the inventory demands of customers and distributors, reducing warehousing space and costs, improving automation and reducing or reallocating headcount that would normally be assigned to performing conventional microbiology testing. Furthermore, many companies have realized significant cost savings or cost avoidances by implementing rapid methods for similar reasons described earlier. In these cases, the payback period for the investment in validating and implementing a rapid method is minimal.

Applications

Practically any conventional microbiology test method can be replaced by an alternative or rapid method. Many microbiology tests supporting the manufacture and distribution of cosmetics include an assessment of the number of organisms present in finished product, raw materials or other samples, whether any of the organisms are objectionable in nature and what the identity of the organism is, for example, to the genus and species level.

Quantitative rapid methods have been used as alternatives to compendial bioburden assays, such as USP 61, *Microbiological Examination of Nonsterile Products: Microbial Enumeration Tests* (1); FDA Bacteriological Analytical Manual (Chapter 23), *Microbiological Methods for Cosmetics* (2); Personal Care Products Council (PCPC; formerly Cosmetics, Toiletries, and Fragrance Association [CTFA]) Microbial Content (M-1) test (3); or ISO Microbial Content Standard Test Methods for Cosmetics (e.g., ISO 21149) (4).

The same quantitative rapid methods may also be used for other types of bioburden studies, including antimicrobial or preservative effectiveness tests, water analyses, environmental monitoring, in-process bioburden assays and raw material testing. For example, firms have validated alternative methods to USP 51, *Antimicrobial Effectiveness Testing* (5); PCPC (CTFA) challenge tests (e.g., PCPC M-3) (6); AOAC 998.10, *Preservative Challenge Efficacy Test of Non-Eye Area Water Miscible Products* (7); and ISO 11930, *Cosmetics – Microbiology – Efficacy Test and Evaluation of Preservation of a Cosmetic Product* (8).

Qualitative rapid methods have been used as alternatives to compendial presence/absence tests, including USP 62, *Microbiological Examination of Nonsterile Products: Tests for Specified Microorganisms* (9) and PCPC (CTFA) M-2, *Examination for S. aureus, E. coli, Ps. Aeruginosa and C. albicans* (10). For example, rapid methods will detect the presence (or absence) of target microorganisms in the original sample, and a variety of growth-based and nucleic acid amplification techniques have been utilized for this purpose.

Qualitative RMMs have also been implemented to quickly detect the presence of microorganisms as a surrogate to performing a quantitative assay. For example, many cosmetic companies have implemented rapid methods for the QC release of finished batches based on a qualitative ATP bioluminescence technology. Specifically, test samples are enriched in media for a relatively short period of time (e.g., 24–48 hours) followed by an ATP assay in which relative light units (RLUs) are measured. The RLU is actually a measure of photons of light arising from the ATP bioluminescent reaction. Enrichment of the sample is required because there is not enough ATP from low levels of bacteria to illicit a detectable level of RLUs. As such, the greater the RLU readings, the higher the number of organisms are in the enrichment medium and this would be indicative of the biological load in the original sample. Conversely, a low RLU level would indicate the original sample had none to minute levels of organisms. Because this method requires an enrichment step, additional considerations must be taken into account, including neutralizing preservatives or other components in the product formulation that might prevent the growth or organisms should they be present. Furthermore, because the assay is qualitative in nature, any positive result (above baseline) may require confirmation testing to demonstrate the sample meets the quantitative release specifications. In this case, a quantitative ATP bioluminescent method may be more relevant; however, current technologies require the sample to be filtered prior to the enrichment step and some cosmetic matrices may not be compatible with this requirement (e.g., the formulation is viscous in nature). ATP bioluminescent rapid methods are described in greater detail in a later section.

In many cases, there is a need to identify microorganisms recovered from finished product testing, in process material and/or raw materials. Most likely, microbial identifications are used to support investigations into out-of-specification findings or other microbiological excursions, root cause analyses and to determine whether organisms in finished product are of an objectionable nature (e.g., potentially harmful based on the type of organism and/or the manner in which the product is used). There are many types of rapid identification technologies, and some of these are described later in this chapter.

Implementation Strategy

There are a variety of options to consider when a firm decides to implement a rapid or alternative microbiology method. The following activities are commonly performed:

1. Review existing microbiological methods and identify opportunities for improvement based on the user's requirements. User requirements will be very specific and the validation plan must demonstrate the requirements can be met. The following examples are provided to understand what might be considered; however, these may change based on the particular requirements for a rapid method:
   a. Faster time to result, where the actual time to result would be defined (e.g., minutes vs. hours vs. days)
   b. Level of sensitivity (e.g., limit of detection or limit of quantification, such as 10 viable cells)
   c. Required sample size
   d. Organisms that must be detected (e.g., bacteria, yeast, mold, aerobes, anaerobes)
   e. Level of automation
   f. A positive return on investment
2. Assess currently available RMM technologies and determine what methods may meet the user requirements and be compatible with the testing product or other test samples.
3. Match compatible RMM technologies with the intended application (e.g., bioburden, detection, identification).
4. Conduct pre-validation activities, including a review of regulatory considerations (e.g., whether a formal submission would be required), business and quality needs, vendor audits, and risk assessments associated with replacing the existing method with an alternative method.
5. Conduct proof-of-concept or feasibility testing to ensure there are no compatibility issues with the anticipated test samples.
6. Develop and execute the validation plan (e.g., design qualification [DQ], installation qualification [IQ], operational qualification [OQ], performance qualification [PQ], method suitability and equivalency studies).

Review of RMM Technologies

It is assumed that the first step in the implementation strategy has been performed; namely, existing microbiological methods have been reviewed and the firm has identified those tests in which a rapid method would provide a benefit. From there, the firm must match the right technology with the intended application while making sure there is a good probability of success that the user requirements will be met and there are no incompatibilities between the test samples and the technology itself. As stated, feasibility studies can be performed with the technology supplier to answer the compatibility question.

It is paramount that the end-user understands potential RMM capabilities in terms of user requirements. For example, a RMM that relies on membrane filtration should not be considered for test samples that are non-filterable. Likewise, if the user requires a time to result within an 8-hour shift, many growth-based RMMs and/or those that require an enrichment step greater than 8 hours would not be good candidates for validation and implementation. To assist the reader in deciding what technologies may work with their samples and required applications, the following technology overview is provided. Although it is not possible to describe all of the rapid methods that are available, particular technologies have been chosen based on their current accepted use in healthcare and personal care industries. However, a more comprehensive review of RMM technologies is provided in PDA's *Encyclopedia of Rapid Microbiological Methods* (11) and the RMM Product Matrix at http://rapidmicromethods.com (12). In fact, the tables summarizing the technologies discussed in this chapter have been adapted from the rapidmicromethods. com website.

Growth-Based Methods

Rapid methods that rely on the growth of microorganisms in liquid or solid conventional media can be used for a variety of applications including bioburden testing, environmental monitoring, sterility testing and microbial identification. Most systems will quickly detect growing organisms or enumerate microcolonies using specialized scientific principles, such as measuring changes in electrical conductivity or impedance, detecting byproducts of respiration (e.g., oxygen consumption or carbon dioxide production), utilizing carbohydrates and other substrates or sensing autofluorescence of microcolonies following excitation from specific wavelengths of light (Table 7.1).

Impedance microbiology is based on the premise that microbial growth results in the breakdown of larger, relatively uncharged molecules into smaller, highly charged molecules (e.g., proteins into amino acids, fats into fatty acids and polysaccharides/sugars into lactic acid). Growth may be detected by monitoring the movement of ions between electrodes (conductance) or the storage of charge at an electrode surface (capacitance). Impedance systems can detect changes in measurable electrical threshold in liquid media (during microbial growth) when microorganisms proliferate in containers that include electrodes. Growth may, therefore, be detected prior to the liquid media showing any signs of turbidity. Impedance systems were utilized as one of the original rapid methods for screening antimicrobials and preservatives in the early 1990s. The Sy-Lab BacTrac system is an example of this technology that is available currently.

Microorganisms, when grown in liquid culture, produce carbon dioxide. In a closed container, microbial growth may be detected by monitoring the changes in the amount of carbon dioxide present. BioMérieux's BacT/ALERT allows carbon dioxide that is generated during microbial growth to diffuse into a liquid emulsion sensor and the resulting color change is the indication for the presence of microorganisms. Many gene and cell therapy companies are looking at this type of system for the rapid release of products that have a relatively short shelf life or that must be implanted or infused in patients within days of manufacturing or compounding. Another example of this type of RMM is the Becton Dickinson (BD) Diagnostic Systems BACTEC FX.

A number of identification technologies measure the ability of microorganisms to utilize biochemical and carbohydrate substrates dehydrated in a microtiter plate format. These types of RMM systems monitor changes in kinetic reactions or turbidity, the latter indicating microbial growth. One technology, the Biolog Omnilog system, includes a tetrazolium violet dye in the same wells that contain a dehydrated carbon source and if a microorganism utilizes that carbon source, the well will turn purple. The bioMérieux VITEK 2 uses an optical system that monitors changes in each well using different wavelengths in the visible spectrum and detects turbidity (microbial growth) or colored products as a result of substrate metabolism. In both systems, the resulting data (normally in the form of positive and negative responses) are compared with an internal database or reference library for that specific platform and a microbial identification is provided.

TABLE 7.1

Growth-based technologies

	Scientific Method	Time to Result	Throughput	Sample Size or Type	Sensitivity	Organisms Detected
Sy-Lab BacTrac	Impedance microbiology, electrical measurement of total viable growth and selective growth	12–72 hrs.	64 per instrument, up to 12 instruments per system	1–10 mL or gm	1 CFU after enrichment	Total aerobic, yeast and mold, coliforms, *E. coli*, lactic acid bacteria, coliforms, *Enterobacteriaceae*, *Salmonella*, *Pseudomonas*, *P. aeruginosa*, *Enterococci*, *Listeria*, *Cronobacter*, *Staphylococcus* (including coagulase positive), *Bacillus cereus*, *Clostridia*, *C. perfringens*.
bioMérieux BacT/ALERT	Growth-based; CO$_2$ detection	24–96 hrs.	480–1,440 per incubation period	1–10 mL or gm	1 CFU after enrichment	Bacteria, yeast, mold
BD Diagnostic Systems BACTEC FX	Growth-based; CO$_2$ detection	8–48 hrs.	240–1,200 per incubation period	1–10 mL or gm	1 CFU after enrichment	Bacteria, yeast, mold
Biolog Omnilog	Growth-based; carbohydrate utilization	2–72 hrs.	50 per day	Cells from colony		>1,226 bacteria and >885 yeast/mold
bioMérieux VITEK 2 Compact	Growth-based; biochemical and carbohydrate utilization	2–18 hrs.	30–60 per day	Cells from colony		>285 bacteria and >48 yeast
Rapid Micro Biosystems Growth Direct	Growth-based; automated detection of cellular auto-florescence	Final results in half the time of conventional agar-based method	280 samples per incubation period	Filterable samples	1 CFU	Bacteria, yeast, mold
Biolumix and Soleris Neogen	Growth-based; CO$_2$ detection and selective growth	3–48 hrs.	32–128 tests at a single temperature per instrument	0.1–5.0 mL	1 CFU after enrichment	Total aerobic, yeast and mold, coliforms, *E. coli*, lactic acid bacteria, *Enterobacteriaceae*, *Salmonella*, *Pseudomonas*, *Staphylococcus*
Bactest Speedy Breedy	Respirometry, pressure sensing	4–20 hrs.	2–4 per day	Up to 50 mL	1 CFU after enrichment	Aerobes, facultative anaerobes, anaerobes, and microaerophilic bacteria; yeast

Source: Adapted from http://rapidmicromethods.com.

Rapid Micro Biosystems' Growth Direct provides a sensitive digital imaging method for detecting microbial growth on agar surfaces. The technology detects the yellow-green fluorescent signal emitted by growing microcolonies when illuminated with blue light. Cellular autofluorescence in this spectral region is a property of all microbial cells due to the presence of ubiquitous fluorescent biomolecules including flavins, riboflavins and flavoproteins. The system will provide a microcolony count in about half the time it would take for the same organisms to growth into a colony-forming unit, the size of which is countable by a laboratory technician.

The Biolumix and Soleris Neogen systems employ a variety of broth media that will encourage the growth of target microorganisms. The vials contain unique dyes in which microbial growth is detected by changes in color or fluorescence. An optical sensor detects these changes, which are expressed as light intensity units. The vials are also constructed with two independent zones: an upper incubation zone and a lower reading zone. The two zones eliminate masking of the optical pathway by the test sample and/or by microbial turbidity.

A relatively new RMM—the Bactest Speedy Breedy—is a portable respirometer that monitors pressure changes relating to gaseous exchanges within a closed culture vessel as a result of microbial respiration. The system provides real-time analysis of positive and negative pressure changes in the vessel headspace, facilitating the detection of viable microorganisms.

Cellular Component-Based Technologies

Cellular component-based RMMs focus on detecting specific cellular components or the use of probes that are specific for microbial target sites of interest. For example, ATP, fatty acids, surface macromolecules, bacterial endotoxin, proteins and nucleic acids have been used as targets for RMMs for the detection, quantification and identification of microorganisms. Similarly, for growth-based technologies too, a wide range of microbiology applications may be realized (Table 7.2).

Bioluminescence is the generation of light by a biological process and is most commonly observed in the tails of the American firefly *Photinus pyralis*. In the presence of D-luciferin and luciferase, bioluminescence occurs when ATP is catalyzed into adenosine monophosphate (AMP). One of the reaction byproducts is light (in the form of photons), which can be detected and measured using a luminometer. Because all living cells store energy in the form of ATP, cellular ATP can be used as a measure of microorganism viability. Current bioluminescent technologies use ATP-releasing agents to extract cellular ATP from microorganisms that may be present in a sample, and following the addition of bioluminescent reagents, can detect the amount of light emitted from the sample. Depending on the technology used, the amount of light emitted can indicate the presence of microorganisms, or may be correlated with actual cell counts. In addition, if a sample is expected to contain very low levels of microorganisms, it may be necessary to allow these microorganisms to replicate (e.g., either in liquid culture or on agar medium) in order to increase the amount of ATP that can be detected. Quantitative and qualitative ATP bioluminescence systems are currently available; for example, the Millipore Milliflex Rapid system is a quantitative technology that detects the ATP arising from micro-colonies that have developed on an agar surface; qualitative technologies provide a measurement of relative light units indicating the presence of microorganisms in the original sample. One qualitative system, the Celsis Advance II system, utilizes an additional substrate, adenosine diphosphate (ADP), which can be converted to ATP in the presence of an enzyme—adenylate kinase; ADP is extracted from cells in addition to cellular ATP. The additional substrate and enzyme reaction helps to increase the total amount of ATP in the reaction by 1,000 times, thereby increasing the sensitivity of the assay.

A different technology used for microbial identification is based on the analysis of fatty acids recovered from microorganisms. The cellular membrane contains lipid biopolymers, and the fatty acid profiles are unique for different types of organisms including bacteria and fungi. In the MIDI Sherlock MIS system, fatty acids that are extracted from a microbial culture are analyzed using gas chromatography and the resulting peaks compared with an internal library or database.

Matrix-assisted laser desorption/ionization (MALDI) mass spectrometry is a recent technology that has been introduced for the identification of microorganisms. Different organisms, when exposed to an energy source, generate a variety of charged molecular weight patterns or spectra. These patterns are

TABLE 7.2

Cellular component-based technologies

	Scientific Method	Time to Result	Throughput	Sample Size or Type	Sensitivity	Organisms Detected
Millipore Milliflex Rapid	ATP bioluminescence; quantitative	24–28 hrs.	60 per day	Filterable samples	1 CFU after growth	Bacteria, yeast, mold
Charles River Laboratories Celsis Advance II	ATP bioluminescence; qualitative	<1–48 hrs.	120 assays per hour	Liquid or solid samples	1 CFU after enrichment	Bacteria, yeast, mold
MIDI Sherlock MIS	Detection of fatty acids for microbial identification	< 15 min. – 2 hrs.	100 per day	Cells from colony		>1,200 bacteria and >200 yeast/mold
Bruker Daltonics MALDI Biotyper	MALDI-TOF mass spectrometry for microbial identification	1–2 min.	30–60 per hr.	Cells from colony or liquid sample		> 2,000 species and > 4,010 strains of bacteria, yeast and mold
bioMérieux Vitek MS	MALDI-TOF mass spectrometry for microbial identification	2 min.	480 every 8 hrs.	Cells from colony		>508 bacteria and >78 fungi

Source: Adapted from http://rapidmicromethods.com.

based on the macromolecules normally expressed on the surface of a particular species. Intact cells from a primary culture are smeared onto a stainless steel target plate and allowed to co-crystallize with a UV-absorbing matrix. After drying, the plate is placed into a mass spectrometer and exposed to a laser. The matrix absorbs energy from the laser, and cellular macromolecules are desorbed, ionized and analyzed. The resulting mass spectra are compared with an internal database to provide a microbial identification. Multiple instruments are currently available to perform this type of analysis to identify bacteria, yeast, mold and Mycobacteria. These include the Bruker MALDI Biotyper (the first instrument that was introduced for microbial identification) and the bioMérieux Vitek MS.

Viability-Based Technologies

Viability-based technologies differentiate viable cells from dead cells and can target specific microorganisms using nucleic acid, enzymatic or monoclonal antibody probes. In many cases, direct labeling of single cells is possible with no cell growth requirement, facilitating time-to-result in hours or even minutes. And because these methods do not require growth, the enumeration of stressed, fastidious, dormant or viable, but non-culturable organisms may be higher than that obtained using conventional, growth-based methods. Applications are fairly broad-based, including quantitative in-process and finished product bioburden testing, water analysis, environmental monitoring and even sterility testing.

A viability-based rapid method may employ the use of flow cytometry. Cells are labeled with a viability marker and passed through a flow chamber, one cell at a time. Fluorescence and light scatter signals are detected and individual cells are counted as they pass through a laser beam. The process of labeling and detecting viable cells in these systems can be accomplished in as little as a few minutes. The sample size required for flow cytometry systems are usually low (e.g., less than 1 mL), and aqueous and many types of non-aqueous samples are compatible with this method. Because this technology can use fluorescent dyes and microbe-specific probes—such as antibodies, rRNA or peptide nucleic acid (PNA)—simultaneous enumeration and detection of target organisms is possible. Existing systems provide a quantitative assessment of the test sample; however, although single cell detection is possible, this is usually not at an acceptable level of accuracy and precision. For this reason, 10–50 cells are the accepted limit of quantification. Examples of available technologies include the bioMérieux Chemunex D-Count and BactiFlow.

Solid-phase cytometry is similar to flow cytometry except that cells are captured on a solid surface such as a 0.45μ filter. The filter is stained with a viability substrate followed by laser excitation, which enables a quantitative result. Single cell quantification, with good accuracy and precision, has been demonstrated by a number of companies.

A common workflow involves passing the test sample through a membrane filter and then labeling the filter with a non-fluorescent viability substrate. Within the cytoplasm of metabolically active cells, the substrate is enzymatically cleaved to liberate a free fluorochrome. Only viable cells with intact membranes have the ability to perform this cleavage and retain the fluorescent label. The entire membrane surface is subsequently laser-scanned, and labeled microorganisms are quantified. The process of labeling and detecting viable cells in this system can be completed in approximately 90 minutes. Some of these types of systems also utilize antibodies and nucleic acid probes to detect and quantify specific microorganisms in a few hours. Examples of solid-phase cytometry systems include the bioMérieux Chemunex ScanRDI and the LumiByte BV MuScan (Table 7.3).

Spectroscopic-Based Technologies

Optical spectroscopy is an analytical tool that measures the interactions between light and the material being studied. Light scattering is a phenomenon in which the propagation of light is disturbed by its interaction with particles. For example, "Mie scattering" is one form of light scattering in which scattered light is proportional to the particle size. Therefore, many particle counters employ Mie scattering to detect, count and size particles in an environment, such as those used in cleanrooms and other microbiologically controlled areas.

Mie scattering is also the basis for a number of rapid methods used to detect, count and size viable cells in the air and water (Table 7.4). When particles from an air or water sample are processed through one of

TABLE 7.3

Viability-based technologies

	Scientific Method	Time to Result	Throughput	Sample Size or Type	Sensitivity	Organisms Detected
bioMérieux Chemunex D-Count/ BactiFlow	Viability staining and flow cytometry	30 min.	15–50 per hr.	Liquids, usually less than 1 mL	10–50 cells with good accuracy and precision	Bacteria, yeast, mold
bioMérieux Chemunex ScanRDI	Viability staining and solid phase cytometry	1.5–3 hrs.	30 per day	Filterable samples	1 cell	Bacteria, yeast, mold, spores
LumiByte BV MuScan	Viability staining and solid phase cytometry; detection of target organisms	10–65 min.	100 per 8 hrs.	Filterable samples; 1 uL to 1L	1 cell	Bacteria, yeast, fungal spores; test kits include *Legionella, Salmonella, Listeria, Chronobacter* and *E. coli*

Source: Adapted from http://rapidmicromethods.com.

TABLE 7.4

Spectroscopic-based technologies

	Scientific Method	Time to Result	Throughput	Sample Size or Type	Sensitivity	Organisms Detected
BioVigilant IMD-A	Intrinsic fluorescence and Mie scattering for air samples	Instantaneous	Continuous or episodic monitoring	1.15 or 28.3 L/min. air	1 cell	Bacteria, yeast, mold, spores
Particle Measuring Systems BioLaz	Intrinsic fluorescence and Mie scattering for air samples	Instantaneous	Continuous monitoring	3.6 L/min. air	1 cell	Bacteria, yeast, mold, spores
TSI BioTrak	Intrinsic fluorescence and Mie scattering for air samples	Instantaneous	Continuous or episodic monitoring	28.3 L/min. air	1 cell	Bacteria, yeast, mold, spores
BioVigilant IMD-W	Intrinsic fluorescence and Mie scattering for water samples	Instantaneous	Continuous monitoring or point sampling	10 mL/min.	1 cell	Bacteria, yeast, mold
Mettler Toledo 7000RMS Microbial Detection Analyzer	Intrinsic fluorescence and Mie scattering for water samples	2 sec	Continuous monitoring	30 mL/min.	1 cell	Bacteria, yeast, mold
mibic Gram[RAY]	Viable staining and imaging LED Raman spectroscopy; quantitative and microbial identification	3–10 min.	300–600 per hr.	Cells from colony, liquid medium, product/raw material, surfaces	1 cell	Database under development

Source: Adapted from http://rapidmicromethods.com.

these systems, particles within a 0.5–20μm range are sized and counted. At the same time, a UV laser that intersects the particle beam will cause biological material, such as microorganisms, to auto-fluoresce, due to the presence of NADH, riboflavin or dipicolinic acid. These types of technologies are highly sensitive and provide viable and non-viable detection and counting results continuously and in real-time. In addition, there is no need for reagents, staining, labeling or cellular growth. Examples of technologies that are specifically designed for air or water sampling include the BioVigilant IMD-A and IMD-W, Particle Measuring Systems BioLaz, TSI's BioTrak system and Mettler Toledo 7000RMS Microbial Detection Analyzer.

Another type of light scattering is Raman, where information about molecular vibrations and rotations of molecules may be ascertained. Rapid methods based on Raman have been developed for the detection of microorganisms in a variety of sample matrices and in air, and because microorganisms have their own unique Raman spectrum, this can be used as a fingerprint for identification. However, most Raman systems will detect both viable and non-viable cells, which would present a challenge for industries in which the viability of microorganisms must be confirmed. One technology vendor has overcome this issue by employing a viability-staining step prior to conducting Raman spectroscopy. The mibic Gram[RAY] instrument allows for a Raman signature to be generated only from particles that have been determined to be viable cells, enabling detection, enumeration and identification within minutes.

Nucleic Acid Amplification-Based Technologies

Nucleic acid amplification-based rapid technologies utilize a number of gene amplification and detection platforms, including polymerase chain reaction (PCR), transcription-mediated amplification, 16S rRNA typing and gene sequencing. Most of these methods will detect the presence of a target microorganism or generate data that can be used to determine the identification of an isolate, from the genus level down to the sub-species and/or strain level (Table 7.5).

To maintain correct RNA structure and ribosome function, the 16S sequence of rRNA is highly conserved at the genus and species level. However, the non-conserved fragments within the rRNA operon (the spacer and flanking regions of the 16S sequence) can be used to differentiate strains within a particular species. One rapid technology makes use of the DNA sequences that encode for the rRNA operon for microbial identification and strain differentiation. In the Hygiena Riboprinter, restriction enzymes (such as EcoRI or PvuII) are used to cut recovered and purified DNA into fragments. The fragments are then separated according to size by gel electrophoresis and immobilized on a nylon membrane (this is commonly referred to as a Southern Blot technique). The double-stranded DNA is denatured to single-stranded DNA, and the membrane is subsequently hybridized with a DNA probe (derived from an *E. coli* rRNA operon). Finally, an antibody-enzyme conjugate is bound to the probe and a chemiluminescent agent is added. Light emitted by the fragments is captured, and the image pattern is compared with patterns stored in the system database. If the pattern is recognized, a bacterial identification is provided. The pattern can also be used to determine if the same strain has been previously observed. This may be helpful when investigating the source of an environmental isolate or a contaminated product.

Most nucleic acid amplification technologies that detect a specific or target microorganism employ PCR as their fundamental scientific principle. Small fragments of DNA (primers) are used to find a specific sequence (target) on a sample of DNA. A heat stable enzyme (e.g., *Taq* DNA polymerase) makes millions of copies of the target sequence, which can then be easily detected and used to determine if a specific microorganism was present in the original sample. A typical workflow is as follows: after the extraction of DNA from microorganisms in a sample, all the reagents necessary for PCR (the specific DNA primer, DNA polymerase and nucleotide bases [A, T, C, G]) plus a fluorescent dye (e.g., SYBR Green, which binds to double-stranded DNA) are hydrated with the DNA sample and processed in a thermocycler. The thermocycler goes through a series of heating and cooling steps to facilitate binding of the primer onto the target DNA sequence (if it is present), followed by elongation of the double-stranded DNA and then amplification of the DNA fragments. Each amplification cycle results in two copies of DNA. This is repeated and the number of copies of DNA per amplification cycle increases exponentially (i.e., from 2 to 4 to 8 to 16, and so on). Real-time quantitative PCR can track the increase in fluorescence from one complete PCR cycle to the next, indicating that the target DNA sequence was present in the test sample because it is being replicated and amplified over time. This would indicate the target microorganism was also present in the original test sample. Additional detection phases may also be employed, in which the temperature of the amplified DNA sample is raised to the point where the DNA strands separate (denature), releasing the fluorescent dye and lowering the signal. This change in fluorescence can be plotted against temperature to generate a melting curve. Similar detection techniques using different types of probes and dyes (e.g., Taqman or FRET probes) are also available, depending on the supplier's system. Because each target organism generates its own specific melting curve related to its endpoint fluorescence detection, the system can determine if a specific target organism was present in the original sample. A number of systems use PCR as the scientific principle for microbial detection; these include the Hygiena BAX system, Pall Corporation's GeneDisc and Roche's MycoTool systems.

Most PCR systems can detect the presence of a single target DNA sequence only at a time; however, some newer technologies can perform multiplex detection assays, meaning they can detect multiple DNA targets simultaneously and in some cases, within the same reaction vessel or tube. This is made possible by using different primers and probes/dyes at the same time.

TABLE 7.5

Nucleic acid amplification–based technologies

	Scientific Method	Time to Result	Throughput	Sample Size or Type	Sensitivity	Organisms Detected
Hygiena Riboprinter	Ribotyping of DNA fragments	8 hrs.	32 per day	Cells from colony		>1,440 bacteria and >8,500 strain or sub-species patterns
Hygiena BAX System Q7	PCR	1.5–2.5 hrs.; 48 hrs. for yeast/mold	96 per 1.5–2.5 hrs.	10–50 µL		*Salmonella, Listeria monocytogenes, Camplyobacter jejuni/coli, E. coli* O157:H7, *Enterobacter sakazakii, Staphylococcus aureus*, yeast and mold, *Vibrio*
Pall Corporation's GeneDisc	qPCR	3–8 hrs. including sample filtration, nucleic acid prep, and PCR	96 per PCR run	1–300 mL	1 CFU after enrichment for 6–24 hrs.; >100 CFU without enrichment	*E. coli, Salmonella, Pseudomonas aeruginosa, Staphylococcus aureus, Candida albicans, Aspergillus brasiliensis*, STEC and non-STEC, *E. coli* O157, *Listeria, Legionella, Enterococcus, Cyanobacteria*
Roche MycoTool	PCR for Mycoplasma detection	< 5 hrs.	40 biological samples per day	1 mL of cell culture	<10 CFU/mL	>150 Mollicutes species
Applied Biosystems MicroSEQ	PCR and gene sequencing for microbial identification	4–5 hrs.	80 per day; higher with greater capacity capillary analyzers.	Cells from colony		>1,800 bacteria, >90 Mycoplasma and >1,100 yeast and mold

Source: Adapted from http://rapidmicromethods.com.

Unfortunately, PCR is not without its limitations. Although the time to result can be as early as a few hours to detect the presence of a particular organism, the potential for false positives is present when the starting material is DNA. DNA is ubiquitous in the environment and residual DNA, or DNA from non-viable cells could result in a positive assay when that target microorganism was never present in the original test sample. Therefore, care must be taken to avoid DNA contamination when performing the test. In addition, the test sample may need to be enriched in media before performing PCR to ensure that any DNA detected and amplified came from the target organism(s) in the original sample under investigation.

To overcome the potential for false positives, a different gene amplification technique called transcription-mediated amplification (TMA) has been developed. TMA targets single-stranded RNA, which is less stable in the environment as compared with DNA. TMA also uses the enzyme RNA polymerase to produce many RNA copies per amplification cycle, as compared with only two copies of DNA from a PCR cycle, representing up to a 10-billion-fold increase of copies in as early as 15–30 minutes. There are a number of additional advantages when using TMA as compared with PCR. For example, PCR requires a series of temperature changes to facilitate amplification whereas TMA is performed at one temperature (e.g., 41°C), eliminating the need to use a thermocycler. There is also improved amplification reliability and sensitivity because there are usually thousands of rRNA copies per cell instead of a single DNA target.

PCR and TMA have been used for the detection of a specific target microorganism. When microbial identification is required, the industry commonly turns to gene sequencing. The use of 16S rDNA is the current standard for taxonomic classification. Therefore, if we can extract DNA from an isolated microbial colony, amplify the DNA using PCR and sequence the first 500 base pairs of the 16S rRNA gene, we can compare the sequence to an internal database to assist with a microbial identification. Current systems accomplish this task using a genetic analyzer and automated workflows. The most commonly used instrument in microbiology labs for this purpose is the Applied Biosystems MicroSEQ.

Finally, it is suggested that gene amplification techniques can be used to estimate the number of microorganisms in the test sample based on the number of cycles it takes to detect the presence of a target sequence. However, there may be too many technical hurdles to overcome to get this to work reliably and repeatedly. For example, in order to detect a wide range of microorganisms, multiple nucleic acid primers would be required. Next, steps would need to be taken to minimize false positives, such as using RNA as the starting material. Third, there would need to be some correlation between the numbers of cycles required to detect the amplified copies to a viable cell count. Until these challenges are adequately addressed, nucleic acid amplification technologies may be limited to the detection of specific microorganisms and for microbial identification purposes.

Micro-Electro-Mechanical Systems (MEMS)

Micro-Electro-Mechanical Systems (MEMS) use the integration of mechanical, electrical, fluidic and optical elements, sensors and actuators on a common silicon substrate through microfabrication technology. Examples include lab-on-a-chip and microfluidics devices, microarrays and biochips, biosensors and nanotechnologies. (Table 7.6).

Lab-on-a-chip technologies are based on an automated, micro- or nano-scale laboratory that enables sample preparation, fluid handling, and analysis and detection steps to be carried out within the confines of a single microchip. The technology is based on microfluidics, and the most familiar consumer application is inkjet printing. Microfluidics allow for the manipulation of minute amounts of liquid in miniaturized systems that are composed of a network of channels and wells that are etched onto glass or polymer chips. Pressure or voltage gradients move pico- or nano-liter volumes through the channels in a well-controlled manner that enables sample handling, mixing, dilution, electrophoresis and chromatographic separation, staining and detection. Currently available lab chips analyze protein, DNA, RNA and whole cells in fluid samples. At least one currently available technology (bioMérieux's DiversiLab) uses a microfluidics chip to separate rep-PCR amplicons (rep-PCR targets short, repeating sequences of unknown function that occur randomly throughout the DNA of an organism). The chip is processed in a bioanalyzer, where the amplicons pass through a laser, causing fluorescence of an intercalating dye. The resulting rep-PCR fingerprints are compared with a database, and a detection result, or microbial identification, is provided.

TABLE 7.6

MEM technologies

	Scientific Method	Time to Result	Throughput	Sample Size or Type	Sensitivity	Organisms Detected
BioMérieux's DiversiLab	PCR for detection and microbial identification	4 hrs.	13 samples per chip in 4 hrs. Each additional chip (13 samples) every 1 hrs.	Cells from colony		>168 bacteria and >1,100 strain or sub-species patterns
Greiner Bio-One CytoInspect	PCR and microarray analysis for Mycoplasma detection and identification	5 hrs.	100 per day	Cell culture		Detection of > 90 species of Mycoplasma and identification of 40 Mycoplasma species

Source: Adapted from http://rapidmicromethods.com.

Microarrays are collections of miniaturized test sites, arranged on solid substrates that permit many tests to be performed at the same time. They are composed of an orderly arrangement of protein or thousands of DNA or RNA fragments on glass, silicon or nylon substrates. This technology evolved from Southern Blot technology, in which fragmented DNA is attached to a substrate and then probed with a known gene or DNA fragment, using fluorescent tags to allow visual detection. Microarrays are usually fabricated using a variety of technologies, including printing with fine-pointed pins onto glass slides, photolithography, inkjet printing or electrochemistry. Other methods may also be used, such as *in situ* synthesis, whereby the probes are synthesized directly on the chip instead of spotting them on the array. Applications for microarrays include nucleic acid sequence identification and measuring expression levels of genes. For example, the entire human genome (~50,000 known genes and gene variants) has been fit on a single chip and microarrays are currently being used to detect influenza A, Avian H5N1 (Bird Flu) and other clinically relevant viral strains.

Microarrays are also being used to detect and speciate Mycoplasma that has been recovered from cell cultures and fermentation processes within the biotech industry. In the Greiner Bio-One CytoInspect system, PCR is performed on DNA from the cell culture and the PCR amplicons are processed in the microarray. If the amplified DNA hybridizes with complementary sequences on the microarray, a positive result for Mycoplasma is confirmed. There is the potential for developing microarrays for target microorganisms relevant to the cosmetic and personal care industries; however, at the time of writing this chapter, commercial technologies had not been developed for this purpose.

Nanotechnology operates at the atomic, molecular, or macromolecular range of approximately 1–100 nanometers to create and use structures, devices and systems that have novel properties. The key to this technology is high-voltage electron-beam (or E-beam) lithography, in which a beam of electrons is scanned across a surface covered with a thin film, called a resist. The electrons produce a chemical change in the resist, which allows the surface to be patterned.

Nanotechnology has allowed us to fabricate nanoarrays, with molecules placed at defined locations on a surface with nanometer spatial resolution. Nanoarray spots can include biological samples such as proteins, DNA, RNA and whole viruses, as well as non-biological samples such as chemical solutions, colloids and particle suspensions. Nanoarrays are the next evolutionary technological step in the miniaturization of bioaffinity tests for proteins, nucleic acids and receptor-ligand pairs. These arrays utilize approximately 1/10,000th of the surface area occupied by a conventional microarray, and over 1,500 nanoarray spots would occupy the area required for a single microarray spot. These technologies utilize surface patterning tools, which are microcantilever-based micro-fluidic handling devices. The droplet volumes these microcantilevers deliver to the nanoarray are in the femtoliter and attoliter range (10^{-12} milliliter and 10^{-15} milliliter, respectively). Nanoarrays offer a number of advantages, including label-free detection (via atomic force microscopy). They work in both solutions and biological liquids, retaining biological activity for subsequent analyses.

Nano-biosensors are now in development that can be wirelessly monitored or probed with a non-contact device to detect a chemical or biological exposure. For example, these biosensors will be used to detect contamination in packaging (e.g., raw materials, food) and in air. There are possibilities for future applications to use these and other MEMS for consumer and healthcare products.

Validation of RMMS

Because rapid methods are considered alternatives to existing or compendial microbiology methods, the end-user is responsible for demonstrating the new method is at least equivalent to, or is non-inferior to, the method intended to be replaced. There are a number of validation documents that provide guidance on method development, method suitability testing, equivalency studies, the use of statistics, feasibility or proof-of-concept studies, training, technology transfer and the establishment of validation plans. Examples of the most commonly used documents are as follows:

- PDA Technical Report #33, *Evaluation, Validation and Implementation of Alternative and Rapid Microbiological Methods* (2013 revision) (13).
- USP ⟨1223⟩, *Validation of Alternative Microbiological Methods* (2015 revision) (14).
- Ph. Eur. Chapter 5.1.6, Alternative Methods for Control of Microbiological Quality (2017 revision) (15).

Each of the documents provides a review of validation strategies, although PDA TR33 is considered to be the most comprehensive in terms of content. Furthermore, the 2015 revision to USP ⟨1223⟩ was a significant departure from its prior version, and in some cases, appears to conflict with some of the guidelines in PDA TR33 and Ph. Eur. Chapter 5.1.6. For this reason, the reader is encouraged to review recent publications (16,17) on this subject.

Generally speaking, the validation process usually starts with feasibility or proof-of-concept studies to demonstrate product or test samples will be compatible with the rapid technology of interest. This also assumes the end-user has already developed user-requirements and has matched the right method for their application(s) as described earlier in this chapter. These activities should be completed before committing to purchase a rapid system. The studies can be performed in-house (after renting an instrument or obtaining an instrument on loan) or at the rapid method supplier's laboratory. Concurrent with these activities, the end-user should audit or assess the supplier no differently from if they were qualifying a new supplier of raw materials or other equipment or services. In addition, a risk assessment should be conducted to identify any new risks or hazards that may be associated with the implementation of a rapid method.

The next step is to develop the validation plan or the roadmap for all of the activities that will be required to demonstrate that the rapid technology is validated and suitable for its intended use. The validation plan should identify all project deliverables, responsible parties for each phase of test execution, review and approval processes and the documentation required to satisfy the expectations of the validation strategy.

A functional design specification (FDS) should be developed that will describe all of the functions and requirements for the RMM system and what will be tested to ensure that the system performs as specified in the end-user's original user requirement specification. The FDS can cover system functionality, configuration, input/outputs, environment, utilities, computer and communication architecture, interfaces, data and security. The FDS should also point to specific test scripts where each requirement will be evaluated and verified against pre-established acceptance criteria (e.g., what will be performed during the IQ, OQ and PQ phases of the validation plan).

Prior to the start of the validation plan, all users should have been appropriately trained in the use of the rapid system and all relevant procedures should be documented and approved.

The IQ establishes the equipment is received as designed and specified, that it is properly and safely installed with the correct utilities in the selected environment, and that the environment is suitable for the operation and use of the equipment. The IQ can be carried out by the RMM supplier (during initial commissioning) and/or by the end-user, especially if the end-user's company requires a more extensive IQ program.

The OQ provides documented verification that the equipment performs effectively and reproducibly as intended throughout the anticipated or representative operational ranges, defined limits and tolerances. The OQ is the focal point for the majority of the computer system validation (CSV), including hardware, software and security testing.

The PQ provides documented evidence that the instrumentation, as installed, consistently performs in accordance with predetermined criteria and thereby yields correct and appropriate results. The PQ will include validating the method, method suitability for the product or test samples to be routinely evaluated and a demonstration of equivalence to the existing method.

Method validation will usually encompass an appropriate selection of test microorganisms and/or other material that are used to demonstrate an appropriate level of accuracy, precision or repeatability, specificity, limit of detection or quantification, linearity, range, ruggedness and robustness. Specific testing requirements will depend on whether the rapid method will provide a quantitative, qualitative or identification result.

Method suitability studies are very similar to what current compendial requirements are for microbiological testing: that the presence of a particular product, material or sample matrix does not significantly impact the performance of the rapid method, which may include background noise, interference, false positive and/or false negatives.

Finally, equivalency testing will determine how similar the new method test results are when compared with the existing method. The new method is run in parallel with the existing method for a specified period of time or number of product batches or test samples and then the results are statistically compared with each other. The end-user should determine the most appropriate strategy for the duration and extent of these studies, which may be influenced by the critical nature of the test method, the material being analyzed, the statistical methods used when interpreting the resulting data, regulatory expectations and/ or other quality requirements.

Once the validation plan has been executed and approved, the RMM may be implemented for routine use. If an identical technology will be transferred to a separate facility from where it was validated, it is usually not necessary to repeat the same qualification test plan in its entirety; however, any product or test sample that was not included in the original validation must be evaluated for Equivalency and Method Suitability. It is up to the end-user to determine the extent of additional testing to be performed as part of the technology transfer plan.

Once the validation plan has been completed and the rapid method is being utilized, procedures should be established to maintain the system in a validated state. This may be accomplished through an approved ongoing maintenance and periodic review program.

The reader is encouraged to review the validation guidance documents already referenced from PDA, USP and Ph. Eur. Additional publications (18–20) that may be helpful to review are provided in the reference section of this chapter.

Return on Investment

The initial costs associated with feasibility studies, validation testing and installation activities for a new, rapid method can be significant. However, it is unfair to focus only on the up-front costs when evaluating a new technology, as there can be substantial long-term cost savings or cost avoidances that may be realized. Therefore, the end-user should develop a comprehensive economic analysis to support the decision to purchase, validate and ultimately implement a rapid method for routine use.

Financial models, such as return on investment (ROI), payback period and net present value may be used to support the decision to purchase a new rapid method. Using one of these models, it is relatively simple to compare the overall costs associated with the conventional method and the proposed RMM, taking into account the potential cost savings by implementing the RMM. And the information obtained should be used to complement the technical and quality justifications for qualifying the RMM. Publications (21,22) on this topic may help the reader in understanding how to practically conduct these types of financial exercises.

Summary

Rapid microbiological methods offer novel solutions for the detection, enumeration and identification of microorganisms. By evaluating and implementing these innovative technologies, the cosmetic industry will help advance the science of microbiology, enhance its understanding of the microbiological state of control for products and manufacturing processes and improve the availability of consumer products by obtaining release test results faster and more efficiently.

To enable these objectives, it is mandatory to understand the current microbiological methods, look at opportunities for improvement, identify the right RMM for the product and testing requirements, establish a robust and meaningful validation plan and execute the plan. The time to move away from 19th-century microbiology and embrace 21st-century approaches is now.

REFERENCES

1. United States Pharmacopeial Convention ⟨61⟩, Microbiological Examination of Nonsterile Products: Microbial Enumeration Tests. 2017; USP 40/NF35: 117–123.
2. U.S. Food and Drug Administration. BAM: Bacteriological Analytical Manual. Chapter 23, Microbiological Methods for Cosmetics. 2017; www.fda.gov/Food/FoodScienceResearch/Laboratory Methods/ucm565586.htm.
3. Personal Care Products Council. M-1, Determination of the Microbial Content of Personal Care Products. Microbiology Guidelines. 2016; 187–193.
4. International Organization for Standardization. ISO 21149:2017. Cosmetics – Microbiology – Enumeration and Detection of Aerobic Mesophilic Bacteria. 2017.
5. United States Pharmacopeial Convention ⟨51⟩, Antimicrobial Effectiveness Testing. 2017; USP 40/NF35: 111–114.
6. M-3 Method for Preservation Efficacy Testing of Water Miscible Personal Care Products, Personal Care Products Council (PCPC).
7. AOAC 998.10, Preservative Challenge Efficacy Test of Non-Eye Area Water Miscible Products.
8. International Organization for Standardization ISO 1930:2012. Cosmetics – Microbiology – Evaluation of the Antimicrobial Protection of a Cosmetic Product. 2012.
9. United States Pharmacopeial Convention ⟨62⟩, Microbiological Examination of Nonsterile Products: Tests for Specified Microorganisms. 2017; USP 40/NF35: 123–130.
10. Personal Care Products Council. M-2, Examination for and Identification of *Staphylococcus aureus*, *Escherichia coli*, *Pseudomonas aeruginosa*, and *Candida albicans*. Microbiology Guidelines. 2016; 195–208.
11. Encyclopedia of Rapid Microbiological Methods, Volumes 1–4 (Miller MJ ed). PDA and Davis Healthcare International Publishing. 2005–2012.
12. Rapid Micro Methods. 2020; http://rapidmicromethods.com.
13. Parenteral Drug Association. Evaluation, Validation and Implementation of Alternative and Rapid Microbiological Methods. Tech Rep No. 33; 2013.
14. United States Pharmacopeial Convention ⟨1223⟩, Validation of Alternative Microbiological Methods. 2017; USP 40/NF35: 1756–1770.
15. European Directorate for the Quality of Medicines & HealthCare. Chapter 5.1.6, Alternative Methods for Control of Microbiological Quality. 2017; Supplement 9.2: 4339–4348.

16. Miller MJ. A Fresh Look at USP ⟨1223⟩, Validation of Alternative Microbiological Methods and How the Revised Chapter Compares with PDA TR33 and the Proposed Revision to Ph. Eur. 5.1.6. *Am. Pharm. Rev.* 2015; 18(5): 22–35.
17. Miller MJ. Rapid Methods Update: Revisions to a United States Pharmacopeia Chapter. *Eur. Pharm. Rev.* 2015; 20(4): 38–43.
18. Miller MJ, van den Heuvel ER, Roesti D. The Role of Statistical Analysis in Validating Rapid Microbiological Methods. *Eur. Pharm. Rev.* 2016; 21(6): 46–53.
19. Miller, MJ. Microbiology Series. Article 2: The Implementation of Rapid Microbiological Methods (Validation Strategies). *Eur. Pharm. Rev.* 2010; 15(2): 24–26.
20. Miller, MJ. Developing a Validation Strategy for Rapid Microbiological Methods. *Am. Pharm. Rev.* 2010; 13(3): 28–33.
21. Miller, MJ. Breaking the Rapid Microbiological Method Financial Barrier: A Case Study in RMM Return on Investment and Economic Justification. *BioPharm. Internat.* 2009; 22(9): 44–53.
22. Miller, MJ. Rapid Microbiological Methods and Demonstrating a Return on Investment: It's Easier Than You Think! *Am. Pharm. Rev.* 2009; 12(5): 42–47.

Biography

Dr. Michael J. Miller is an internationally recognized microbiologist and subject matter expert in pharmaceutical microbiology and design, validation and implementation of rapid microbiological methods. He is currently the President of Microbiology Consultants, LLC (http://microbiologyconsultants.com). In this role, he is responsible for providing scientific, quality, regulatory and business solutions for the pharmaceutical, biotech, personal care and other regulated industries. He is also the owner of http://rapidmicromethods.com, a website dedicated to the advancement of rapid methods.

Dr. Miller has held numerous R&D, manufacturing, quality and business development leadership roles at Johnson & Johnson, Eli Lilly and Company and Bausch & Lomb. He has authored over 100 technical publications and presentations in the areas of microbiology, ophthalmics, disinfection and sterilization, and is the editor of PDA's *Encyclopedia of Rapid Microbiological Methods*.

Dr. Miller is the chairperson for revising PDA Technical Report #33, *Evaluation, Validation and Implementation of New Microbiological Testing Methods*. He also advises the USP on matters related to rapid sterility testing. Dr. Miller holds a PhD in Microbiology and Biochemistry from Georgia State University and a BA in Anthropology and Sociology from Hobart College.

8

Prevention of Microbial Contamination during Manufacturing

Donald J. English

Introduction

Every cosmetic or personal care manufacturer has the responsibility to ensure the microbiological safety of their finished products. This goal is accomplished by ensuring that their product formulations are free from the numbers and types of objectionable microorganisms that may affect either the product quality and/or the health of the consumer. However, it is not unusual for these product formulations to have some type of a microbial bioburden or content (1). This microbial bioburden should not be harmful to either the product's esthetics or the consumer especially if they have a pre-existing condition such as being immunocompromised or otherwise sensitive to a particular microorganism by having a disease, open wounds, or organ damage (2).

The source of a microbial bioburden from a manufacturing facility in a non-sterile product formulation could be one or all of the following: facility itself, manufacturing systems, equipment, and cleaning/sanitization processes.

Facility

Design and Overall Layout

The design and overall layout of a manufacturing facility should minimize the risk of a non-sterile finished product being contaminated with either high numbers of microorganisms or contain the presence of a microbial pathogen or objectionable microorganism. The facility design and overall layout should accomplish the following:

- Minimize the risk in preventing the improper flow of raw ingredients, packaging and finished product.
- Permit effective cleaning and sanitization of manufacturing equipment and the facility where appropriate materials of construction and design are used in order to prevent build-up of dirt, dust and product residues.
- Ensure the effective maintenance of the facility and equipment.
- Take all precautionary steps to avoid the possibility of having an adverse effect on the microbial quality of finished products.

Facility HVAC Systems

Temperature control such as air conditioning and heating from a heating, ventilation and air-conditioning (HVAC) is generally required for the comfort of manufacturing personnel. However, the design of HVAC systems for a manufacturing area must be specific for each area served. Several design aspects for an air system must be considered including the quality of the incoming air, temperature, humidity, air exchange rate, desired air purity, location of incoming/exhaust air vents or ducts and duct work for the control of airflow patterns.

Air Filtration

Besides removing particulates, the facility air intakes should be fitted with a screen to prevent insects from entering the interior of the building. The degree of air filtration will depend upon the quality of the incoming air and the area to be served. Areas in which raw ingredients are handled may require low efficiency air filtration while manufacturing/filling areas will usually require more highly purified air. Most air handling systems will use a primary filter in order to provide a lower filtration level. Secondary and tertiary filters are used to provide high filtration levels. Location of these filters should be downstream of the air handling units (e.g., fans). Electrostatic precipitators can be used in place of a final filter to remove particulate matter (e.g., 0.5–1.0 microns) from the air. These filters should be maintained or changed with new filters on a regular schedule.

Air Treatment

On the basis of geographical location, time of the year and types of non-sterile finished products that are being manufactured, it may be necessary to either humidify or dehumidify the air. Relative humidity control is desirable for manufacturing in either tropical climates or for the production of pressed powders in order to prevent mold proliferation due to the absorption of environmental water vapor by formulation binders. Air humidifying or dehumidifying systems need to be properly maintained in a clean and sanitary manner. To prevent proliferation of microorganisms, water collection pans and drains of these systems should be monitored and maintained.

Air Exchange

A facility air supply system will need to be balanced in order to have proper air exchange rates for the areas served. Facility clean areas should be under a slightly higher air pressure than adjoining areas. Clean air in the slightly positive areas will restrict the flow of contaminated air from dirty areas via openings. To maintain slightly positive air pressure, it is important to prevent air filters from becoming overloaded such that the incoming air flow is restricted. Any unplanned openings such as cracks in the walls could also alter the exchange rate.

Energy Conservation

To save energy, it is common practice today to turn off a HVAC facility system at night, on weekends and during holidays. When work is planned, it is important that the HVAC system be turned on again to allow enough time to bring the air quality back into conformance with requirements.

Makeup Air

Some HVAC systems will use 100% makeup or fresh air from outside of the facility. However, many facility HVAC systems will use either re-circulated air or will add a portion of fresh air to the re-circulated air. In either case, it is important that the air intake ducts be located far away from the facility exhaust air ducts or loading dock in which either facility exhaust air or truck fumes can be drawn into the air supply. For those facilities that have a Quality Control Analytical Laboratory, it is also important for those air exhaust ducts to be located away from the air intake ducts to prevent chemical vapors from re-entering the facility. If the air is being re-circulated, and depending on the airborne contamination, a High Efficiency Particulate Air (HEPA) filter may need to be installed in the air stream for the removal of contaminants. These HEPA filters should have an EN1822 classification of H13 (3).

For the manufacturing of non-sterile product formulations, the use of a classified area is not required (3). If a manufacturing area is going to be classified, these areas should be in static mode only when the facility is cleaned. A minimum classification of an ISO 14644-1 Class 8 or Grade D from the Europe Commission's cGMPs is recommended for use because higher air classifications such as Grades A, B and C might not be possible to obtain when measuring 0.5 and 5.0 micron particles (4). Furthermore, the temperature, relative humidity and ventilation should be appropriate for each of the facility manufacturing areas and should not adversely affect the quality of non-sterile finished products during their manufacturing and storage.

Floors

According to the U.S. Food and Drug Administration's (FDA) Good Manufacturing Practice (GMP) Guidelines/Inspection Checklist for Cosmetics, FDA 21 CFR Part 211 current Good Manufacturing Practice for Finished Pharmaceuticals, Subpart C-Buildings and Facilities, and the EU Guidelines to Good Manufacturing Practices, Chapter 3, one basic requirement is that all floor finishes be smooth, free of cracks, free of joints and are easily cleanable (5–7).

A smooth surface that is free of cracks and joints prevents dust from accumulating and the collection of water in these areas in which microorganisms could proliferate. In addition, the floors should have a slight sloop to them in order to have proper water drainage. Furthermore, the flooring material should extend a short distance up every wall that it touches. In general, floors in a manufacturing facility should be constructed on a concrete base in which a smooth, durable, and non-penetrable material can be added on top in order to provide a surface that is slip-resistant to an operator and is also able to withstand cleaning and disinfectant solutions.

Types of Flooring Systems

There are three types of flooring systems that are used to provide a smooth finish in a manufacturing facility: polymer-modified cement terrazzo, resinous and welded vinyl or rubber sheet (8). The use of a polymer-modified cement terrazzo flooring system eliminates employing a traditional 2-inch sand bed to isolate the substrate from the terrazzo finish. The use of this modified cement matrix allows for a 3/8-inch thick resin-based terrazzo to be directly placed on the concrete slab. The terrazzo is a mixture of aggregates embedded in an epoxy or some other polymer that is ground to a smooth polish to serve as a top coat that seals the terrazzo and provides appropriate protection from chemical exposures. The second type of flooring system is a resinous flooring system. It consists of a polymeric material such as epoxy, polyurethane or acrylic with epoxy. This type of system is applied in multiple layers and no grinding is required. The third flooring system is a vinyl or rubber rolled sheet in which the seams are either heated or chemically welded together. A benefit in using this type of flooring system is the ergonomic comfort by the cushioning provided when standing on it. However, the downside of this type of flooring system is the increased possibility of delamination from the substrate or tearing and gorging when heavy loads are moved across it.

Drains

Floors should have a slight slope to the floor drains. This will help ensure proper water drainage. It is also recommended that each of the drains be constructed and maintained well so that they remain unclogged and prevent the backflow of wastewater from cleaning and sanitization processes. Single point trapped drains with grates containing holes should be constructed from stainless steel and be an adequate size to accommodate the required drainage rate to prevent the accumulation of standing water on manufacturing and filling floors (9). However, it is recommended that trench drains be used in the entries of wash bays from production areas. These trench drains should be shallow with a semi-circular cross section and sloped to allow for proper drainage. In addition, the connection of the manufacturing drainage system to the sewage system of the facility should include a suitably-sized air break or other mechanical device in order to prevent back siphonage from the sewage system into manufacturing areas (10). The drains of the facility should be kept clear of debris in order to allow proper water drainage into the drain.

It is recommended that floor drains be allowed to dry out completely between water exposures without leaving traps of dried materials within the drain, if possible in a production environment. Instead, some companies will periodically pour a disinfectant solution down the drain and flush with potable water to reduce the number of microorganisms that are present in a drain and to eliminate the possibility of odors being generated by resident drain microorganisms. Generally, microbial monitoring of floor drains is not recommended because microorganisms always will be present due to the wet and soiled environmental conditions supporting microbial survival and proliferation.

Walls, Ceilings, Windows and Doors

Walls should be free from cobwebs, dampness, condensation and mold, and properly maintained without flaking paint, damaged tiles, and improper grouting between tiles, cracks and open joints. From a micro-biological design consideration, it is recommended that all walls and ceilings be smooth, non-porous and free from cracks and open joints (9). These smooth surfaces should be covered in a non-friable concrete or plaster and be painted with a waterproof or water-resistant paint to allow for proper cleaning and sanitization. All walls and ceiling seams should be sealed. The junctions between walls, floors ceilings and windows should be a concave coved to eliminate difficult-to-clean right angles and where dust could collect. Any cracked, damaged or peeling wall and ceiling surfaces should be repaired or replaced as soon as possible. Kick plates or wall shielding should also be used to prevent damage where doors, corners or walls could be subjected to contact with either heavy equipment or pallets of raw ingredients for use in manufacturing.

Projections on walls and ceilings should be kept to a minimum in order to maintain a smooth and easy-to-clean surface. Suspended ceilings should be used wherever possible (9). Ceiling titles should be covered with an impervious layer such as polyvinyl chloride (PVC) and designed in such a way that the tiles clip into a frame to reduce the possibility of dislodgement in which contamination could occur. Light fixtures and air vents should also be flush with the ceiling surface. Suspended piping and overhead utilities from the ceiling should be kept to a minimum. Where possible, overhead piping and utilities should be located behind a ceiling overhead, but should be readily accessible for maintenance and repairs. Exposed overhead roof beams, pipes and duct work should be avoided. When this is not possible, exposed overhead pipes and duct work need to be mounted so that they do not touch the walls or ceiling to allow for thorough cleaning. Any exposed overhead pipes and ducts should be free of dust, rust, mold, flaking paint, cobwebs and extraneous material. Ceilings should be kept free from condensation to prevent the growth of mold and water from dropping into non-sterile finished products.

Windows should be non-opening and flush with the wall surface when ventilation is adequate (10,11). Ledges for non-opening windows should be avoided because they are subject to dust accumulation and moisture deposition during cleaning and sanitization processes. If windows are open to the outside environment, they should be properly screened to prevent entry of insects (10).

Doors should be tight fitting and maintained in good condition and free of mold, flaking paint and periodically cleaned. Doors leading into manufacturing areas, other than emergency exits, should be fitted with self-closing devices, air curtains or plastic strips. External doors should be constructed to prevent the entry of rainwater into the facility and should be rodent proof (i.e., gaps not exceeding 6 mm) and be self-closing or protected by an internal lobby with a self-closing door.

Equipment Placement

Placement of processing and filling equipment in a manufacturing facility should avoid overhead unprotected pipes, conveyers or other difficult-to-clean equipment. Leakage, condensate formation or lubricant drippings from overhead unprotected pipes, conveyers or other difficult-to-clean equipment can be a source of microbial contamination in a product formulation. In addition, processing and filling equipment should be raised from the floor or otherwise constructed so that the floors underneath this equipment can be cleaned and sanitized.

Traffic and Material Flow

The design of the manufacturing facility should allow for one-way, sequential flow of materials and personnel to eliminate the possibility of cross-over or the need for facility personnel to transit through one area to reach their place of work. Separate pathways should be provided for personnel to move around the facility without interfering in product production. The movement of materials and personnel should also be designated to restrict entry into facility manufacturing areas.

The facility should have sufficient space to allow the manufacturing areas to be segregated from storage, laboratory, restrooms and administrative and eating areas. Also, there should be separate areas for the manufacturing and packaging of different types of product formulations (e.g., powders, nail enamels, creams, lotions, etc.). Raw ingredients should enter the processing areas of the facility from a single set entry area. Any materials that are brought into the manufacturing area should be clean prior to entry for the removal of dust and dirt that may contain microorganisms. Secondary packaging materials should be removed before they enter the raw ingredient dispensing area or the manufacturing area.

Facility storage areas should have sufficient capacity and appropriate design to allow for effective segregation of raw ingredients, packaging components and finished products that are either released for use for manufacturing or are under quarantine while waiting for the completion of Quality Control analytical, packaging component and microbiological release testing. The quarantine area for incoming raw ingredients and packaging components should be of an appropriate design establishing sufficient space for storage and a sampling area for incoming receipts.

External raw ingredient bulk delivery or unloading areas for tanker trucks or rail cars must be clearly identified and designed to prevent errors in transferring the delivered material into correct bulk storage tanks.

Manufacturing Systems

In a manufacturing facility, it is common to find the following systems present: compressed air, vacuum and process water. Compressed air systems are mostly used to blow away product residues from manufacturing equipment, remove debris and insects from packaging components (e.g., jars and tubes), remove excess cleaning solutions and dry surfaces or components after cleaning or sanitization. Vacuum systems are either dry or wet. A wet vacuum system is used to remove excess or pooled cleaning solutions and water from equipment, floors and other surfaces. A dry vacuum system is used in those areas where dry ingredients are used or in the manufacturing of powder product formulations. A process water system is used to provide purified water for the manufacturing of product formulations and cleaning/sanitization of manufacturing equipment.

Compressed Air Systems

Examples of direct and indirect contact points for compressed air in a non-sterile finished product manufacturing facility can range from such activities that occur during compounding (e.g., sparging/ mixing), packaging, pressurization or blanketing bulk finished product in holding tanks before filling, and equipment drying after cleaning and sanitization. Because the uses of compressed air within the industry can vary greatly, there is no set design standard in place (12).

It is well known that air contains water vapor, particles and microorganisms. Hence, contaminants in a compressed air system will consists of microorganisms, solids, liquids and vapors. These contaminants can enter a compressed air system at the compressor intake, or can be introduced into the air stream by the system itself. By compressing the air, the concentration of water vapor, particles and microorganisms will increase. During the compression process, the air is heated. As the compressed air flows through the compressed air distribution system, the heated compressed air will cool and the concentrated water vapor will condense into a liquid. Inlet air for an air compressor will often contain 5–50 microorganisms per cubic feet per minute (CFM) along with moisture and particular matter (13). A 75 Horse Power (HP) air compressor with a capacity of 300 standard cubic feet per minute (scfm) can take in between 100,000 and 1 million microorganisms each hour.

Air is compressed by either a lubricant-free or lubricant-injected air compressor. The air compressor is a contamination source for the following: water aerosols, condensed liquid water, liquid oil, oil aerosols, atmospheric dirt and microorganisms. After compression, the air is stored in a wet air receiver/reservoir or compressed air tank. The compressed air tank provides a wet, warm, dark environment in which mesophilic aerobic bacteria and fungi are able to survive and proliferate. It is not unusual to detect the presence of *Pseudomonas aeruginosa* or *Candida albicans* in a compressed air tank. The compressed air tank can potentially contaminate a distribution system with water vapor, microorganisms, atmospheric dirt, oil vapor, water aerosols, condensed liquid water, liquid oil, oil aerosols, rust and pipe scale. Furthermore, piping, fittings and controls that are located downstream of this compressed air tank are ideal harborage sites for microbial biofilms especially when they are fed with food grade compressor oils that inevitably migrate downstream (14).

Design

When designing a compressed air system, point-of-use filtration is the best defense in preventing the introduction of microorganisms whenever compressed air comes into direct or indirect contact with the non-sterile finished product. However, point of use filtration does not eliminate harborage sites and microbial biofilm build-up within the system. To help in controlling the development of microbial biofilms within a compressed air system, three stages of filtration are used (15). The first stage of filtration involves the removal of liquid and wet particulate matter from compressed air in the compressed air tank by a coalescing filter with an automatic drain. The second stage of filtration is the removal of oil and water aerosols by using a second coalescing filter with an automatic drain. After each of these coalescing filters, water vapor is removed from compressed air by using an air dryer. Drying the air to a low dew point is an effective way to inhibit microbial growth (16). After elimination of water vapor, oil vapors will need to be removed from the compressed air by an adsorption type of filter because oil vapors cannot be removed by an oil coalescing filter. After this absorbing filter, the compressed air is passed thru a particulate filter for the removal of 1–3 micron particles. After the particulate filter, the compressed air can be stored in a dry air receiver for eventual use in the manufacturing areas. The third stage of filtration occurs at the point-of-use by using microbiological filters 0.22 microns in pore size. The first and second stage compressed air filters should be changed every 6–12 months. Point-of-use microbial retentive filters should be changed every 3–6 months or as necessary based on the point-of-use compressed air quality microbial test results (14).

Vacuum Systems

Most non-sterile product manufacturing facilities will use a centralized vacuum system, but they may also be portable. A vacuum system could serve as a potential site for microbial contamination because vacuum lines are generally not sanitized, and the presence of diluted product, dirt and water condensation may provide the necessary nutrients for the proliferation of microorganisms.

To prevent vacuum lines from being a contamination source, a backflow device should be installed. This will prevent the introduction of microbial contamination back into finished product. The backflow of collected product residues, dirt, dust and water condensation can be checked by this device.

Process Water Systems

It is important to control the microbial quality of process water because it is a major ingredient in aqueous non-sterile product formulations and is used during cleaning and sanitization of manufacturing equipment. If process water is contaminated with high levels of microorganisms and/or contains certain types of microbial species such as Gram-negative bacilli, it could cause adverse physical changes to the product such as phase separation, malodors and color changes and may pose a health risk to the consumer. In addition, a high microbial load in process water for a non-sterile finished product formulation could overwhelm the preservative system causing it to become inadequately preserved versus consumer use or even result in gross contamination of the finished product.

Overall Design Considerations

Source water for a process water system should be potable or drinking water in compliance with the National Primary Drinking Water Regulations (NPDWR) (40 CFR 141) issued by the U.S. Environmental Protection Agency (EPA) or the drinking water regulations of the European Union, Japan or the World Health Organization (16–18). The design of a process water system consider the chemical components. Typically analyzed by the supplier during the design phase, source water must be addressed in order for the system to produce deionized water that complies with the USP Purified Water monograph. The following chemical tests may be conducted: silica content, water hardness (e.g., levels of calcium and magnesium ions), total dissolved solids, soluble organic impurities, bicarbonate ions, suspended solids (e.g., inorganic or organic origin) and dissolved gases such as ammonia, carbon dioxide, hydrogen sulfide and sulfur dioxide (19,20). Depending upon the chemical test results of the source water, the presence or absence of the following components can be installed in the generation section of a process water system: (16,19,21,22).

- Deep-bed filtration
- Activated carbon bed
- Water softeners
- Reverse osmosis
- Cation/anion/mixed bed ion exchange columns or continuous electrodeionization (EDI).

Deep-bed filtration or multimedia/sand filters are used to remove suspended material such as particulate matter, colloidal matter, and heavy molecular weight matter such as naturally occurring organic matter. The installation of an activated carbon bed is used to absorb chlorine, chloramines and organic material from a potable or drinking water source. Water softeners are used to remove calcium, magnesium and other cations that can cause water hardness. A reverse osmosis unit is a purification technology in which a semi-permeable membrane is used to remove both multivalent and monovalent ions from water. Depending upon the water quality, reverse osmosis units be either a single or a double pass. In a double-pass reverse osmosis unit, two individual reverse osmosis units are operated in a series in which one unit will provide the feedwater to the second unit. Cation/anion/mixed bed ion exchange columns or electrodeionization unit (EDI) unit is used to remove cations and anions from water that had not been removed by the reverse osmosis unit.

Microbial Design Considerations

The microbiological quality of process water may vary and can be influenced by conditions of manufacturing such as pH, temperature, equipment and the presence of chemicals. Seasonal variations in the source or feedwater for a process water system can also have an effect on the microbial and chemical quality of the process water. To ensure the microbial quality of the process water, the following design considerations need to be taken into consideration (17,20,22,23).

- Water distribution lines should be sloped for proper drainage over the entire length of pipe run (e.g., 1% or greater such as 2%) (23,24,25).
- The entire process water and storage system should be designed for proper re-circulation with a continuous, turbulent flow of a minimum of 1–2 meters/second to reduce stagnation and the possibility of biofilm development.
- Pipe diameter for water distribution water loop lines should be a maximum of 1.0–1.5 inches in order to help maintain an adequate flow rate.
- Elbows, tees and bends should be kept to a minimum.
- U-bends should be avoided unless they are inverted so as to eliminate pockets of water that can stagnate to cause the development of microbial biofilms. Unused valves and branch lines (dead legs) should be removed to prevent similar water stagnation and biofilm development. A dead leg is determined by using the mathematical formula of $X < 2D$, where X is the length of the line and D is the diameter of the line. If the diameter of a line is 25 millimeters and the length of X is greater than 50 millimeters (2 times D), a dead leg is present and must be removed.
- Sanitary types of unions and valves should be used in the system to prevent the formation of water pockets that cannot drain and dry out when they are closed.
- For water distribution loops and storage tanks, the recommended material of construction is 316L stainless steel. The 316L stainless steel piping should be used for the water distribution loop with joints be orbitally welded (26,27).
- 316L stainless steel surface finishes of the water storage tank and distribution loop should have a sanitary finish greater than 150 grit or have a roughness average of less than 0.8 (19). Most finishes currently used are 189 or 249 grit. Having a smooth stainless steel surface, it aids in the prevention of developing a microbial biofilm.
- Stainless steel is subject to chemical attack by deionized water which removes the iron from the stainless steel. Iron is a microbial growth factor. To prevent this chemical attack, 316L stainless steel surfaces of water storage tanks and distribution loop lines must be passivated. Passivation is a chemical process by which iron is removed from the stainless steel surface and chromium and nickel of the stainless steel are oxidized by the passivating agent (e.g., nitric acid, citric acid or its mixed chelants) forming an impervious layer of chromium oxide and nickel oxide. This chromium oxide and nickel oxide layers protect the underlying 316L stainless steel against contact with and corrosion by deionized water.
- If the 316L stainless steel storage tank is replaced or the distribution loop piping is modified in which new 316L stainless steel piping is added, the whole system should be re-passivated.
- The use of plastic piping as a material of construction for a distribution loop is cheaper than the use of 316L stainless steel. However, it should be noted that the ranking of plumbing materials for inhibiting the development of a microbial biofilm is as follows: stainless steel > Polytetrafluoroethylene > Polypropylene > chlorinated Polyvinyl chloride (PVC) > Unplasticized PVC > High Density Polyethylene (HDPE) > plasticized PVC (28–31).

- With the exception of Polyvinylidene fluoride (PVDF) or Polytetrafluoroethylene (PTFE) and 316L stainless steel, plastic piping is known to be intolerant to the use of heat and ozone as a water system sanitizer (32). PVC piping is also incompatible with most chemical sanitizers. In addition, plasticizers (phthalates) can be leached from PVC piping and are able to serve as a microbial food source for the development and maintenance of a microbial biofilm. Furthermore, PVC piping joints cannot be heat welded but must be joined with couplings that use a solvent to partially dissolve the joints to form a rough weld unlike the smooth welds of stainless steel, PVDF and PTFE. These rough PVC welds are known to be excellent sites for the development of a microbial biofilm. If PVDF and PTFE piping is planned for use to distribute heated water, it needs to be supported and expansion sections will need to be built into the design because it will expand. Furthermore, PVDF and PTFE piping carrying hot water will need to be insulated.

Possible Sources of Microbial Contamination

There are indigenous, exogenous and manipulative microbial contamination sources in a process water system. The indigenous microbial contamination sources can be from the feedwater, air from unfiltered vents on water storage tanks and compressed air used to open and close valves. Exogenous microbial contamination sources can be from new ion exchange resins, new activated carbon beds, new equipment and fittings, regenerants such as softener brines and airborne dust. Manipulative microbial contamination sources could be from operator hygiene and operator technique such as assembly and sampling of the purified water system.

Sources of Microbial Growth Requirements in Process Water

For microorganisms to survive and proliferate in a process water system, certain microbial requirements need to be present such as oxygen, organic carbon, nitrogen, phosphorous, sulfur and trace minerals (33). Depending upon the water level, a source of oxygen is the air that passes in and out the vents that are present on the top of the water storage tank. Sources of organic carbon for microbial growth in a process water system include system feedwater, pipe plasticizers, pump and gauge lubricants, microbial by-products, personnel, degraded deionized resins, gaskets and membrane filter surfactants. The primary source of nitrogen for growth in a process water system is the system feedwater containing nitrates, nitrites and microbial by-products. A source of phosphorous and sulfur is the system feedwater (e.g., phosphates and sulphates), microbial by-products and membrane surfactants. Trace minerals originate from feedwater, system piping and membrane filter extractables.

Microbial Contamination in Process Water Systems

Because process water is not sterile, it is not unusual to detect microorganisms in samples taken from various process water system sites. However, coliform bacteria and the United States Pharmacopeia (USP) indicator microorganisms such as *Escherichia coli*, *Staphylococcus aureus* and *Salmonella* species should not be isolated from purified water samples. There are several reasons for not detecting their presence in process water samples, including the fact they are sensitive to the antimicrobial action of chlorine when the potable or drinking source water is chlorinated (16). In a study that was conducted over a 14-year test period, none of these microbial species had been isolated from the source water for a purified water system. Instead, the following types of Gram-negative bacterial species were isolated from the potable source water for a process water system: *Pseudomonas fluorescens*, *Brevundimonas vesicularis*, *Ralstonia pickettii*, *Pseudomonas stutzeri* and *Sphingomonas* species (34). Risk of system contamination with these is limited as the ambient temperature (e.g., 15.0–20.0°C) of a circulating process water system is sub-optimal for their growth, and each requires a highly nutritious environment to survive and proliferate.

Common characteristics of process water system microbial isolates are as follows: nutritionally versatile (e.g., heterotrophic), aerobic, ability to grow in low nutrient conditions, and resistant to low levels of chlorine. The following Gram-negative bacillus species have been recovered from process water systems: *Pseudomonas aeruginosa, Ralstonia pickettii, Pseudomonas fluorescens, Bradyrhizobium* species, *Sphingomonas* species, *Flavobacterium* species, *Burkholderia cepacia* complex, *Moraxella* species, *Stenotrophomonas maltophilia* and *Flavimonas oryzihabitans* (34–37).

Although process water microbial contamination may be planktonic or floating or drifting in water, the majority of process water bacteria reside in a surface biofilm somewhere within the system. Biofilms are mixed bacterial communities embedded in a polysaccharide slime layer of the biofilm. Biofilms are typically formed in low or high turbulence liquid environments (38). The morphological shape of the microbial biofilm in a process water distribution system will be influenced by the process water flow rate. In water that is stagnant or has a low flow rate, the morphological shape of a microbial biofilm tends to be tall, fluffy and columnar allowing for the detachment of planktonic bacteria for additional colonization (39). In flow paths of high turbulence, the morphological shape of the microbial biofilm tends to be solid streamline patches that are more difficult to remove (40). In addition, a fewer number of planktonic bacteria are removed due to shedding, and new surfaces are colonized to a lesser extent in a process water system with a high turbulent flow rates (39).

Reasons for Microbial Contamination Issues in Process Water System Components

The following process water system components are known sites for microbial contamination issues: deep-bed filtration units, activated carbon beds, water softeners, reverse osmosis units and cation/anion/mixed-bed ion exchange columns. Deep-bed filtration units offer a high surface area for absorption of microbial nutrients and deposition of microorganisms allowing formation of microbial biofilms with subsequent shedding.

Activated carbon beds are usually installed after the deep-bed filtration. They have a high degree of bacterial adherence and shedding due to a high surface area (e.g., 1,000 meters^2/gram). If the incoming feedwater is chlorinated, chlorine and chloramines are removed in the upper portion of this activated carbon bed and this allows bacterial proliferation in the lower portion of the unit. In addition, these beds are known to absorb organic compounds that can serve as bacterial nutrients for microbial proliferation within the unit. Accumulated organic compounds in activated carbon beds source organic nutrients downstream to other process water system components.

In water softeners, microorganisms can increase and may serve as a contamination source in downstream water system components. Periodically, water softeners should be regenerated by using a brine solution. A brine solution is not a sanitizer, and the brine tank may itself serve as a haven for microbial proliferation.

Reverse osmosis units are not absolute in removing all microorganisms. Small numbers of bacteria can penetrate and are able to multiply downstream during stagnant periods.

Microbial contamination problems occur in cation/anion/mixed bed ion exchange columns because they are continuously inoculated with microorganisms from upstream components. Due to a large surface area and the ability to contain nutrients, growth of microorganisms will occur in these columns. Periodically, the resins in these columns need to be regenerated by using either sulfuric or hydrochloric acid. Rechargeable canisters or redundant units after regeneration are stored moist and stagnant where microorganism can proliferate with the passage of time.

Instead of using cation/anion/mixed ion exchange columns to remove water cations and anions, an Electronic Deionization (EDI) unit can be used. An in-line ultraviolet (UV) light (e.g., 253 nanometer wavelength) is recommended to be positioned downstream of the EDI unit and upstream of the final filtration system (41). If bacteria are present in the water from the EDI unit, they will collect on the downstream side of the membrane filtration system and proliferate to form a microbial biofilm. With the presence of a biofilm, there is the potential for back growth into the EDI unit. Installing an UV light after the EDI can inactivate low levels of bacteria in the water and prevent the possible formation of a microbial biofilm on the downstream side.

In the process water distribution loop, microbial contamination could occur in purified water storage tanks and the piping system because these areas will have a reduced water flow and sufficient microbial nutrients will be present to allow for microbial growth. If dead legs and/or inadequately sloped lines are present in the distribution loop, water can stagnate. In addition, cracks in welds and gaskets, poorly fitting flanges and gaskets and threaded joints or connections could provide potential lodging spots for microbial proliferation.

Microbial Control Measures

There are several microbial control measures for a process water system. For example, personnel who routinely operate and maintain a process water system should be adequately trained and this training needs to be documented. To prevent the accumulation of microbial nutrients and the formulation of microbial biofilms within a process water system, all of the surfaces need to be smooth and clean. To reduce the possibility for the development of a microbial biofilm, process water should have a continuous, turbulent flow (e.g., 1–2 meters/second). This will eliminate low flow or stagnant water areas in water storage tanks and the distribution loop. In addition, the process water needs to re-circulate continuously in the distribution loop, storage tanks, deionizers, softeners and carbon beds. Within storage tanks, spray balls need to be used on the re-circulating loop back into the storage tank. Furthermore, the temperature of the re-circulating water in the water storage tank and distribution loop can be maintained at 80°C, a temperature more than sufficient to kill all microorganisms with the exception of spores and extremely thermophilic microorganisms. Most waterborne microorganisms will not grow at temperatures of 60.0–80.0°C, and psychrophilic and mesophilic microorganisms do not grow at a temperature above 50.0°C (42,43). Most thermophilic microorganisms will not grow at temperatures above 73.0°C (44).

Periodic draining, flushing or backwashing can be used to remove nutrients and mitigate biofilm formation in deep-bed filters, carbon beds and water softeners. For deep-bed filters, a back purge or backwashing is used to remove particles and microbial nutrients from the unit. In carbon beds, organic and particulate matter will accumulate and a pressure drop will occur. Back flushing with water in a carbon bed can remove the microbial nutrients and particulate matter. Because microorganisms will proliferate in a carbon bed, a back flush of 90°C water or a steam flush can be used to sanitize the unit. However, a steam flush cannot be used if PVC piping is used.

To regenerate cation ion exchange columns, sulfuric or hydrochloric acid is used. Use of sulfuric or hydrochloric acid and 4% sodium hydroxide solution as regenerates for cation and anion ion exchange columns kills bacteria and disrupt microbial biofilms.

Brine solutions are used to regenerate water softeners but do not have antimicrobial activity, and a brine makeup tank can serve as a source of microbial contamination for water softeners. To reduce the possibility of being a microbial contamination source, the brine solution should be maintained in a clean area or immediately prepared before use. To sanitize a water softener, periodic flushing with 65.0–90.0°C hot water or calcium hypochlorite can be added to the salt supply of the water softener.

Microbial Control Methods

To help control the levels of microbial bioburden in process water, it is recommended that at least two or more of the following microbial control methods be used for routine process water treatment:

- **Chlorination at 0.5–2 parts per million (ppm) (19,27,32).**
  If well water is being used as the source water for a process water system, it needs to be treated and tested to confirm that it is in compliance with local potable or drinking water standards. A sodium hypochlorite solution is often used as the chlorine solution for adding residual chlorine to the well water to meet potable water standards (45).

  For chlorine to work as an antimicrobial treatment for generating potable or drinking water, it is important to know that the concentration of hypochlorous acid (HOCL) and hypochlorite ion (OCL⁻) in the treated water is pH dependent (46). The antimicrobial activity of chlorine residuals can be inactivated if the water contains trace organic residuals or a pH level above 8.5. It should be noted that chlorine may react with ferrous and manganese ions in water and hence may not serve as a disinfectant. To maximize the amount of Hypochlorous acid HOCL and Hypochlorite ion OCl⁻ content, the pH of the source water needs to between 5 and 7.

For sodium hypochlorite solution to work as a water disinfectant, it is important to maintain an appropriate temperature (46). The rate of decomposition of undiluted hypochlorite solutions (e.g., 10–15%) doubles with every 10°F rise in storage temperature. Thus, a stored container of undiluted solution of sodium hypochlorite exposed to temperatures greater than 20.0°C will not be as effective in controlling the presence of microorganisms in potable or drinking water. Undiluted solutions of sodium hypochlorite must be stored under temperature-controlled conditions (e.g., 20.0–25.0°C) to prevent chemical degradation.

It should be noted that medium wavelength UV light (e.g., 185–254 nanometers) can mitigate the antimicrobial efficacy of chlorine (21).

- **UV light (254–265 nanometer wavelength) (16,19,21,32).**
  If UV light at 254–265 nanometers is going to be used as a microbial control method in a process water system, it is important that the energy output of the lamp be periodically verified. Most manufacturers of UV lamps recommend replacement every 8,000 working hours, at approximately one year (45). In addition, the cell housing must be periodically cleaned to allow UV light to penetrate flowing water. The absorbed UV dose in process water will act as a disinfectant depending upon the depth and turbidity of the water, flow rate, lamp intensity and temperature. Because UV light at a 254–265 nanometer exposure is not 100% effective in reducing the microbial load of process water, it is recommended that it is used in conjunction with micro-filtration (47,48). Microbial contamination issues will occur if (1) the incorrect UV lamp is used (e.g., 184–256 nanometer vs. 254–265 nanometer wavelength), (2) the energy output of the UV lamp is not periodically verified in maintaining efficiency and (3) the UV lamp is not changed after reaching the recommended hours of exposure by the manufacturer.

- **Micro-filtration, with a 0.45 micron or smaller pore size.**
  Micro-filtration can be used to remove microorganisms from water. For this, process water should be filtered using a synthetic filter media. To remove microorganisms from process water, it is recommended that an in-line water filter cartridge in the distribution loop and a barrier filter on water storage tank vents be used. If a filter is being used in conjunction with ozone, the filter cartridge should be composed of polytetrafluoroethylene (PTFE) and polyvinylidene difluoride (PVDF) because they are the most resistant to ozone in comparison to filter cartridges that are composed of either nylon/polyester or polysulfone/polypropylene (19). Nylon/polyester and polysulfone/polypropylene filter cartridges are known to react and absorb ozone from ozonated water.

  To ensure that microscopic holes do not form in the filter cartridge during usage, the pressure differential across the filter should be periodically monitored, which will confirm that the filter is still intact to have effective filtration.

  If an incorrect filter pore size is used, microbial contamination of the process water could result from microorganisms passing through the filter. If the filter cartridges are not changed periodically, microorganisms will eventually be able to pass through by one of the following ways: grow-through, blow-through and go-through. Grow-through occurs after an extended period of time when microorganisms start proliferating on and within the membrane cartridge. By binary fission, new smaller cells will eventually be able to penetrate the filter pore passageways of the filter (49). When filtering water, bacteria will collect on the upstream filter cartridge side. Blow-through or blowgun effect occurs when the filtration process is interrupted and bacterial cells are able to grow in the filter cartridge pores. When the filtration process is re-started, these bacterial cells within the pores are then injected into the sterile downstream side of the filter cartridge by the differential pressure from the resumed water flow (50). Go-through occurs when microorganisms germinate with an L-form cell shape due to a cell wall defect where their rigidity is reduced to the point that they have a minimal surface interaction with the surface of the membrane filter matric and are able to transverse through the filter pores without sticking to the membrane (19). It is speculated that the formation of L-shaped bacteria can occur in process water systems as a response to either the presence of low nutrient conditions or to exposure to sub-lethal UV light doses.

- **Heat, at ≥ 80.0°C (19,32,51).**
The use of heat is an effective means of controlling microorganisms in process water. Process water can be heated to a temperature of 80.0°C in a storage tank or by passing it through a heat exchanger located in the distribution loop (17). Hot water at 80.0°C is re-circulated in a distribution loop and this hot water can be placed directly into a vessel for the production of aqueous product formulations. However, there are several disadvantages to the use of heat as a microbial control method: expense due to energy requirements, time required to attain high temperatures throughout the system, and the safety hazard of personnel exposure to hot water.

- **Ozone, at 0.1–1.0 milligram (mg)/milliliter (mL) or 0.1–1.0 parts per million (52).**
Ozone as a microbial control measure should be used only in process water storage tanks and distribution loops that are composed of 316L stainless steel due to its excellent compatibility (52). The use of ozone is not suitable in water that contains more than 0.5 parts per million ppm of manganese because ozone is able to convert soluble manganese to an insoluble form (53). The solubility of ozone in water is inversely proportional to the temperature of the water (i.e., the lower the water temperature, the more readily ozone will be dissolved). In addition, high water temperatures will accelerate decomposition rate of ozone to oxygen—from approximately 20 minutes to a matter of a few seconds. For a maximum concentration of dissolved ozone in water, it is important to control the temperature of the water (e.g., 15.0–25.0°C) by installing an active cooling system (19,52). Ozone's lethality is considered to be excellent against planktonic bacterial cells by having a direct attack against unprotected cell walls and membranes. However, once bacterial cells are embedded within a microbial biofilm and protected by its slimy exopolymer layer, the effectiveness of ozone in killing bacteria in a biofilm is significantly diminished.

Ozonated water should not be used for the manufacturing of product formulations due to its reactivity with product ingredients. UV radiation at a wavelength of 254–265 nanometers can be used to remove ozone from water, but the UV radiation intensity of 100,000 μW-sec/cm^2 must ensure the complete destruction of ozone because ozone might be converted to oxygen and hydroxyl free radicals (52,54). It should be noted that UV light used for performing water disinfection has a light intensity of only between 30,000 and 35,000 μW-sec/cm^2, not sufficient to inactivate the presence of ozone in water. To inactivate ozone in process water before usage in manufacturing, UV lights will need to be installed at either the point-of-use or after the storage tank where ozone is injected. UV lights for the destruction of ozone should never be installed immediately after the ozone generator. There is a potential issue in using ozone as a microbial control method because it can be irritating to the eyes, nose and throat, and when inhaled it could cause damage to the lungs. Because of theses safety issues, ambient ozone monitors are recommended for use in the manufacturing facility for detecting the presence of ozone gas leakage in the environment. To maintain the effectiveness of ozone destruction, the UV light should be replaced approximately every 6 months (41). Re-circulated ozonated water should go directly back into the water storage tank of the distribution loop. Ozonated water should never be re-circulated back to ion exchange resin beds and most membrane filters in the generation portion of a process water system due to its incompatibility. If ozonated water is re-circulated back to these units, it must first be de-ozonated with UV light that is upstream of these units.

If ozone is being used, ozonated water tanks must be de-rouged every 2–3 years due to the highly oxidative environment that ozone creates. In addition, it is recommended that the 316L stainless steel distribution loop piping is rouged at least on an annual basis. If the distribution loop piping is not derouged on an annual basis, the usage of an ongoing "side stream" monitoring program should be established to determine the degree of rouging (41). A typical location for determining the degree of rouging is the first elbow/tee downstream of the purified water distribution pump. As a minimum, de-rouging and re-passivation should be considered every 2 years.

Equipment

Sanitary Design Considerations

Manufacturing equipment sanitary design considerations and construction elements are described by the food industry and regulatory authorities (55–60). The following are essential sanitary design principles:

- Equipment should be constructed to ensure effective/efficient cleaning and to prevent microorganisms ingress, survival and proliferation on both product and non-product equipment contact surfaces.
- Materials used for the construction of equipment must be composed of inert materials such as 316L stainless steel or polypropylene that are not reactive, additive or absorptive of the product, cleaning agents and sanitizers.
- 316L stainless steel surfaces with a 140 grit or better finish must be passivated to minimize the possibility of the stainless steel from reacting with the product. If plastics or polymers are used, care must to be taken to ensure that the product does not leach materials. All product equipment contact surfaces will need to be free of sharp corners and crevices that can harbor product residues and microorganisms.
- All parts of the equipment should be readily accessible for inspection, maintenance, cleaning and sanitization without the use of tools.
- Equipment should be self-draining to ensure that liquid does not accumulate, pool or condense that can harbor or promote the growth of microorganisms.
- Hollow areas of equipment such as frames and rollers must be eliminated wherever possible or permanently sealed. Items such as bolts, studs, mounting plates, brackets, junction boxes, nameplates, end caps, sleeves and other items must be continuously welded to the surfaces and not attached via drilled and taped holes.
- To prevent harborage of product residues and microorganisms, equipment parts should be free of niches such as pits, cracks, corrosion, recesses, open seams, gaps, lap seams, protruding ledges, inside threads, bolt rivets and dead ends. Welds and joints should be ground and polished smooth. For stainless steel, sanitary welding techniques such as orbital or gas tungsten arc welding is recommended. For plastic pipes, chemically welded joints should be smooth.
- Maintenance enclosures and human machine interfaces such as push buttons, valve handles, switches and touchscreens must be designed to ensure that product residues or water does not penetrate or accumulate in and on the enclosure or interface.
- If equipment requires additional sub-systems such as drainage or automated cleaning systems, it should not create a sanitary design risk by causing the creation of soils or causing improper operational conditions.
- To allow for easy cleaning under and around equipment, placement of machinery should be at least 4 inches from walls. Floor-mounted equipment should be at least 6 inches from the floor (60). Table-mounted equipment should be sealed to a table or be no less than 4 inches from the counter top (61).

Types of Equipment

Processing Tanks/Vessels/Mixers

Processing tanks/vessels/mixers are used to compounding product formulations and should be designed and constructed to allow easy cleaning (58). The following items require attention: vent filter, hygienic pressure relief valve, inlet piping, domed top, curved sides, mixing blade and shaft, conical bottom and hygienic base valve (9).

To prevent the ingress of airborne microorganisms and dust, a vent filter on top of a processing tank/vessel/mixer should be fitted to allow the entry and exit of air from the interior during compounding. This vent should have a sterile 0.22-micron filter cartridge and should be checked regularly. If it becomes wet during processing, it needs to be changed. To prevent over-pressurization of a sealed processing vessel or tank, a hygienic pressure relief valve or bursting disc will need to be used. During compounding in processing tank/vessel/mixer equipment, liquid raw ingredients should be added by using an angled inlet pipe to prevent excessive foaming and splashing. Openings to processing tanks/vessels/mixers should be lipped and covered with a shoe box type design to divert the potential contamination away from the top when product compounding takes place (60). Top rims of the equipment should be constructed and fabricated in such a way that they avoid the collection of water droplets or dust. To prevent the build-up of water condensation (which can be a source for the growth of microorganisms) and product residues (which can serve as a source of microbial nutrients), the top of the processing tank/vessel/mixer must be domed. This will allow drainage of the water condensation and easy cleaning of product residues from this area. The sides of the processing tank/vessel/ mixer also need to be curved to ensure ease of cleaning for removing product residues. The mixing blade and shaft need to be a welded or single piece that consists of a smooth finish and the absence of joints in order to provide an easier surface for cleaning and to eliminate areas where product could become entrapped to provide harborage for microorganisms and nutrients for microbial proliferation. To ensure proper drainage, the bottom of the processing tank/vessel/mixer should be conical in shape so that finished bulk product material will not collect at the bottom or water will not become stagnant in which microorganisms could proliferate. At the bottom of the processing tank/vessel/mixer, a sanitary valve should be present to ensure easy cleaning and eliminate the possibility of product residues being retained. Clean-in-place (CIP) systems are usually installed in processing tanks/vessels/mixers for the removal of product residues that are not easily accessible by performing manual cleaning.

Valves

Manufacturing equipment should include sanitary valves to avoid the presence of non-sanitary cavities. Diaphragm and butterfly valves are recommended. Diaphragm valves can be easily cleaned-in-place. Butterfly valves do not retain water and finished product after cleaning. Furthermore, butterfly valves can be taken apart for cleaning but can also be cleaned-in-place. Ball valves are not sanitary because they have non-sanitary cavities or dead spaces where water and/or finished product can be retained after cleaning and a microbial biofilm could develop.

Pumps

Pumps are used to move liquids of various viscosities from one location to another in a facility, to homogenize, and to re-circulate product (58). The following sanitary design and fabrication considerations are required to prevent microbial contamination: easy accessibility and complete disassembly for cleaning and sanitization, vertical inlet and outlet for the drainage of finished product from the interior portions, bypasses and pressure relief valves designed to prevent water or product retention. The following pumps are of a sanitary design: diaphragm and peristaltic or lobe pumps (61). Centrifugal, gear and mono pumps are non-sanitary due to the possible retention of finished product after cleaning. These have been implicated in numerous microbial contamination issues of finished products (9). It should be noted that centrifugal pumps are commonly used in process water systems for moving water.

Different types of materials are used in the pump construction. Because of wear, pump bearings and shaft seals should be periodically disassembled and inspected for evidence of lubricant leakage or product retention. The integrity of gaskets and impellers in pumps should also be inspected.

Storage Vessels

Fixed and portable storage tanks are used to store bulk finished product after compounding in a processing vessel/tank/mixer and are connected directly to a filling line to fill finished product packages. Many of the sanitary design principles that are followed for fabricating processing vessel/tank/mixers are also followed for fabricating fixed and portable storage tanks. Portable storage vessels usually do not have a dome top because these units are small enough to allow for easy access of the interior ceiling for cleaning and sanitization. All storage tanks should have close-fitting lids or be totally sealed with the only access possible via a manway (62). In large fixed storage tanks, side entry manways should be avoided as they require the use of gaskets that may contact bulk finished product.

The use of plastic intermediate bulk container (IBC) or other types of plastic containers for storing bulk finished product is an unsanitary practice. The container exit point is usually 1 or 2 inches (e.g., 2.54–5.08 centimeters) above the flat bottom of the container. This location makes it impossible to completely remove product residues and water due to improper drainage. Remnant water can become stagnant and allow microbial proliferation. If intermediate bulk containers are used, they be lined with a plastic form fitting disposable liner. These plastic form-fitting disposable liners are cube-shaped with a bottom discharge valve. Bulk finished product is filled into the liner through a top opening. The disposable liner and valves can be removed from the intermediate bulk container after usage and disposed. The intermediate bulk containers do not have to be cleaned and sanitized.

Filters, Strainers and Sieves

Filters, strainers and sieves are used with raw ingredients and bulk finished product to achieve desired particle size, break up agglomerates, eliminate foreign materials and remove excess material in suspension (58). The material of construction for these items can be either 316L stainless steel or non-reactive fabrics. Filtration media (e.g., screens, bags, cartridges and filter aids) will need to be selected and evaluated for the ease of cleaning.

Transport Piping

Transport piping is used to move bulk finished product from one location to another in a manufacturing facility. Transport piping systems will consist of the following parts: pumps, filters, fittings (e.g., elbows, Ts, reducers), valves and educators (58). Transport pipes should be of 316L stainless steel and include sanitary fittings. Other materials used in transfer piping have been shown to have the potential for microbial biofilm build-up and are difficult to clean. Transport piping should be seamless and continuously welded wherever possible in order to reduce the number of sanitary connections (9). The length of the pipe runs should be minimized to facilitate cleaning and sloped to be self-draining (e.g., $>/=1\%$). Sagging of transport piping prevents effective cleaning and sanitization and offers areas for product build-up. To prevent sagging, the piping must be supported along its entire length. In addition, there should be a minimal number of T fittings in the line. Transport pipelines also need to be designed to avoid dead legs, right angles and vertical bends because they can become microbial contamination reservoirs. When stainless steel pipes are joined together, sanitary welding techniques such as tungsten inert gas (TIG) orbital welding should be used to avoid the creation of difficult-to-clean crevices and rough surfaces where microorganisms and bulk finished product can accumulate. In-line filters should be designed for easy cleaning, sanitization and inspection. If an in-line filter is not cleaned routinely, it can become a source of microbial contamination. When valves are used to control the flow from the main piping into a secondary pipeline, they should be seated as close as possible to the entry point to prevent dead spots (58). All fixed piping and valves should be clearly identified as to their contents and the direction of flow. Often, a color coding system is used to differentiate pipelines from one another in order to prevent mix-ups during production.

Piping Joints

The following piping joint types should be avoided in order to prevent microbial contamination issues: taped and threat, socket and flanged joints (9). Threading of threaded joints and misaligned pipe sections of a flanged joints provide areas difficult to clean for product accumulation. To prevent product accumulation, sanitary fittings such as tri-clamp or a dairy joints should be used. Tri-clamp joints use a sealing ring in brining two pipe sections together with a joint clamp. In a dairy joint, a sealing "O" ring or gasket is used to connect two pipes with one end of the pipe having an external thread and the other an external sealing ring to tighten together.

Gaskets

Gaskets are used to establish mechanical seal which fills the space in piping connections. Gasket sanitary design considerations require construction with materials of inert chemical composition compatible with cleaners, sanitizers and product formulations that do not react with or absorb product preservatives. It is well known that plasticizers can leach from certain types of PVC and inactivate phenolic preservatives, while low to medium density polyethylene can be permeable to oil-soluble preservatives such as parabens. Polyurethane can reduce the antimicrobial activity of phenolic and quaternary ammonium preservatives (63). Benzyl alcohol is known to interact with polyethylene and polystyrene (64). Benzalkonium chloride and benzethonium chloride can be absorbed by polyethylene, polypropylene, polystyrene and PVC (65). Parabens can be absorbed into rubber. In addition, parabens and phenols can be absorbed into nylon and plasticized PVC (66). Teflon™ (polytetrafluoroethylene) and Viton™ (synthetic rubber and fluoro-polymer elastomer) are acceptable materials for gasket composition (62). Gaskets should be non-porous in order to prevent the entry of microorganisms into pores and holes. When using gaskets, it is important to establish a proper seal during the installation to prevent the accumulation of bulk finished product in the connection.

Hoses

Hoses are used to transfer bulk finished product or process water from one location to another in a facility. They are favored due to flexibility and convenience. There are several hose sanitary design considerations: they should be composed of material that is compatible with finished product and can be used with cleaners and sanitizers. Common materials for hose construction are reinforced food grade rubber or Neoprene, TYGON® or reinforced TYGON®, polyethylene or polypropylene and nylon (58). Hoses should have sanitary fittings at each of the ends and be as short as possible. After cleaning and sanitization, hoses should be hung to drain and dry when not in use. After drying, ends of the hose should be either covered or capped in order to prevent the introduction of dust and dirt.

Filling Equipment

Filling equipment can be double or multi-nozzle, in-line or rotary head, and there are some common sanitary design considerations in each of these variations. All filling equipment should be designed in such a way that they are easy to clean and sanitize. The equipment should also be designed for fast and easy dismantling. If a clean-in-place (CIP) system is not part of the filling equipment, product hoses from the hopper and filling nozzles will need to be dismantled for cleaning and sanitization. The use of drip pans and water lubricated belts should be avoided. If compressed air is used on a filling line, microbial air filters and airline dryers should be installed in order to prevent airline condensates from contaminating finished product during the filling operation. To receive bulk finished product from a transport pipeline, filling line hoppers should be conically shaped to allow for proper drainage of product to and avoid water retention after cleaning and sanitization. Conveyors, turntables or other areas, where open product package containers are exposed to the manufacturing facility air, should be fully enclosed to prevent entry of airborne dust. After cleaning and sanitization, filling line hoppers should be covered to prevent the introduction of microbial contamination during storage.

Gauges and Meters

Equipment gauges and meters are used to measure and/or record temperature, pressure, flow, pH, viscosity, speed and volume of bulk finished product, intermediates or raw ingredients. Gauges and meters are generally not disassembled for cleaning but installed in equipment to accomplish easy cleaning. To accomplish this, design considerations include a means for minimizing product contact with the working parts of the instrument and for preventing build-up of product residues and diluted cleaning solutions. These can cause malfunction and the possibility of microbial growth within the instrument. Furthermore, it is important to ensure that the connections of gauges and meters to manufacturing equipment do not create dead ends or areas where bulk finished product can accumulate and not be accessible to cleaning and sanitizing solutions. Gauge and meter connections should be close coupled (e.g., gauge and meter connections to manufacturing equipment should not be more than the length of one pipe diameter) (60).

Cleaning and Sanitization

Cleaning and sanitization of manufacturing equipment is an extremely important preventive measure to ensure the microbiological quality and safety of non-sterile finished product formulations. Equipment should be cleaned and sanitized before they are used in the manufacturing of finished products. Depending on the product formulation (e.g., colognes, perfumes, lipsticks, lip balms, nail enamels) equipment may need to be cleaned, but not sanitized because the risk of being microbiologically contaminated is low (67).

Cleaning

Cleaning is the process of physically and/or chemically removing dirt, dust, grease, product residue or other contaminants from equipment surfaces (68). A cleaning procedure reduces the possibility of product-to-product contamination. Without performing proper equipment cleaning, sanitization (i.e., reducing the microbial bioburden to an acceptable level) is almost impossible to achieve. Water quality (pH, conductivity, water hardness and total organic carbon (TOC)) is also an important factor for cleaning the equipment. Water pH may affect the cleaning ability of some cleaners. If water has a high conductivity level, there is the possibility of introducing chemical contaminants to surfaces. If an alkaline cleaning agent is used, water hardness ions may precipitate out as calcium carbonate observed as a white residue. If the TOC in water is not controlled, organic residues can cause contamination of equipment surfaces.

Considerations for Cleaning

A cleaning procedure needs to be designed and developed for each piece of equipment. The following parameters will need to be determined prior to cleaning procedure implementation: operational parameters, factors affecting cleaning and relevant equipment specifics.

The following operational parameters will need to be specified in each cleaning procedure: contact time for cleaning agent, action of the cleaning agent, cleaning agent concentration and temperature of the cleaning agent. These operational parameters are referred to as TACT (Time, Action, Concentration and Temperature) and are interrelated and will have a direct relationship to the success of each of the cleaning cycle phases for a piece of equipment:

- *Time* is defined as the length of time for each cleaning procedure step.
- *Action* is the mechanism used to deliver the cleaning agent. These action mechanisms can be characterized as soak, scrubbing, impingement or turbulent flow. For example, agitation often enhances the chemical actions of cleaning agents and helps to increase the effectiveness of the cleaning process, for example, by shortening the required contact time. Manual cleaning typically includes soaking or scrubbing as the action mechanism to achieve cleaning. Automated cleaning cycles typically employ the use of impingement and/or turbulence as the mechanism of cleaning. In automated cleaning cycles, spray devices such as spray balls are used that have a minimum and maximum flow rate requirements, and piping should be flushed at a velocity that is more than sufficient to assure adequate coverage of equipment surfaces and turbulence.
- *Concentration* of a cleaning agent must be specified in cleaning Standard Operating Procedures (SOPs). Cleaning agent selection for a piece of equipment should be based on the consideration of soil types, ease of removal and the need for chelating agents. Chemical cleaning agents are usually

supplied by vendors in a concentrated form or need to be diluted by using deionized water. A low concentration of a cleaning agent may result in the failure of removing the soil from equipment surfaces whereas a high concentration may result in the difficulty of removing cleaning agent residues from equipment surfaces and may require excessive rinsing. To remove cleaning agent residues from equipment surfaces, rinsing with potable or drinking water is permissible, but the usage of a final rinse with deionized water may be necessary in order to prevent interference of potable water residues with the antimicrobial activity of chemical sanitizers. For automated cleaning procedures, the easiest means of verifying the removal of highly alkaline (e.g., ammonium hydroxide, sodium phosphate, etc.) or acidic (e.g., hydrochloric acid, acetic acid, citric acid) aqueous cleaning agents is by performing a conductivity test on a collected final deionized water rinse sample. However, it should be noted that conductivity measurements cannot be performed on a collected potable or drinking water rinse sample due to the presence of chlorine. If alkaline/acidic cleaning agents or chemical detergents with surfactants are used, TOC analysis of the rinse water must be used to verify their removal from equipment surfaces before sanitizing.

- Optimal *temperature* differs depending on the stage of the cleaning process. Initial solvent rinses are typically performed at ambient temperatures to minimize the effects of degradation of the cleaning solution and to maximize the dilution effects. Cleaning solutions may be heated to increase their effectiveness. A final rinse with deionized water may be performed at high temperatures (e.g., >80.0°C) to increase the solubility of any remaining residues and to increase the drying rate after rinsing.

Product characteristics and condition can affect cleaning processes and must be known before designing an equipment cleaning procedure. For example, is the condition of a product residue wet or dry? A wet product residue on an equipment surface may be easier to remove by using a water rinse than a dry product residue. The chemical composition of a product formulation will affect water solubility and the difficulty of residue removal from equipment surfaces. If the product residues on an equipment surface are difficult to remove, the equipment cannot be cleaned adequately and contaminating product residue will be introduced into the next product formulation that is manufactured.

In designing an equipment cleaning protocol, the following equipment specifics must incorporated: automated cleaning pathways, the sequence of manual or automated cleaning steps and flow rate during each of the steps.

Equipment Surface Considerations

The surface of equipment is an important consideration when developing an equipment cleaning procedure. An improper equipment surface finish may prevent the removal of soil. Rough surfaces enable easier soil contact and their cracks and crevices may prove difficult for a cleaning agent to penetrate for soil removal. For process, transfer and storage equipment, 316L stainless steel with 140 grit or a type 2B finish is recommended for the proper removal of soil from the surface.

Application Cleaning Methods

There are four basic application cleaning methods that are in use today: spraying, soaking, mopping and wiping (69). Spraying is used to remove soils from equipment surfaces, and this can also be used to wet surfaces. The cleaning action for spraying equipment surfaces is enhanced by using detergents. Soaking involves the immersion of utensils or small equipment parts into tubs or tanks containing a detergent solution. A mopping system is used to remove residues from walls and floors. For walls, mopping is done from the highest surface point to the lowest surface point. For floors, mopping is done from the cleanest to the dirtiest area. To clean a surface by performing mopping, the surface needs to be wetted. However, mopping by itself does not provide adequate wetting like spraying because the wringing of mop heads and the inability for mop heads to hold a sufficient amount of liquid will compromise the level of surface wetting. Wiping is performed by using a pre-saturated cloth or a dry wipe that is wetted with a cleaning agent to clean surfaces. Wiping is usually performed on smaller surfaces that need cleaning such as door handles and small pieces of equipment.

Types of Cleaning Equipment Procedures

There are several types of cleaning procedures for equipment including clean-in-place (CIP), clean-out-of-place (COP), manual and semiautomatic. CIP systems consist of various tanks and piping for delivering a cleaning solution. There may be a pre-rinse and final rinse tank. Sprayballs are used in CIP systems and these can be stationary or moving (e.g., rotating, oscillating) to provide coverage for the physical impingement of a cleaning solution onto equipment surfaces. CIP systems are automated and are found in processing vessels, storage tanks and some filling lines. A CIP procedure typically does not involve personnel intervention (except to select a cycle and to start/stop the operation) and are usually programmable (i.e., use various types of cleaning cycles). When designing a CIP procedure, the following parameters must be considered: volume of cleaning agents, volume of rinse water, flow rates, temperature of wash and rinse solutions, duration of wash and rinse cycles, pressure of solution, operating ranges and detergent concentration.

A COP procedure is primarily for smaller equipment components and portable process equipment typically disassembled due to the difficulty of cleaning as installed. The disassembled parts are transported to a designated cleaning or wash area where the cleaning procedure is performed using either manual or automated methods. Manual or physical procedure for cleaning involves scrubbing, scraping or spraying to remove product residues from equipment surfaces. A semi-automated cleaning procedure uses both manual and automated cleaning steps by combining the sprayballs and manual cleaning methods. Examples of a semi-automated procedure includes the removal of gaskets/fittings for manual cleaning prior to the CIP of a tank and disassembly of a pump or filter housing prior to cleaning in an automated COP system.

Cleaning Equipment and Systems

Low pressure systems are suitable for removing gross or loosely adhered product residues and for rinsing away cleaning solutions. A high pressure system is very efficient for removing adhered residues from equipment surfaces. Low and high pressure systems will often use chemical additives to help in soil removal.

Steam generators can be used to deliver high velocity steam or sprays with or without chemical additives. They are effective in removing product residues, films, oils, and fats from equipment surfaces, but steam can be very hazardous to personnel.

Foam generators can provide a stream of chemical foam at ambient temperature under air pressure of about 100–400 psi. Foam provides a longer contact time between a cleaning agent and soil. By using a generator, it reduces the amount of cleaning solution that is required to clean a surface. Foam application prevents splashing of cleaning solutions where irritating fogs and vapors can form. In addition, foam can be used to clean the undersides and other hard-to-reach equipment surfaces.

Compressed air can be used to blow away powder product residues, remove excess cleaning solutions and dry equipment surfaces or components.

Wet vacuum systems are used to remove excess or pooled cleaning solutions and water from equipment, floors and other surfaces. Dry vacuum systems are necessary in those production areas where dry raw ingredients are used or where powder product formulations are manufactured. Dry vacuum systems are used to remove dry residues, powders and soils and are required in those situations in which wet methods cannot be used.

Re-circulation wash tank systems consist of an immersion tank in which jets are used to re-circulate a cleaning solution at an elevated temperature across and through the tank for small immersed pieces of equipment. These combine a cleaning agent, hot water and the physical sheer force of circulation remove soil.

Automatic washer includes a cabinet or tunnel washer that can pre-rinse, wash, rinse, sanitize and cool items and dry items.

For transfer pipelines, pigging systems are used to clean the piping of product residues. Pipeline pigs are devices made of a non-porous material for the recovery of bulk finished product and to clean product pipelines (68). To clean, a pipeline pig is placed into the pig launcher and water is used to push the pig and any finished product bulk out of the transfer piping until the pig enters into the piping system's receiving station. From the receiving station, the pipeline pig is transferred into the receiving end pig launcher and compressed air is used to push the pig back through the pipeline for the removal of any remaining water. Thorough cleaning and sanitization of the pigging system and the pig must be ensured. When not in use, pigs must be handled and stored under sanitary and dry conditions.

Manual or special cleaning of equipment and its parts may require special types of cleaning devices and supplies including scrappers, non-metallic abrasive pads, squeegees, soft or stiff bristle brushes, brooms, wiping, cloths, buckets, sinks, pallets, ladders and stools. Steel wool and metal scouring pads can shed metal particles that can become incorporated into the product. Wire brushes, steel wool and metal scoring pads should never be used on production equipment due to their possibility of causing scratches to the equipment, especially on the surfaces that come into contact with bulk finished product. Barely visible minute equipment scratches can constitute a perfect place for microbial proliferation.

Selection of Cleaning Agents

The choice of a cleaning agent for pieces of manufacturing equipment should be based on the knowledge and understanding of the surface to be cleaned (e.g., metal, glass, plastic, etc.), the soil types (e.g., organic, inorganic, oils, heavy soils, light soils, etc.), the intended cleaning method (e.g., manual, soaking, CIP, power spray wand, etc.) and the level of cleanliness (acceptance criteria) required.

In general practice, one of the following cleaning agents should be used: hot water, steam, potable water, organic solvents, alkaline cleaners, acid cleaners and detergents. Hot water can be used as the sole cleaning agent for water soluble residues. However, depending on product types, equipment and other related factors such as water solubility of product residues and safety for those associated with the use of steam, the use of hot water or steam may not be appropriate. Steam usage may "bake on" soil rather than remove it. The final water rinse of the cleaning process should be deionized water. Potable or drinking water can also be used to rinse product residues from equipment surfaces. If hard potable water is used, alkaline cleansers may react with the water hardness ions (e.g., calcium ions) and may precipitate out as calcium carbonate to form a white residue on the equipment surface. If a hard potable water rinse is used, the equipment surfaces must be rinsed with deionized water before using an alkaline cleanser.

Organic solvents such as isopropyl or ethyl alcohol can be used for cleaning, but the issue of alcohol vapor flammability must be addressed.

Alkaline cleansers such as sodium hydroxide, ammonium hydroxide, potassium hydroxide or borax solutions are used as an alkaline wash to remove soils such as oils, fats, grease particulates and films (68). The alkalinity of sodium hydroxide solutions may enhance the solubility of organic process residues and in some cases facilitate hydrolysis, but it can also facilitate the precipitation of salts or oxides of such ions as calcium, magnesium and iron if these ions are present during the cleaning process.

Acid cleaners (e.g., hydrochloric acid, sulfuric acid, phosphoric acid, acetic acid, citric acid) may be used for the removal of soils and inorganic salts and soluble metal complexes such as metal oxides (68). To broaden the spectrum of equipment soils to be removed, the addition of an acid washing step in the cleaning procedure after a caustic wash/rinse may overcome precipitation and build-up of inorganic compounds and improve rinsing.

Formulated detergents are multi-component cleaning agents that take advantage of several different cleaning mechanisms and provide a broad spectrum of effectiveness. A formulated alkaline detergent might prove effective for improved wetting and soil penetration, emulsification and chelation of calcium, iron oxide or other inorganic ions and may facilitate the dispersion of particulates. Detergents used in cleaning procedures can be amphoteric, cationic or nonionic. Depending upon the pH, amphoteric surfactants may be either anionic or cationic and they are very compatible with builders, acids and alkalis that are used in detergents. However, anionic surfactants are highly sudsing, and excess foaming is undesirable for surface cleaning. Furthermore, excess foam leaves a residue that produces a tacky surface which will cause a likely re-soiling problem. Cationic surfactants are not typically used alone as cleaning agents. Non-ionic surfactants in detergents are particularly effective for removing oily soil residues and many are low sudsing.

The final step in any cleaning procedure is to rinse the equipment with deionized water to remove any residues of the cleaning agent from the equipment surface.

Validation of Cleaning Procedures

Equipment cleaning procedures should be validated for the removal of product residues or cleaning agents, but there are several challenges in developing a manufacturing cleaning validation program. These include use of non-dedicated manufacturing equipment, Over-The-Counter (OTC) drug product formulations based upon FDA OTC monographs versus non-OTC product formulations and the number of different product formulations produced in a facility.

To overcome these challenges, a risk-based approach has to be taken. A matrix should be developed by which   product formulations are grouped together into different product categories based on product composition and types of manufacturing equipment (70,71). Examples of grouping criteria for different product formulation can range from what actives are being used in OTC drug product formulations, the main ingredient in a non-OTC drug product formulation besides water, whether the formulation is an oil-in-water or water-in-oil emulsion. Also, different equipment types can be classified based, for example, on their processing, filling and storage, whether similar cleaning procedures are used between each piece in an equipment group, and whether the equipment in a group is similar but not 100% identical in design and construction. After group formation, a risk-based matrix is constructed by equipment group versus product group in order to minimize testing and to determine which group is the worst case for cleaning.

Cleaning Acceptance Criteria

To validate the removal of product residues or cleaning agents, visual or chemical analytical methods can be used and determine cleaning acceptance criteria for manufacturing equipment. To develop a visual cleaning acceptance criterion, a visual limit for the presence of product residues must be established under specific viewing conditions by adding solutions of the residue at different concentrations (e.g., micrograms ($\mu g/cm^3$) to equipment surface material coupons and have a panel of trained observers determine the lowest observable level of the product residue that can be detected visually. However, it should be recognized that this lowest observable level specification depends on factors such as the nature of the residue and equipment surface, lighting, viewing distance, viewing angle, the visual acuity of the observer and the subjectivity of the observer.

To determine the cleanliness of an equipment surface, there are two chemical analytical methods: specific and non-specific. A specific analytical test method involves the measurement of the concentration that is present on an equipment surface such as the drug active ingredient from an OTC drug product formulation, intermediates or degradation products of drug active ingredient, any preservative used in the product formulation or cleaning agent. The sampling method could involve collecting a rinse water sample or swabbing a surface of equipment to detect the presence of an active ingredient, preservative or cleaning agent. Rinse water sampling involves taking a sample of the final deionized water rinse. Swabbing involves using either a wipe or a swab that is moistened with deionized water and then sampling a defined surface area (e.g., 10 cm × 10 cm). For specific analytical test methods, High Performance Liquid Chromatography (HPLC), ion selective electrodes, flame photometry, derivative UV spectrometry and Thin Layer Chromatography can be used (71).

Non-specific test methods for determining the cleanliness of a surface involve conductivity or TOC analysis. By collecting a rinse water sample after cleaning, conductivity can be carried out if deionized water is used as the final equipment rinse. If the final equipment rinse is potable water, the presence of chlorine and salts in potable water will give a false conductivity reading indicating that the equipment is not cleaned. The conductivity of the deionized rinse water should be no more than twice the conductivity reading of the deionized water that had been used for rinsing. TOC analysis is an alternative to conductivity as a non-specific test method for determining the cleanliness of an equipment surface. TOC analysis can be used to detect the presence of any residue (e.g., ingredients and cleaning agents) remaining on equipment surfaces which contains carbon. Sampling for the presence of TOC can be done by direct surface sampling (e.g., swab) or indirect surface sampling (e.g., rinse water). If swabs are used to take direct TOC equipment samples, it should be noted that very clean swabs or wipes are required for taking the sample to prevent a false positive TOC reading. If a rinse water sample is going to be collected, deionized water should be used.

Cleaning Operator Training

Operator training for cleaning is critical in maintaining the microbial quality of non-sterile finished products. Operators should be trained on the requirements of equipment cleaning SOPs. Only trained associates should be assigned cleaning responsibilities. Proper training consists of understanding relevant SOPs, demonstration of the correct procedure by a trained operator and successful demonstration of the correct procedure by the trainee. All training must be documented.

Sanitization

Sanitization is a process carried out to reduce the number and type of viable microbial contaminants on a physically-clean surface to acceptable or insignificant numerical levels (68). Rough surfaces, bad welds and other equipment defects are difficult to sanitize. Water quality with its pH, hardness and microbial bioburden is also an important factor in performing sanitization of facility and equipment surfaces. For example, pH of the water and water hardness may have an adverse effect on the antimicrobial activity of chemical sanitizers. If the microbial quality of the water is not controlled, it may serve as a source of microbial bioburden on facility and equipment surfaces. All cleaning agents must be thoroughly rinsed from equipment surfaces by using deionized water prior to the use of a chemical sanitizer because some cleaning agents are not compatible with some chemical sanitizers. For example, residues of an anionic cleanser may react with a chemical sanitizer containing a cationic surfactant, and the antimicrobial activity of the sanitizer is inactivated.

Sanitization of equipment can be accomplished by soaking utensils and small equipment parts in tubs of sanitizer or by spraying or fogging of sanitizer over large surface areas. Fogging involves the generation of a chemical sanitizer mist to cover large areas of equipment surfaces, but it can be used only with closed equipment systems. In addition, fogging of chemical sanitizers should be done using only those chemical sanitizers for which the manufacturer had provided label instructions on how to perform a fogging sanitization procedure for their material.

Types of Chemical Sanitizers

Common types of chemical sanitizers are as follows: acid anionics, alcohols, chlorine, glutaraldehyde, hydrogen peroxide, peroxy-hydrogen peroxide, phenolic compounds and quaternary ammonium compounds.

Acid anionics are anionic surfactants or acids that have antimicrobial activity with a typical use concentration of 100 ppm. The advantage of using this is that they are stable, non-corrosive, non-staining, have a low odor, their antimicrobial activity is not affected by hard water and are able to remove and prevent the formation of mineral films. The disadvantage as a sanitizer is that they are pH sensitive, have poor antimicrobial activity against yeast and mold and are high foaming.

Ethyl and isopropyl alcohol solutions are bactericidal and fungicidal but not active against spores (72). In general, isopropyl alcohol is considered to be slightly more efficacious against bacteria (73). A 60–70% ethyl or isopropyl alcohol concentration can be used as a sanitizer, but it is limited because of flammability risks. The contact time for a 60–70% ethyl or isopropyl alcohol solution as a sanitizer is 15 minutes. The advantage of using alcohol as a sanitizer is that no equipment rinsing is required due to its evaporation from equipment surfaces. It can also be used to dry small pieces of manufacturing equipment and is often used for manufacturing equipment that is involved in making liquid anhydrous product formulations. The disadvantage of alcohol is that it is not sporicidal and flammable vapors might form if used in large amounts. Because of their lipid solvency and low surface action, many alcohols can also be used as cleaning agents besides as a sanitizer (72).

Chlorine can be used a sanitizer with sodium and calcium hypochlorite. Sodium and calcium hypochlorite ionize in water and produce Na^+ or Ca^+ ions and the hypochlorite ion OCL^-, and an equilibrium is established with HOCL (74). Between a pH of 4.0 and 7.0, chlorine will exist predominantly as hypochlorous acid which is the active moiety of chlorine (75). Care must be taken to limit acidity as chlorine gas can be evolved if the pH falls too low. Chlorine is bactericidal, fungicidal and sporicidal (76,77). To use chlorine as a sanitizer, a concentration of greater than 100 ppm with a 30-minute contact will need to be ensured (78). The advantages of chlorine is that it has excellent antimicrobial activity, can be used in cold water and it is easy to verify the removal of its residues from equipment surfaces. The disadvantages of chlorine are that it has an odor, is less sensitive as a sanitizer as the pH increases and the hypochlorite ion predominates, sensitive to light exposure and temperature increases, its antimicrobial activity is inactivated by organics and it may react with metal surfaces by pitting stainless steel surfaces.

Glutaraldehyde is a dialdehyde that has bactericidal, fungicidal and sporicidal activity (75,79). An activated 2% alkaline glutaraldehyde solution is used as a disinfectant. The advantages are that it has a broad spectrum of antimicrobial activity, is active in the presence of organic matter and is noncorrosive toward metals and rubber. The disadvantages are that it is sensitive to acidic pHs and alkaline solutions of glutaraldehyde have poor stability in maintaining the antimicrobial activity for storage periods greater than 2 weeks (80,81). Furthermore, glutaraldehyde can cause sensitivity reactions on unprotected skin and its vapors are an inhalation irritant. The following types of personnel protective equipment are recommended if glutaraldehyde is used: nitrile or butyl rubber gloves, safety goggles, disposable water-proof aprons and charcoal-impregnated face masks.

Hydrogen peroxide also can be used as a sanitizer because it has bactericidal, fungicidal and sporicidal activity and can be purchased as a 35% stable solution, though it is not widely used (82). Hydrogen peroxide use concentration and contact time is between 1% and 35% and 30 minutes. The disadvantage is that it is highly reactive and is less stable in the presence of light.

Peroxy-hydrogen peroxide compounds such as peroxyacetic acid and peracetic acid can be used as sanitizers. Peracetic acid is a mixture of acetic acid and hydrogen peroxide. When dissolved in water, peracetic acid disintegrates into hydrogen peroxide and acetic acid which will eventually degrade into water, oxygen and carbon dioxide. Peracetic acid is considered to be a more potent sanitizer than hydrogen peroxide (75). The advantages of using peroxy-hydrogen peroxide compounds are that they have bactericidal, fungicidal and sporicidal activity, are non-corrosive to stainless steel and aluminum, are tolerant to organic soil and break down into acetic acid and water. The disadvantages are that they are corrosive to soft metals (iron, copper, zinc, brass, galvanized steel, etc.), have a pungent odor and their antimicrobial activity will vary against different fungal species.

Phenolic compounds such as phenyl and/or chlorinated phenols can be used alone as a sanitizer, but are more frequently used together with anionic detergents to produce disinfectant-detergents that have bactericidal and fungicidal activity, but are considered to be low-to-intermediate-level disinfectants (83). The use concentration and contact time for phenolic sanitizers is 1:200 dilution for 10 minutes. The advantages are that they are able to clean, deodorize and have a broad spectrum of antimicrobial activity. The disadvantages are that they must be formulated, rinsing of equipment surfaces is required to remove residues, use solution may become unstable within 2–3 hours after preparation, organic matter reduces antimicrobial activity and alkaline pHs will inactivate antimicrobial activity. However, *Pseudomonas* species are known to be somewhat resistant to the antimicrobial activity of phenolic compounds (84).

Quaternary ammonium compounds consist of cationic surfactants. They are most frequently used in combination with a nonionic detergent as a disinfectant-detergent or detergent-sanitizer. However, nonionic detergents usually do not clean as good as the more caustic cationic detergents. Quaternary ammonium compounds are more bactericidal against non-spore-forming Gram-positive bacteria, less active against Gram-negative bacteria and are not sporicidal, but are sporostatic (inhibitory to spore germination or outgrowth) (76,85,86) The typical use concentration for a quaternary ammonium compound sanitizer is 200 ppm. The advantages are that they can clean and deodorize at the same time, are most effective at neutral or slightly alkaline pHs, are odorless and are very stable. The disadvantages are that they are not sporicidal, their antimicrobial activity can be inactivated by anionic cleaners, use of hard water for preparing use concentrations will adversely affect the antimicrobial activity, rinsing is required to remove equipment surface residues and are less effective against pseudomonads (87,88).

Types of Physical Sanitizers

Heat is the most efficient physical sanitizer. The most common physical sanitizers are steam and hot water. Using deionized water as the boiler feedwater, clean steam can be generated which will serve as a physical sanitizer. If plant steam is generated by using non-deionized water as the boiler feedwater, it must meet local regulatory requirements governing the presence of boiler water additives or, in the absence of local regulatory requirements, the requirements listed in the FDA Code of Federal Regulations (see 21 CFR 173.310). If steam is being used, the minimum contact time is 10–15 minutes and the temperature of the exiting equipment condensate water must be 100°C. If 80.0–100.0°C hot water is used, a 20-minute contact time with an exit temperature of at least 70.0°C is recommended. If hot water at a lower temperature (e.g., 65.0–80.0°C) is used, a 30-minute contact time with an exit temperature of 60.0°C is recommended.

The advantages heat sanitization are penetrating into small cracks and crevices, non-corrosivity, are non-selective, broad spectrum of antimicrobial activity, lack of residues on equipment surfaces, disruption of microbial biofilms and ready availability. However, there are some challenges to using heat sanitization. For example, heat may cause condensation problems because of the high humidity conditions that are created. If purified water is not being used to generate clean steam, there is the possibility of boiler additive residues being present on equipment surfaces after the completion of the sanitization procedure and the potential residual effects will need to be assessed. High energy costs are usually offset by reduced labor costs when compared to the cost in using chemical sanitizers.

Considerations for Sanitization

Before conducting equipment sanitization, there are several considerations that need must be addressed such as rough surfaces such as bad welds or other surface defects which can make it difficult to sanitize due to the improper product residue removal, cleaning agent residues to be removed from an equipment surface by rinsing with deionized water, if an anionic cleanser is used with a cationic surfactant sanitizer, the sanitizer's antimicrobial activity can be inactivated due to their incompatibility, water used to prepare chemical sanitizer use-concentration must have a low microbial burden level to avoid the consumption of the sanitizer; and hard water ions can inactivate the antimicrobial activity of quaternary ammonium compound sanitizers. Furthermore, it is important to follow manufacturer instructions on how to prepare and use their chemical sanitizer. For using physical sanitization methods such as steam or hot water, it is important for the operators to use the proper contact times and temperatures to accomplish sanitization.

Sanitization Acceptance Criteria

Prior to the validation of sanitization procedures for manufacturing equipment, chemical sanitizer residue and microbial bioburden limits will need to be established. To validate the removal of chemical sanitizer residues from equipment surfaces after rinsing with deionized water, analytical test specification will need to be established for detecting the presence of an allowable sanitizer residue limits (68). This can be accomplished by using an analytical test method to detect the specific active ingredient in a chemical sanitizer or by using non-specific test methods such as conductivity or TOC analysis on collected equipment deionized rinse water samples. Microbial bioburden limits for validation of sanitization procedures for equipment surfaces is generally based upon the Quality Control microbial release test specifications for non-sterile finished product formulations.

Sanitization Process Operator Training

Operator training to perform equipment sanitization is critical. Operators should be trained on the requirements of equipment sanitization SOPs. Furthermore, only trained operators should be assigned to perform sanitization responsibilities. Proper training for equipment sanitization consists of trainee personnel obtaining an understanding of relevant SOPs, demonstration in how to perform the sanitization procedure by a trained operator and successful demonstration in performing the sanitization procedure by the trainee. All training in equipment sanitization must be documented.

Operator training for manual sanitization methods should include qualification and/or re-qualification of the operator based upon measuring sanitizer residue and microbial bioburden levels on equipment surfaces that have been sanitized. Operator training should be done on a more frequent basis for manual sanitization procedures in comparison to automated sanitization procedures in order to prevent drift or slight accidental changes in how the sanitization procedure is conducted. After training has been completed, it is important to conduct periodic microbial and chemical sanitizer residue monitoring to ensure that the operators who are conducting equipment sanitization procedures are still in continued compliance with the SOPs.

Rotation of Sanitizers

If a physical sanitization method such as hot water or steam is being used, there is no need to conduct rotation with a chemical sanitizer. However, there has been a debate for many years concerning the possible development of resistance of microorganisms to the antimicrobial activity of chemical sanitizers, disinfectants and sporicides based upon a parallel theoretical relationship to resistance found with antibiotics (89). However, there is no conclusive evidence in the scientific literature to substantiate the recommendation for rotating between different types of chemical sanitizers, disinfectants or sporicides (90,91). Resistance to antibiotics is typically acquired by a single mutation that blocks a very specific antimicrobial action of an antibiotic. Chemical sanitizers, disinfectants and sporicides have numerous effects on the metabolism of a microorganism ranging from inhibition of protein synthesis to the disruption of cell wall formation. The development of microbial resistance to sanitizers, disinfectants and sporicides is less likely because they are more potent agents than antibiotics, have multiple sites of antimicrobial action and are applied in high concentrations against low populations of microorganisms. Thus, the selective pressure is low for the development of antimicrobial resistance to chemical sanitizers, disinfectants and sporicides (92). Because of this, many companies have moved away from rotating with two different chemical sanitizers or disinfectants. Instead, the routine practice is to use either a single chemical sanitizer or a sanitizer/disinfectant which is rotated with the usage of a sporicide to prevent the development of microbial bioburden levels consisting of mostly spore-forming microorganisms.

Summary

In conclusion, there are many factors that are involved in preventing microbial contamination during manufacturing of non-sterile finished product formulations. If even one of the factors described is ignored, it may cause a finished product to be rejected for having a microbial content that may be harmful to the user or compromise product esthetics with malodors, phase separation, color changes or the presence of visible microbial colonies. By maintaining a manufacturing facility in a sanitary state, it is possible to manufacture reliably and consistently non-sterile finished product formulations that are considered to be microbiologically clean with low microbial bioburden levels (e.g., < 100 CFU/gram) and absence of objectionable microorganisms.

REFERENCES

1. Anon. General Chapter ⟨1115⟩ Bioburden control of nonsterile drug substances and products. United States Pharmacopeia & National Formulary USP 40 – NF 35. The United States Pharmacopeial Convention, Rockville, Md. 2017.
2. Anon. General Chapter ⟨1111⟩ Microbiological examination of nonsterile products: acceptance criteria for pharmaceutical preparations and substances for pharmaceutical use. United States Pharmacopeia & National Formulary USP 40 – NF 35. The United States Pharmacopeial Convention, Rockville, Md. 2017.
3. Anon. Annex 5 Supplementary guidelines on good manufacturing practices for heating, ventilation and air-conditioning systems for non-sterile pharmaceutical dosage forms, World Health Organization. WHO Technical Report Series No. 961, 2011; 215–260.
4. Anon. General Chapter ⟨1116⟩ Microbiological evaluation of clean rooms and other controlled environments. United States Pharmacopeia & National Formulary USP 40 – NF 35. The United States Pharmacopeial Convention, Rockville, Md. 2017.
5. Good Manufacturing Practice (GMP) Guidelines/Inspection Checklist. www.fda.gov/cosmetics/guidanceregulation/guidancedocuments/ucm2005190.htm, 2008.
6. 21 CFR Part 211 Current Good Manufacturing Practice for Finished Pharmaceuticals, Subpart C-Buildings and Facilities, 211.42, (c), (10, (i). Code of Federal Regulations, Title 21, Volume 4, Revised April 1, 2017.
7. EU Guideline to Good Manufacturing Practice, Chapter 3 – Premises and Equipment, European Commission, Brussels, Belgium, August 2014.
8. Bohn, E. How to select the appropriate flooring system for your GMP facility. www.pharmaceutical online.com/doc/how-to-select-the-appropriate-flooring-system-for-your-gmp-facility-0001.
9. CTPA GMP. *A Practical Guide for the Cosmetic Industry*. London, United Kingdom: Cosmetic, Toiletry and Perfumery Association. 1999.
10. Anon. Annex 2. Premises (Facility). In: *PCPC Quality Assurance Guidelines* (Nikitakas, J.M., ed.). Washington, DC: Personal Care Products Council. 2014.
11. ISO 22716 Cosmetics-Good Manufacturing Practices (GMP) – Guidelines for Good Manufacturing Practices, Geneva, Switzerland. 2007.
12. Mehltretter, N. How to select the right compressed air system, Pharmaceutical Manufacturing, 2015.
13. Scott, L. Compressed Air GMPs for GFSI Food Safety Compliance. www.airbestpractices.com/standards/food-grade-air/compressed-air-gmps-gfsi-food-safety-compliance.
14. Scott, L. Reducing contamination risks of compressed air in food plants: benchmarking good manufacturing practices. Haverhill, Ma.: Parker/Balston White Paper. 2012.
15. Anon. High quality compressed air from generation to application; a guide to ISO 8573.1:2001 Air Quality Classes. www.domickhunter.com.
16. Anon. General Chapter ⟨1231⟩ Water for pharmaceutical purposes. United States Pharmacopeia & National Formulary USP 40 – NF 35. The United States Pharmacopeial Convention, Rockville, Md. 2017.
17. U.S. Food & Drug Administration. 2014. Guide to inspection of high purity water systems. www.fda.gov/ICECI/Inspections/InspectionGudies/ucm074905.htm.
18. U.S. Environmental Protection Agency. 1998. National primary drinking water regulations: disinfection and disinfection byproducts. 40 CFR Parts 9, 141, and 142. www.epa.gov/safewater/mdbp/dbpfr.pdf.
19. Meltzer, T. *Pharmaceutical Water Systems*. Littleton, Colo.: Tall Oaks. 1997.
20. *USP Purified Water Monograph, United States Pharmacopeia & National Formulary*. USP 40 – NF-35, Rockville, Md. 2017.
21. Collentro, W.V. *Pharmaceutical Water: System Design, Operation and Validation*. New York: Interpharm/CPC. 1999.
22. Anon. Microbiological quality of process water. In: *Personal Care Product Council Microbiology Guidelines* (Krowka, J., Lang, B., eds.). Washington, DC: Personal Care Product Council. 2016.
23. ASME BPE. *Bioprocessing Equipment. American Society of Mechanical Engineers*. New York: Three Park Avenue. 2009.
24. Dick, A. C&S Practical experience vs. validation/how to make hygienic equipment non-hygienic and vice et versa. Presentation. PDA Conference on Pharmaceutical Microbiology, October 18, 2011.

25. Pasmore, M., Fry, R. Controlling biofilms in drug manufacturing equipment. In: *Biofilm Control in Drug Manufacturing* (Clontz, L., Wagner, C.M., eds.). River Grove, Il.: PDA Davis Healthcare. 2012: 165–203.

26. ASME BPE. *Bioprocessing Equipment 2–12, Part MJ, Materials Joining*. New York: American Society of Mechanical Engineers. 2014; 118–122.

27. Collentro, W.V., *Pharmaceutical Water System Design, Operation, and Validation,* 2nd Edition. New York: Informa Healthcare. 2011.

28. Rogers, J., Dowsett, A.B., Dennis, P.J., Lee, J.V., Keevil, C.W. Influence of plumbing materials on biofilm formation and growth of Legionella pneumophilia in potable water systems. *Appl. Envir. Microbiol.* 1994; 60 (6): 1842–1851.

29. Perez-Ibarrece, M., Castellano, P., Leclereq, A., Vignoto, G. Control of Listeria monocytogenes biofilms on industrial surfaces by the bacteriocin-producing Lactobacillus sakei CRL1862. *FEMS Microbiol. Lett.* 2006; 363 (12); 1–6.

30. Meyer, B. Approaches top prevention, removal and killing biofilms. *Int. Biodeter. Biodeg.* 2003; 50 (4): 249–253.

31. Rozej, A., Cydzik-Kwiathowska, A., Kowalska, B., Kowaslski, D. Structure and microbial diversity of biofilms on different pipe materials of a model drinking water distribution system. *World J. Microbiol. Biotechnol.* 2015; 31 (1): 37–47.

32. Soli, T.C. Design and sanitization of water systems to prevent contamination. In: *Designing and Controlling Water Systems* (Madsen, R.E., Moldenhauer, J., eds.). Parenteral Drug Association, Bethesda, Md. 2014.

33. Mittelman, M.W. Biofilm development in purified water systems. In: *Microbial Biofilms* (Lapin-Scott, H.M., Costerton, J.W., eds.). New York: Cambridge University Press. 2003; 133–147.

34. Sandle, T. Characterizing the microbiota of a pharmaceutical water system – A metadata study. *SOJ Microbiol. Infec. Dis.* 2015; 3 (2): 1–8.

35. Penna, V.T., Martins, S.A., Mazzola, PG. 2002. Identification of bacteria in drinking and purified water during the monitoring of a typical water purification system. *BMC Public Health.* 2002; 2–13.

36 Kulakov, L.A., McAlister, M.B., Ogden, K.L., Larkin, M.J., O'Hanolan, J.F. Analysis of bacteria contaminating ultrapure water in industrial systems. *Appl. Envir. Microbiol.* 2002; 68 (4): 1548–1555.

37. Mcalister, M.B., Kulakov, L.A., O'Hanlon, J.F., Larkin, M.J., Ogden, K.L. 2002. Survival and nutritional requirements of three bacteria isolated from ultrapure water. *J. Ind. Microbiol. Biotechnol.* 2002; 29 (2): 75–82.

38. Clontz, L. Microbial contamination control considerations in biopharmaceutical production. In: *Biofilm Control in Drug Manufacturing.* (Clontz. L., Wagner, C.M., eds.). River Grove, Il.: PDA DHI. 2012; 75–116.

39. Florjanic, M. Kristl, J. The control of biofilm formation by hydrodynamics of purified water in industrial distribution system. *Int. J. Pharm.* 2011; 405 (1-2): 16–22.

40. Purevdorj, B., Costerton, J.W., Stoodley. P. Influence of hydrodynamics and cell signaling on the structure and behavior of Pseudomonas aeruginosa biofilms. *Appl. Envir. Microbiol.* 2002; 68 (9): 4457–4464.

41. Collentro, W.V. Compendial water systems, maintenance and monitoring considerations, Pharmaceutical Processing. Nov/Dec 2013: 14–19.

42. Gounot, A.M. Psychrophilic and psychrotropic microorganisms. *Experientia.* 1986; 42 (11–12): 1192–1197.

43. Niemela, S.I., Sivela, C., Luoma, T., Tuouinen, O.H. Maximum temperature limits for acidophilic, mesophilic bacteria in biological leaching systems. *Appl. Envir. Microbiol.* 1994; 60 (9): 3444–3446.

44. Brock, T.D. Life at high temperatures. *Science.* 2012; 230 (October 11,1985): 132–138.

45. International Society for Pharmaceutical Engineering (ISPE). *Approaches in Commissioning and Qualification of Pharmaceutical Water and Steam Systems.* ISPE, Tampa, Fla. 2014.

46. Dychdala, G.R. Chlorine and chlorine compounds. In: *Disinfection, Sterilization and Preservation,* 5th Edition. (Block, S.S., ed.). Philadelphia, Pa.: Lippincott, Williams & Wilkens, 2001: 135–157.

47. Meulemans, C.C.E. The basics principles of UV-disinfection of water. *J. Int. Ozone Assoc.* 1987; 9 (4): 299–313.

48, Kowlaski, W. *Ultraviolet Germicidal Irradiation Handbook, UVGI and Surface Disinfection.* New York: Springer. 2009.

49. Christian, D.A., Meltzer, T.H. The penetration of membranes by organisms grow-through and its related problems. *Ultrapure Water* 1980; 3 (3): 39–44.
50. Wallhausser, K.H. Grow-through and blow-through effects in long-term sterilization processes. *Die Pharmaceutische Industry* 1983; 45 (5): 527–531.
51. Spinks, A.T., Dunstan, R.H., Coombes, P., Kuczera, G. 2003. Thermal destruction analyses of water related pathogens at domestic hot water system temperatures. *28th International Hydrology and Water Resources Symposium: About Water; Symposium Proceedings*, Barton, A.C.T: Institution of Engineers, Australia. 2003; 2: 323–333. http://search informit.com.au/documentSummary;dn=35961 1640707146;res=IELENG.
52. International Society of Pharmaceutical Engineering [ISPE]. *Good Practice Guide: Ozone Sanitization of Pharmaceutical Water Systems.* Tampa, Fl.: ISPE. 2012.
53. Rice, R.G., Robson, G., Miller, W.M., Hill, A.G. Uses of ozone in drinking water treatment. *Amer. Water Works Assoc.* 1981; 73 (1): 49–57.
54. Nebel, C., Nenel, T. Ozone: the process water sterilant. *Pharm. Manufact.* 1984; 1 (2): 16–22.
55. Sanitary Equipment Design Principles-Checklist & Glossary, Foundation for Meat & Poultry Research and Education, AMI Foundation, Washington, D.C. October 2014.
56. IFPA Sanitary Equipment Design Buying Guide & Checklist – Guideline, Definitions, Illustrations and Instructions for the Use of the Sanitary Design Checklist for Equipment Used in Processing Fresh-cut Fruits and Vegetables. International Fresh-cut Produce Association, Alexandria, Va. 2003.
57. 3-A Sanitary Standards. 3-A Sanitary Standards Symbol Administrative Council, Cedar Rapids, Iowa. 2014.
58. Anon. Annex 3 Equipment Part II-Processing. In: *PCPC Quality Assurance Guidelines.* (Nikitakas, J.M., ed.). Washington, DC: Personal Care Products Council. 2014.
59. USDA Guidelines for the Sanitary Design and Fabrication of Dairy Processing Equipment. U.S. Department of Agriculture, Washington, D.C. 2001.
60. Schmidt, R.H., Erickson, D.J. Sanitary Design and Construction of Food Equipment. FSHN0409, 2017. http://edis.ifas.ufl.edu.
61. Food and Drug Administration. 2004. Food Code. www.fda.gov.
62. Clegg, A., Perry, B.F. Control of microbial contamination during manufacture. In: *Microbial Quality Assurance in Cosmetics, Toiletries and Non-Sterile Pharmaceuticals,* 2nd Edition. (Baird, R.M., Bloomfield, S.F., eds.). Bristol, Pa.: Taylor and Francis. 1996: 49–66.
63. Cowan, R.A., Steiger, B. Why a preservative system must be tailored to a specific product. *Cosmet. Toilet.* 1977; 92 (3): 15, 16, 18–20.
64. Anger, C.B., Rupp, D., Lo, P. Preservation of dispersed systems. In: *Pharmaceutical Dosage-Forms: Disperse Systems.* Vol. 1, 2nd Edition. (Lieberman, H.A., Rieger, M.M., Baker, G.S., eds.). New York: Marcel Dekker. 1996: 377–435.
65. Kakemi, K.K., Sezaki, H., Arakawa, E., Kimura, K., Ikeda, K. Interaction of parabens and other pharmaceutical adjuvants with plastic containers. *Chem. Pharm. Bull. Jpn.* 1971; 19 (12): 2523–2529.
66. Dean, D.A. *Packaging of Pharmaceuticals: Packaging and Closures. Practical Packaging Series.* Leicestershire: Melton Mobbray; Institute of Packaging. 1992.
67. ISO 29621:2017 Cosmetics – Microbiology – Guidelines for the risk assessment and identification of microbiologically low-risk products, ISO, Geneva, Switzerland.
68. Anon. Cleaning and Sanitization. In: *Personal Care Product Council Microbiology Guidelines.* (Krowka, J., Lang, B., eds.). Washington, DC: Personal Care Product Council. 2016.
69. Anon. Section 9 Cleaning and Sanitization; Technical Report No. 70 Fundamentals of Cleaning and Disinfection Programs for Aseptic Manufacturing Facilities. Parenteral Drug Association, Bethesda, Md. 2015: 24–34.
70. Mazonakis, N.E., Karathanassi, P.H., Panagiotopoulos, D.P., Hamosfakidi, P.G., Melissos, D.M. Cleaning validation in the toiletries industry. *Analytica Chimica Acta.* 2002; 467 (1–2): 261–266.
71. Nassani, M. Cleaning validation in the pharmaceutical industry. *J. Valid. Technol.* August 2005; 38–58.
72. Ali, Y. Dolan, M.J, Fendler, E.J., Larson, E.L. Alcohols. In: *Disinfection, Sterilization, and Preservation,* 5th Edition. (Block, S.S., ed.). Philadelphia, Pa.: Lippincott Williams & Wilkens. 2001: 229–253.
73. Coulthard, C.E., Skyes, G. Germicidal effect of alcohol. *Pharma. J.* 1936; 137: 79–81.
74. Bloomfield, S.F. Chlorine and iodine formulations. In: *Handbook of Disinfectants and Antiseptics.* (Ascenzi, J.M., ed.). New York: Marcel Dekker. 1996: 133–158.

75. McDonnell, G., Russell, A.D. Antiseptics and disinfectants: activity, action and resistance. *Clin. Microbiol. Rev.* 1999; 12 (1): 147–179.

76. Russell, A.D. Bacterial spores and chemical sporicidal agents. *Clinic. Microbiol. Rev.* 1990; 3 (2): 99–119.

77. Gupta, A.K., Ahmad, I., Summerbell, R.C. Fungicidal activities of commonly used disinfectants and antifungal pharmaceutical spray preparations against clinical strains of *Aspergillus* and *Candida* species. *Med. Mycol.* 2002; 40 (2): 201–208.

78. Pfuntner, A. Sanitizers and disinfectants: the chemicals of prevention. *Food Safety Magazine*, August/September 2011; 16, 18, 19, 77.

79. Scott, E.M., Gorman, S.P. Glutaraldehyde. In: *Disinfection, Sterilization, and Preservation*, 5th Edition. (Block, S.S., ed.). Philadelphia, Pa: Lippincott Williams & Wilkens, 2001: 361–381.

80. Gorman, S.P., Scott, E.M. Potentiation and stabilization of glutaraldehyde biocidal activity utilizing surfactant-divalent cation combinations. *Int. J. Pharm.* 1979; 4 (1): 57–65.

81. Gorman, S.P., Scott, E.M. Effect of inorganic cations on the biocidal and cellular activity of glutaraldehyde. *J. Appl. Bacteriol.* 1979; 47 (3): 463–468.

82. Block, S.S. Peroxygen compounds. In: *Disinfection, Sterilization, and Preservation*, 5th Edition. (Block, S.S., ed.). Philadelphia, Pa: Lippincott Williams & Wilkens, 2001: 185–204.

83. Goddard, P.A., McCue, K.A. Phenolic compounds. In: *Disinfection, Sterilization, and Preservation*. (Block, S.S., ed.). Philadelphia, Pa.: Lippincott Williams & Wilkens, 2001; 255–281.

84. Paulus, W., Genth, H. Microbiocidal phenolic compounds: a critical examination. *Biodeter.* 1983; 5 (September 1981): 701–712.

85. Cook, F.M., Pierson, M.D. Inhibition of bacterial spores by antimicrobials. *Food Technol.* 1983; 37 (11): 115–126.

86. Russell, A.D., Jones, B.D., Millburn, P. Reversal of the inhibition of bacterial spore germination and outgrowth by antibacterial agents. *Int. J. Pharm.* 1985; 25 (1): 105–112.

87. Sundheim, G., Langsrud, S., Heir, E., Holck, A.L. Bacterial resistance to disinfectants containing quaternary ammonium compounds. *Int. Biodeter. & Biodeg.* 1998; 41 (3-4): 235–239.

88. Rorvik, L.M., Aase, B., Langsrud, S., Sundheim, G. Occurrence of and a possible mechanism for resistance to a quaternary ammonium compound in Listeria monocytogenes. *Int. J. Food Microbiol.* 2000; 62 (1-2) 57–63.

89. PDA Technical Report #70, Fundamentals of Cleaning and Disinfection Programs for Aseptic Manufacturing. Parenteral Drug Association, Bethesda, Md. 2015.

90. Martinez, J.E. The rotation of disinfectant principle: true or False? *Pharm. Technol.* 2009; 33 (2): 58–71.

91. Sutton, S. Disinfectant rotation: a microbiologist's view. www.microbiol.org/wp-content/uploads/2010/07/suttton. *Controlled Environ.* 2005. 8u.7.0 pdf. *Control. Envir.* July 2005: 9–14.

92. Anon. General Chapter ⟨1072⟩ Disinfectants and Antiseptics. United States Pharmacopeia & National Formulary. USP 40 – NF 35. The United States Pharmacopeial Convention, Rockville, Md. 2017.

9

Microbial Monitoring of a Manufacturing Facility

Introduction

Control of microorganisms within a manufacturing facility is a critical quality parameter of cosmetic/personal care products industry. These products is not expected or required to be sterile, but the presence of excessive numbers of microorganisms or pathogenic/objectionable microorganisms is not acceptable. Good manufacturing practices (GMPs) are typically established to put in place controls that prevent microbial contamination during manufacturing. In order to confirm microbiological control, microbial monitoring is performed on critical portions of a manufacturing facility including environmental air, equipment and facility surfaces, and manufacturing systems.

Microbial Air Monitoring

Microbial quality of ambient air in a cosmetic/personal care manufacturing facility can have an adverse effect on the microbial quality of finished products, and it is common for companies to conduct extensive microbial air sampling to determine the state of control of the environmental air within the manufacturing facility. Design of an air monitoring program is based on several considerations including the type of microbial air sampling to be performed, identification of air sampling sites, relevant air sampling specifications, and actions to be taken if specifications are exceeded.

Air Sampling Methods

Microbial air sampling methodology includes both qualitative and quantitative protocols. Qualitative or passive microbial air sampling relies on the placement of settling or sedimentation plates which contain a microbial growth agar such as Soybean-Casein Digest Agar Medium, which is used in open Petri dishes that are placed in critical locations (1). Settling plates are easy to use, economical, and versatile as any microbial growth agar can be used. Their small size allows for convenient placement along filling lines, and continuous air monitoring longer than 4 hours at a sampling site can be performed by changing Petri dishes (2). Utilities (e.g., electrical or vacuum) are not required and using settling plates is not disruptive to the immediate environment or work operations, and settling plates are not as prone to variation as air sampling equipment (3). If a single type plate of one microbial growth medium (e.g., Soybean-Casein Digest Agar Medium) is going to be used for determining both bacterial and fungi counts, incubation should be first at 20.0–25.0°C for 72 hours and then transferred to incubator at 30.0–35.0°C for 48 hours (4). Sabouraud Dextrose Agar (SDA), Potato Dextrose Agar (PDA), or Rose Bengal Agar with or without chloramphenicol can be used as a second microbial growth agar for the recovery of fungi in air samples. The addition of chloramphenicol prevents the growth of bacteria. Fungi settling Plates are typically incubated at 20.0–25.0°C between 72 hours and 5 days. A primary disadvantage of settling plates is its lack of quantitation as a microbial count cannot be correlated with an exposed sample volume of air. In addition, counts are affected by the size of particles, temperature, flow/volume of air passing across the agar surface, and movement and operation in the immediate vicinity of plates. Further, plates can become desiccated if left exposed for a long period of time and can be particularly susceptible to handling, transport, and laboratory contamination (4).

Quantitative air sampling can be accomplished with mechanical instruments that determine microbial numbers per specific volumes of air. However, individual sampling dynamics are such that the microbial test results from one type of air sampler are not reproducible with a different type of air sampler (5). Impaction and centrifugal are the most common types of mechanical air samplers. The Slit-to-Agar Air Sampler is one type of impaction air sampler and is powered by a controllable vacuum source. Air is sampled through a standardized opening or slit, and the air is impacted directly onto the surface of a microbial growth agar on a slowly rotating Petri dish. A second type of impaction air sampler is the Sieve Impactor. It is a unit that consists of a container designed to accommodate a 100×15 millimeter (mm) Petri dish containing a sterile microbial growth agar. In this unit, the cover is perforated with holes of specific diameter. A known volume of air is drawn through the cover under vacuum, and microorganisms are directly impacted onto the agar surface of a Petri dish. Advantages of an impaction air samplers include: a large volume of air that can be sampled, a time–concentration relationship can be obtained, airflow can be calibrated, a remote sampling probe can be used in those areas difficult to access, can be used for compressed air or gas sampling, and no serial dilution or plating is required. Disadvantages of impaction air samplers include: some units require an external vacuum source, an electrical power source may be required, some equipment may be large and cumbersome to move between sampling sites, some units require using 150×15 mm instead of the 100×15 mm Petri dishes, and the unit cannot be sterilized by autoclaving.

Centrifugal air samplers use a propeller or turbine housed in an open drum to sample a known volume of air. The collected air is then accelerated by centrifugal force toward the inner wall of the drum lined with a flexible plastic strip containing a microbial growth agar that is impacted by sampled airborne particle (1,6). Centrifugal air samplers have been reported to selectively recover larger particles resulting in higher airborne counts than other types of air samplers (5). The advantages of centrifugal air samplers are as follows: convenience of operation, portability, a self-contained electrical power supply, autoclavable head assembly, large volumes of air can be sampled, and airflow can be calibrated. Disadvantages include use of specialized microbial growth agar strips requiring additional handling, direct calibration of sampling volume is not possible, and the use of the unit will cause a disruption of the airflow in a laminar flow hood.

Whether a company decides to use a qualitative or a quantitative air sampling method, it is important that one method be consistently applied and every air sampling site be identified. Air sampling sites should be chosen based on microbiological risk to the finished product and consideration should be given to the sites of manufacturing process risk such as difficulty of set-up, extended processing time, and interventions (7). Each sampling site should be described within a Standard Operating Procedure (SOP) and with enough detail to allow for reproducible, specified air sampling. A map is often used for the identification of air sampling sites. Furthermore, it is important that within this air sampling SOP, sampling parameters are described to include frequency, timing and duration of sampling, air volume to be sampled, and specific sampling equipment and techniques. Response to microbiological findings should be driven by alert and action levels and appropriate response to deviations when an alert or action levels are reached for an air sampling site (4).

Location, Frequency, and the Number of Air Sampling Sites

Location, frequency, and the number of sites for air sampling should be based on a qualification that identifies those sites most useful for conducting routine air monitoring. International Organization for Standards (ISO) 14644-1 (7) describes a method for determining the number of sampling sites:

$$N_1 = \sqrt{A}$$

Where: N_1 is the minimum number of sampling sites (rounded up to a whole number) and
A is the area of the room or zone in square meters (m^2).

After determining the number of air sampling sites in a qualification study, the location of these air sampling sites will need to be determined. This is carried out based on data from replicate qualification studies and is used to determine sampling sites most relevant to the microbial quality of the air and the finished product. There are several useful guidance documents from the Parenteral Drug Association, Food and Drug Administration, the EU and the United States Pharmacopeia (2,8,9). However, the most important consideration in selecting a routine air sampling site is the proximity to the non-sterile product and whether air might be in contact with an open product formulation (e.g., raw ingredient weigh outs, batch processing, and product filling areas).

Alert and Action Levels

Microbial air sampling test data from several qualification studies can be used to establish alert and action levels for each air sampling site. After the passage of two or more calendar weather seasons, it is useful to re-establish alert levels for each air sampling site at the 95th percentile based upon observed microbial count readings. From this time period, the action level can also be established by using the 99th percentile of the observed microbial counts at each sampling site. After the establishment of these alert and action levels, it is recommended that air sampling data for each site be tracked and trended in real-time. These data will be useful for the investigation of possible subsequent excursions in the microbial counts and for potential reconsideration of alert and action levels.

Identification of Recovered Air Microbial Isolates

In addition to microbial counts, it is important to identify microbial isolates to detect changes in trends. For example, a shift in the types of microflora indicates deviation from the "norm". In general, microflora present in air samples are associated with either human skin (e.g., Gram-positive cocci) or the environment (e.g., Gram-positive bacilli and fungi) (10). If a Gram-negative bacillus is isolated from an air sample, it is probable that the air sample had been taken in facility wet areas such as wash bays due to the generation of water aerosols. Typical microbial species that can be isolated in air samples from a manufacturing plant environment include species of the genera *Bacillus, Corynebacterium, Paenibacillus, Cutibacterium (Propionibacterium), Staphylococcus, Micrococcus, Streptococcus, Kocuria, Pseudomonas, Alternaria, Aspergillus, Cladosporium, Epicoccum,* and *Penicillium species* (10–13).

Microbial Monitoring of the Facility

Floors

Microbes typically found on dry floors are Gram-positive bacilli, Gram-positive cocci, and fungal spores. This flora is derived largely from microorganisms carried or deposited from footwear and from incoming materials and equipment. If Gram-negative bacilli are found, it can be assumed that water is present somewhere on the floor to allow for its survivability. To conduct a surface sampling of a floor, most people will use contact plates, such as a Replicate Organisms Detection and Counting or RODAC™

Plate (14). RODAC™ contact plates are 65 mm diameter plates containing a microbial growth agar that in application are pressed against a solid flat surface to be sampled. The surface area sampled by a RODAC™ contact plate is approximately 25 square centimeters (cm^2). There are also flexible films and contact slides useful for sampling flat surfaces including the Hycon® Contact Slide and the flex paddle surface monitoring slide. Due to potential residuals of disinfectant agents, it is recommended that growth agar media be supplemented with a disinfectant neutralizing agent such as Lecithin and Polysorbate (Tween) 80. It is very common to see the usage of contact plates with either Soybean-Casein Digest Agar Medium with 4% Tween 80 and 0.5% Soy Lecithin or Dey/Engley Neutralizing Agar. Dey/Engley Neutralizing Agar contains the ingredients that neutralize disinfectant residues: sodium thioglycollate, sodium thiosulfate, sodium bisulfite, polysorbate (Tween) 80, and Lecithin (Soybean) (15). These are not without disadvantages. For one, low concentrations of sodium bisulfite can inhibit the growth of *Staphylococcus aureus* (16). The developers of this medium also reported the inhibitory nature of low sodium bisulfite concentrations and had recommended that Dey/Engley Neutralizing Broth (vs. both broth and agar) be used only as a diluent (17,18). Similarly, sodium thiosulfate can inhibit the growth of staphylococci (19), and sodium thioglycollate can inhibit the growth of *Staphylococcus aureus, Pseudomonas aeruginosa,* and spore-forming bacteria (18,20). On the basis of these inhibitory properties, Dey/Engley medium is not recommended as a recovery microbial growth agar in a contact plate due to diversity of microorganisms that may be present on a floor surface potentially including isolates sensitive to these neutralizing agents. After exposure to agar via contact plate application, the area of contact should be sprayed with a 60–70% ethyl or isopropyl alcohol solution and wiped to remove agar medium residues.

Walls and Ceilings

Microbial monitoring samples are not taken of the ceilings due to room height and the more relevant measure would be air monitoring. However, sampling of flat wall surface can be useful and can be performed using either RODAC™ contact plates, flexible films, or contact slides as described in the sampling the floors of a manufacturing facility. Microorganisms recovered from walls will be similar to those present in microbial air samples.

Microbial Monitoring of Manufacturing Systems

Compressed Air

Monitoring compressed air should be done on a weekly basis. A single microbial test in a year is not sufficient because compressed air systems are dynamic and the compressor air intake is subject to microbial, particulate, and moisture variations throughout the year. Unfortunately, there is no standard method for evaluating the microbial content of compressed air (21). The challenge in conducting monitoring of compressed air is decompression prior to culture.

A simple method to determine the microbial quality of a compressed air sample is to directly impact air onto a microbial growth agar. However, the level of impact stress from the impaction velocity of the cells into the microbial growth agar will have an adverse effect in the recovery of microorganisms (22). To prevent this, compressed air line pressure (e.g., 160 pounds per square inch or greater) can be reduced to a flow rate of approximately 1 cubic foot per minute by using a built-in or external regulator and attached flow meter. Compressed air at 1 cubic flow per minute is then impacted into a sterile Petri dish containing a microbial growth agar. Devices used to take compressed air samples include Slit-to-Agar Air Sampler, Andersen Impactor, and the Compressed Air Microbial Testing Unit (CAMTU) (21,23). In the CAMTU, compressed air is decompressed above a disk in the unit that is suspended over an open sterile Petri dish with microbial growth agar. Microorganisms are propelled from the decompressed air onto the surface of a microbial growth agar and the driven air exits the unit through channels under the Petri dish.

Soybean-Casein Digest Agar Medium is typically used in estimating the microbial count of compressed air. For the recovery of fungi, SDA, PDA, or Rose Bengal Agar can be used. In addition to colony counts recorded after incubation, it is recommended that representative microbial isolates be identified to the species level. Because room air is being drawn into the inlet of air compressor, it is not unexpected to detect the same types of microorganisms encountered in air sampling including Gram-positive bacilli and cocci, Gram-negative bacilli, and fungi that had been isolated in room air samples.

Process Water

Water Sampling

Process water systems should be monitored at an appropriate frequency to ensure control and that it produces process water at an acceptable quality. Process water samples for microbial analysis should be taken from locations within the generation through the distribution portions of the system to identify sources of microbial contamination and identify problem areas in a process water system (24). The following areas of the generation and distribution portions of the process water system need to be addressed in testing (25).

- Incoming source water for the process water system (if well water is being used as the source water and being treated, analytical and microbial testing should be conducted to confirm compliance with local potable or drinking water standards).
- After the activated carbon bed.
- After the water softener unit.
- After the reverse osmosis unit.
- Before and after being in the water storage tank.
- After cation/anion/mixed bed ion exchange columns or Electrodeionization (EDI) unit.
- After each ultraviolet light.
- After each microbial retentive filter.
- At each use-point in the water distribution loop.

Prior to sampling from use-points, the outlet must be sanitized and flushed with process water to remove any sanitizer residues. If a hose at a use-point is being used during production to deliver process water to a processing vessel, the same "sanitize and flush" process should be completed on the hose before a sample is taken from the hose for microbial analysis. As a general practice, it is important to flush 5–10 gallons of process water from each use-point prior to use in manufacturing in order to purge the system of any possible microbial build-up in the use-point value.

Timeliness in conducting microbial enumeration testing on collected process water samples is an important consideration. For example, the number of planktonic bacteria present in a collected process water sample will usually drop as time passes by either die off or due to deposition to sample container walls (24). By contrast, potential presence of low concentrations of organic compounds may promote microbial growth within the collected water sample. In either case, the number of recoverable bacteria in a collected process water sample can change with time. Therefore, it is the best practice to test the sample within 1 hour of collection (26). If this is not possible, water samples should be refrigerated a maximum of about 12 hours to maintain the microbial attributes until analysis could be conducted (24).

Enumeration Methods

Most cosmetic/personal care companies apply microbial enumeration limits of Purified Water from the USP for process water—100 Colony-Forming Units (CFU)/milliliter (mL) (27).

Because process water system microbial isolates are nutritionally stressed, they do not grow reliably on high-nutrient recovery microbial growth agars such as Soybean-Casein Digest Agar Medium. Because of this, a low-nutrient recovery microbial growth agar such as R2A or Plate Count Agar are used in pour plate and membrane filtration enumeration procedures of process water system samples (28,29).

Microbiological test results of a process water system should be monitored for trends to indicate whether there is an increasing microbial count at each system use-point. If high microbial counts are expected to be present at either a sampling or use-point, a pour plate procedure may be used (28). In general, the microbial counts at the process water distribution loop use-points will have microbial counts of <1 CFU/mL. To increase sensitivity necessary to obtain trend data, a 100-milliliter aliquot from a sampling point can be filtered through a sterile filter membrane then placed on a microbial growth agar and incubated (29). In addition to conventional pour plate or membrane filtration techniques, a rapid detection technology termed Online Water Bioburden Analysis (OWBA) is available. OWBA technology determines microbial counts in real time through the application of light induced fluorescence (30). Light induced fluorescence (LIF) is a spectroscopic technique that is capable of detecting compounds that will fluoresce. Microorganisms will fluoresce due to the presence of fluorophores such as tryptophan, nicotinamide adenine dinucleotides (NADH), and flavins (31). In this application, a small portion of a process water sample stream is diverted to the analyzer's flow cell through which a laser is directed. These potential microbial chemical markers will fluorescence and that light signal is detected by a photomultiplier tube. The quantity of particles in the water is also determined by a second sensor in the analyzer via Mie scattering. Data from the two detectors are then processed to accurately distinguish between microorganisms and non-microbial particles, and the microbial count is determined in real time. This technique does not eliminate culture-based microbial testing of process water but allows reduction in the frequency of such testing. Such real-time data enables the rapid identification and correction of deteriorating conditions in the operating parameters of the process water system.

Identification of Recovered Microbial Isolates

For recovered process water microbial isolates, it is important to perform phenotypic (e.g., biochemical) or genotypic identification to the genus/species level, especially to identify waterborne objectionable microorganisms detrimental to the product or process water quality (24). Identifying the potential source of microbial contamination is also mandatory. Although specifications regarding certain microbial species as objectionable are discretionary, this consideration typically ranges from the absence of species such as *Pseudomonas aeruginosa* and *Burkholderia cepacia* complex to the absence of all Gram-negative bacilli.

Alert and Action Levels

For each process water system sampling point, an alert and action level for the number of microorganisms should be established based on historical microbial enumeration test results and should be periodically reviewed. These levels serve as guidance indicators to ensure that the system doesn't drift from its normal operating parameters (32). Microbial alert levels for process water refer to a microbial count that is still within the microbial test specification but is higher than normal for that sampling point. Microbial action levels for process water refer to a microbial count that is higher than the alert level, but is still within the microbial test specification. A microbial action level that is equivalent to the process water microbial enumeration specification should be ruled out because it leaves no room for conducting remedial maintenance on the system that could be used to avoid an excursion that is above the process water microbial test specification. Action levels are events that constitute a warning that the system has drifted from its normal operating range and corrective action needs to be taken to bring the system back into its normal operating range.

Microbial Monitoring of Equipment Surfaces after Sanitization

The microbial quality of the physical surfaces of the manufacturing equipment can have a direct impact on the microbial quality of a non-sterile finished product formulation. Microbial monitoring of manufacturing equipment surfaces is typically conducted after the completion of the cleaning and sanitization processes.

Sampling Methods

There are several sampling methods for conducting microbial monitoring of equipment surfaces ranging from direct contact, swab, rinse water, and ATP Bioluminescence (33,34). The type of sampling method to be used will depend upon the geometry of the surface to be sampled such as whether it is flat, curved, grainy, or smooth. It is also important to determine the chemical condition of the surface in order to address materials such as chemical sanitizer/disinfectant residues, oils, salts, or finished product films still present on the surface that may interfere with the microbial test results.

Direct Contact Method

Direct contact sampling method can be used to monitor the microbial quality of an equipment surface that is flat and smooth by using RODAC™ plates, agar paddles, or flexible agar films which contain a solid microbial growth agar (35). For these sampling devices, a selective or a non-selective microbial growth agar such as Soybean-Casein Digest Agar Medium can be used that may or may not contain a sanitizer/disinfectant neutralizing agent. To sample a flat and smooth equipment surface, the agar surface of these sampling devices are pressed against the surface to be sampled and subsequently incubated and microbial counts recorded. After sampling, it is recommended that the surface area that had been sampled is cleaned by using a 60–70% ethyl or isopropyl alcohol solution to remove any remaining agar residue.

Use of RODAC™ plates or flexible agar films allows enumeration and recovery for speciation the of microbial colonies in a 25 cm^2 area can be determined. However, it should be noted that these sampling devices will not recover 100% of the microbial bioburden that may be present on an equipment surface. The advantages in using direct contact sampling devices include ease of use, quantitative estimation, versatility in the application of different types of microbial growth agar, and—for flexible agar film— effective sampling of curved surfaces.

Swab Method

Sampling of an irregular or smooth equipment surfaces can be accomplished using sterile swabs. Like direct contact sampling devices, swabs will not recover the total microbial bioburden from an equipment surface. To sample a surface, the following types of absorbent materials can be used as a swab: sterile tip applicators such as Dacron™, cotton wool and calcium alginate, sterile cotton balls, sterile cotton gauze, and sterile Speci-Sponge Bags (Whirl-Pak®). The usage of sterile sponges, cotton balls, and gauze are recommended in ISO 18593: 2004 for sampling large surface areas (>100 cm^2) (36).

There are essentially two swab methods for sampling equipment surfaces: qualitative (presence or absence) and quantitative. To perform both a qualitative and a quantitative surface swab method, a sterile swab is moistened with sterile diluent that may contain a sanitizer/disinfectant neutralizing agent. The moistened swab is used to wipe a given equipment surface dimension (e.g., 25 cm^2 or 2-inch × 2-inch area) by reversing the direction between successive stokes while rotating the swab between the fingers. This can be facilitated with the use of a sterile template cut to these dimensions. In a qualitative method, the used swab is streaked across the surface of a microbial growth agar in a Petri dish or immersed in a liquid microbial growth medium. After incubation, streaked agar Petri dishes or liquid microbial growth media are examined for the presence or absence of microbial growth. In a quantitative method, the used swab can be placed into a solution to remove the collected microorganisms by either vortexing or shaking. A calcium alginate swab can be used in a quantitative method. After taking a surface sample, the used calcium alginate swab is dissolved in either a 1% sodium citrate solution or in a 1% sodium hexametaphosphate in ¼-strength Ringers solution to free microorganism that had been collected in the fibrous strands of the calcium alginate swab. Aliquots of the solution are either pour plated by using the appropriate microbial growth agar or filtered through a membrane filter that is transferred to either a microbial growth broth–impregnated pad or to a Petri dish with a microbial growth agar. After incubation, the number of colonies for each sampling site is counted and reported as the number of CFU per swab or surface area.

Swab-based sampling is inexpensive, easy to perform, suitable for taking samples from either irregular or flat surfaces, can be used to take samples of a highly contaminated surfaces, and can be either qualitative or quantitative. However, microorganisms may become trapped in the swab fibers and fatty acids from cotton swabs (37,38), or elutes for calcium alginate swabs (39,40), may inhibit the growth of microorganisms. Such factors can impact the quality of the aseptic sampling technique and processing of the samples can adversely affect the microbial test results and require additional manipulation to culture the sample. Furthermore, poor reproducibility in using swabs between operators has been reported and attributed to different pressures applied to the surface (41). Regarding recovery rates, only a proportion of the total bacterial population present on a surface can be recovered by swab sampling (42,43).

In performing swab sampling, it is necessary to address two factors that may confound test results. The first factor is the presence of sanitizer/disinfectant residues on equipment surface sampling sites that could inhibit the recovery of microorganisms. For this, a sanitizer/disinfectant neutralizer can be used to neutralize the antimicrobial activity of the residue. The second factor is the time between sampling and processing of the swab for microbial analysis. It is recommended that used swabs be processed soon after collection to prevent overgrowth or desiccation of microorganisms. In the case of significant delay (e.g., shipment to an off-site laboratory for processing and analysis), collection swab in transport medium or vehicle may be used to maintain viability of microorganisms. This procedure is typically used for clinical specimens and suffers potential issues in application for equipment surface monitoring. Loss of microbial viability has been observed during transport depending upon the microbial species recovered, system type, and temperature (44–54). For clinical specimens, a 4–6 log reduction in the viability of recovered microorganisms may not be a problem since it is highly likely that the transport swab would initially contain greater than 10^6 CFU in comparison to equipment surface swab samples containing less than 1,000 CFU. It has also been reported that certain types of microorganisms are able to proliferate in the media of a transport system (55). If delay is anticipated in sample processing, appropriate validation testing should be conducted to address potential effects of time and transport.

Rinse Water Method

To sample hard-to-access interior equipment surfaces (e.g., processing vessels, storage tanks, etc.) that cannot be reached by using a swab or direct contact method, a rinse water sampling technique is used (35). To perform a rinse water method of an interior equipment surface, a volume of sterile water is introduced to flush the interior surfaces of the equipment. A 100-milliliter aliquot of the sterile rinse water is collected as it exits from the flushed equipment. This rinse water aliquot can be tested for microbial count by using a pour plate, membrane filtration, or Most Probable Number (MPN) method to yield a quantitative microbial test result. The advantages in using a rinse water method is that inaccessible areas of manufacturing equipment can be accessed, large interior surface areas can be sampled, and quantitative microbial results can be obtained. Disadvantages of sampling rinse water include lack of suitability for many equipment assessments, not suitable for many applications, extensive manual manipulation is required, and aseptic sample collection and processing techniques which can affect microbial test results.

ATP Bioluminescence Method

In the food industry, an ATP Bioluminescence method is used for the detection of food residues and bacteria on equipment surfaces after cleaning and sanitization. However, its application in this context is somewhat limited as foods have a higher acceptable microbial level in comparison to non-sterile product formulations. The advantage of ATP Bioluminescence assay is its rapid detection of contamination. However, in application to surface monitoring, results are not quantitative, sensitivity is poor (greater than 1,000 CFU/sampling site), and non-microbial ATP on an equipment surfaces will provide a false positive signal (56).

The ATP Bioluminescence hygiene monitoring assay uses a swab pre-moistened with a cationic reagent that lyses microbial cells obtained by swabbing surfaces, releasing microbial ATP. The swab is placed into a luminometer in which a firefly reagent is added to measure the amount of Relative Light Units (RLUs) that are proportional to the amount of ATP present. A low RLU level from a swab indicates minimal microbial contamination.

ATP Bioluminescence hygiene monitoring assay has been compared in several studies to traditional hygiene monitoring methods. Although, some studies have indicated a good correlation between the results for ATP and traditional methods, other studies have reported poor correlation (57–61). The use of an ATP Bioluminescence hygiene monitoring assay may or may not be appropriate in a manufacturing facility depending upon the total aerobic microbial plate count specification of finished products.

Frequency of Microbial Monitoring of Sanitized Equipment

Frequency of microbiological monitoring of equipment surfaces is dependent on the manufacturing process, product susceptibility to microbial contamination, facility design, and historical profiles of environmental sampling test data.

For example, microbial monitoring of equipment surfaces is not necessary for manufacturing equipment that is used in a hot manufacturing process (e.g., greater than 65°C temperature) for lipstick, lip balms, and cream blush product formulations as the manufacturing temperature is self-sterilizing (62). Similarly, manufacturing equipment used for products containing greater than 23% alcohol (e.g., colognes, perfumes, hair sprays) does not require monitoring because they are self-preserving (62). Non-sterile product formulations containing greater than 5% process water, 100% anhydrous liquid (e.g., mineral oil), and anhydrous pressed or loose powder product formulation are susceptible to microbial contamination during manufacturing. For these, microbial monitoring of equipment surfaces should be conducted after sanitization if the procedure has not been validated. If the equipment sanitization procedure has been validated, periodic microbial monitoring can be performed to ensure continuing control. The selection of equipment microbial monitoring sites by direct contact or swabbing methods is based upon conducting a Hazard Analysis Critical Control Points (HACCP) risk assessment process for identifying those critical control points (CCP) that are the most difficult to sanitize (63–65).

Unlike many non-sterile pharmaceutical drug product formulations, compositions of cosmetic/personal care product formulations are always dynamic, changing with the innovation of new formulas. Instead of validating the sanitization procedure for each product formulation, it is common practice in the industry that the validation is conducted to address specific manufacturing equipment.

Microbial Test Specifications for Sanitized Equipment

Cosmetic/personal care product manufacturers will need to establish the maximum numerical test specifications for each of the sanitized equipment sampling sites in order to determine whether a microbial level at a site would have an adverse effect on the product quality. One way is to conduct a risk assessment to determine what could be the maximum number of CFU that could be present at an equipment surface sampling site that would have an adverse effect on product quality. The second way is to use the Class D/ISO 8 surface specification after sanitization of 50 CFU/24–30 cm^2 contact or swab area as the maximum numerical specification for an equipment sampling site (2,8,66). Whatever way is chosen to establish the maximum CFU limit for an equipment sanitization sampling site, microbial alert and action levels are often established by trending microbial data in which alert limits are established by using 95th percentile values, where the action limits are established by using 99th percentile values (8). Besides establishing a numerical limit for a monitoring site for sanitization, it is not unusual to see the establishment for the absence of certain microbial species such as *Pseudomonas* species, *Burkholderia cepacia* complex species, *Staphylococcus aureus*, and *Candida albicans*.

Summary

A microbiological monitoring program for a manufacturing facility environmental air, compressed air, process water and sanitization of facility surfaces and equipment is a tool for ensuring that the microbiological quality of non-sterile cosmetic/personal care product formulations are safe for usage by the consumer. Furthermore, personnel who are involved in taking these samples should have received adequate instruction and training in conducting microbial monitoring in a facility.

With appropriate application of monitoring protocols that are described in the chapter and appropriate response, a manufacturing facility can be maintained under microbiological control.

REFERENCES

1. Anon. General Chapter (1116) Microbiological Evaluation of Clean Rooms and Other Controlled Environments. United States Pharmacopeia & National Formulary USP 40 – NF 35. The United States Pharmacopeial Convention, Rockville, Md., 2017.
2. EU Eudralex. The Rules Governing Medicinal Products in the European Union, EU Guidelines to Good Manufacturing Practice Medicinal Products for Human and Veterinary Use; Annex 1 Manufacturing of Sterile Medicinal Products (Corrected Version). European Commission. Brussels. November 25, 2008 (Revised).
3. Yao, M., Mainelis, G. Investigation of cut-off sizes and collection efficiencies of portable microbial samplers. *Aerosol Sci. Technol.* 2006; 40 (8): 595–605.
4. Sutton, S. Microbiology topics: the environmental monitoring program in a GMP environment. *J GXP Compl.* 2010; 14 (3): 22–30.
5. Nakhla, L.S., Cummings, R.F. A comparative evaluation of a new centrifugal air sampler (RCS) with slit air sampler (SAS) in a hospital environment. *J Hos. Infec.* 1981; 2 (3): 261–266.
6. Buddemeyer, J. Selecting an active air sampling methodology. *Cont. Environ.* 2005; 8 (7): 19–23.
7. ISO, ISO 14664-1 Cleanrooms and Associated Controlled Environments. Part 1: Classification of Air Cleanliness. Geneva, Switzerland. 1999.
8. PDA Technical Report #13, Fundamentals of an Environmental Monitoring Program, Parenteral Drug Association, Bethesda, Md., 2014.
9. FDA, Guidance for Industry: Sterile Drug Products Produced by Aseptic Processing – Current Good Manufacturing Practice. 2004.
10. Sandle, T. A review of cleanroom microflora: types, trends and patterns. *PDA J Pharma. Sci. & Technol.* 2011; 65 (4): 392–404.
11. Wu, G, Liu, X-h. Characterization of predominant bacteria isolates from clean rooms in a pharmaceutical production unit. *J Zhejiang Univ. Sci. B.* 2007; 8 (9): 666–672.
12. Park, H.K. Han, J.-H, Joung, Y., Cho, S.-H, Kim, S.-A, Kim, S.B. Bacterial diversity in the indoor air of pharmaceutical environment. *J. App. Micro.* 2013; 116 (3): 718–727.
13. Cundell, A. Mold monitoring and control in pharmaceutical manufacturing areas. *Amer. Pharm. Rev.* 2016, 19 www.americanpharmaceuticalreview.com/Featured-Atricles/190686-Mold-Monitori.
14. Clontz, L. Validation of nonsterile pharmaceutical manufacturing facilities and water system. In: *Microbial Limit and Bioburden Tests, Validation Approaches and Global Requirement.* CRC Press, New York, 1998: 19.
15. Difco Manual, 11th Edition, *Difco Laboratories, Division of Becton Dickinson and Company.* Sparks. Maryland. 1998.
16. Wallhausser, K.H. Appendix B antimicrobial preservatives used by the cosmetic industry. In: *Cosmetic and Drug Preservation, Principles and Practice* (Kabara, J.J. ed.). Marcel Dekker, New York, 1984: 605–745.
17. Engley, F.B., Dey, B.P. A universal neutralizing medium for antimicrobial chemicals. Chemical Specialties Manufacturers Association. Proceedings of 56th Mid-Year Meeting. 1970.
18. MacKinnon, H. The use of inactivators in the evaluation of disinfectants. *J. Hyg. Camb.* 1974; 73 (2): 189–195.
19. Kayser, A., vander Ploeg, G. Growth inhibition of staphylococci by sodium thiosulphate. *J. Appl. Bacteriol.* 1965; 28 (2): 286–293.

20. Hibbert, H.R., Spencer, R. An investigation of the inhibitory properties of sodium thioglycollate in media for the recovery of bacterial spores. *J. Hyg. Camb.* 1970; 68 (1): 131–135.

21. Landsborough, L. Comparison of the compressed air microbial testing unit to a standard method of bioaerosol sampling. www.airbestpractices.com/industries/pharmaceutical/comparison-compressed-air-microbial-testing-unit-standard-method-bioaeroso.

22. Stewart, S.L., Grinshpun, S.A., Willeke, K., Terzieva, S., Ulevicius, V., Donnellly, J. Effect of impact stress on microbial recovery on an agar surface. *Appl. Environ. Microbiol.* 1995; 61 (4): 1232–1239.

23. Sandoval, M. Compressed Air: Choosing the Correct Microbial Sampling Method. 2018. www.ifsqn.com/food-safety-quality-articles/_/compressed-air-and-microbial-sampling-methods.

24. Anon. General Chapter ⟨1231⟩ Water for pharmaceutical purposes. United States Pharmacopeia & National Formulary USP 40 – NF 35. The United States Pharmacopeial Convention, Rockville, Md., 2017.

25. Anon. Microbiological quality of process water. In: *Personal Care Product Council Microbiology Guidelines* (Krowka, J., Lang, B., eds.). The Personal Care Product Council, Washington, D.C., 2016.

26. Anon. Section 9060B. Preservation and Storage. In: *Standard Methods for the Examination of Water and Wastewater,* 20th Edition. (Clesceri, L.S., Greenberg, A.E., Eaton, A.D. eds.). American Public Health Association, Washington, D.C., 1998.

27. USP Purified Water Monograph. United States Pharmacopeia & National Formulary. USP 40 - NF-35, Rockville, Md., 2017.

28. 9215B. Pour plate method, 9215 heterotrophic plate count. In: *Standard Methods for the Examination of Water and Wastewater,* 20th Edition. (Clesceri, L.S., Greenberg, A.E. Eaton, A.D. eds.). American Public Health Association, Washington, D.C., 1998; 9–34 and 9–38.

29. 9215D. Membrane filter method. In: *Standard Methods for the Examination of Water and Wastewater*, 20th Edition. (Clesceri, L.S., Greenberg, A.E., Eaton, A.D., eds.). American Public Health Association, Washington, D.C., 1998: 9–40 and 9–41.

30. Cundell, A., Luebke, M., Gordon, O., Matefly, J., Haycocks, N. Weber, J.W. et al. Novel concept for online water bioburden analysis: key considerations, applications, and business benefits for microbiological risk reduction. *Ame. Pharma. Rev.* 2013, May/June: 16 (4); 26–31.

31. Ammor, M.S. Recent advances in the use of intrinsic fluorescence for bacterial identification and characterization. *J Fluores.* 2007; 17 (5): 455–459.

32. U.S. Food & Drug Administration. Guide to inspection of high purity water systems. 2004. www.fda.gove/ICECI/Inspections/InspectionGudies/ucm074905.htm.

33. Dyer, R.L., Frank, J.F., Johnson, B., Hickey, P. Fitts, J. Microbiological tests for equipment, containers, water and air. In: *Standards Methods for the Examination of Dairy Products,* 17th Edition. (Wer, H.M., Frank, J.F., eds.). American Public Health Association, Washington, D.C., 2004: 325–340.

34. Lemmen, S.W., Hafner, H., Zolldan, D., Amedick, G., Lutticken, R. Comparison of two sampling methods for the detection of Gram-positive and Gram-negative bacteria in the environment: moistened swabs versus Rodac plates. *Int. J Hyg. Environ. Heal.* 2001; 203 (3): 245–248; UECI/inspections/inspectionguides/ucm074922, p 5.

35. Anon. Microbiological evaluation of the plant environment. In: Personal Care Product Council Microbiology Guidelines. (Krowka, J., Lang, B., eds.). The Personal Care Product Council, Washington, D.C., 2016: 11–29.

36. Anon. Microbiology of food and animal feeding stuffs – horizontal methods for sampling techniques from surfaces using contact plates and swabs. Geneva, Switzerland. 2004. ISO 18593:2004.

37. Pollack, M.R. Unsaturated fatty acids in cotton wool plugs. *Nature.* May 29, 1948; 161 (4100): 853.

38. Nieman, C. Influence of trace amounts of fatty acids on the growth of microorganisms. *Bacteriol. Rev.* June 1954; 18 (2): 147–163.

39. Nagaoka, S., Murata, S., Kimura, K. Mori, Hojo, K. Antimicrobial activity of sodium citrate against *Streptococcus pneumoniae* and several oral bacteria. Lett. Appl. Micro. November 2010; 51 (5): 546–551.

40. Post, F.J., Krishnamurty, G.B., Flanagan, M.D. Influence of sodium hexametaphosphate on selected bacteria. *Appl. Microbiol.* 1963; 11 (5): 430–435.

41. Yamaguchi, N. Ishidoshiro, A., Yoshida, Y., Saika, T., Senda, S., Nasu, M. Development of an adhesive sheet for directing counting of bacteria on solid surfaces. *J. Microbiol. Meth.* 2003; 53 (3): 405–410. doi: 10.1016/S0167-7012(02)00246-4.

42. Carpentier, B. Sanitary quality of meat chopping board surfaces: a bibliographical study. *Food Microbiol.* 1997; 14 (1): 31–37.

43. Moore, G., Griffth, C. A comparison of surface sampling methods for detecting coliforms on food contact surfaces. *Food Microbiol.* 2002; 19 (1): 64–73.

44. Baron, E.J., Vaisanen, M.L., McTeague, M., Strong, A., Norman, D., Finegold, S.M. Comparison of the Accu-CultShure systems and a swab placed in a B-D Port-A-Cul tube for specimen collection and transport. *Clin. Infect. Dis. 16 (Suppl. 4).* 1993; S325–S327.

45. Book, I. Comparison of two transport systems for recovery of aerobic and anaerobic bacteria from abscesses. *J. Clin. Microbiol.* 1987; 25 (10): 2020–2022.

46. Citron, D.M., Warren, Y.A., Hudspeth, M.K., Golstein, E.J.C. 2000. Survival of aerobic and anaerobic bacteria in purulent clinical specimens maintained in the Copan Venturi Transystem and Becton Dickinson Port-A-Cul transport systems. *J. Clin. Microbiol.* 2000; 38 (2): 892–894.

47. Hindiyeh, M., Acevedo, V., Carroll., K.C. Comparison of three transport systems (Starplex StarSwabII, the new Coapn Vi-Pak Amies Agar gel collection and transport swabs, and BBL Port-A-Cul) for maintenance of anaerobic and fastidious aerobic organisms. *J. Clin. Microbiol.* 2001; 39 (1): 377–380.

48. Human, R.P., Jones, G.A. Evaluation of swab transport systems against a published standard. *J. Clin. Pathol.* 2004; 57 (7): 762–763.

49. Perry, J.L. Assessment of swab transport systems for aerobic and anaerobic organism recovery. *J. Clin. Microbiol.* 1997; 35 (5): 1269–1271.

50. Roelofsen, E., Van Leeuwen, M., Meijer-Secvers, G.J. Wilkinson, M.H.F., Deggener, J.E. Evaluation of the effects of storage in two different swab fabrics and under three different transport conditions on recovery of aerobic and anaerobic bacteria. *J. Clin. Microbiol.* 1999; 37 (9): 3041–3043.

51. Rosa-Fraile, M., Camacho-Munoz, E., Rodriquez-Granger, J. Liebaba-Marlos. Specimen storage in transport medium and detection of group B streptococci by culture. *J. Clin. Microbiol.* 2005; 43 (2): 928–930.

52. Stoner, K.A., Rabe, L.K., Hillier, S.L. Effect of transport time, temperature, and concentration on the survival of group B streptococci in Ames transport medium. *J. Clin. Microbiol.* 2004; 42 (11): 5385–5387.

53. Teese, N., Henessey, D., Pearce, C., Kelly, N., Garland, D.S.G. Screening protocols for group B streptococcus: are transport media appropriate? *Infect. Dis. Obstet. Gynecol.* 2003; 11 (4): 199–202.

54. Van Rensburg, E., Du Preez, J.C., Kilian, S.G. Influence of the growth phase and culture medium on the survival of *Mannheimia haemolytica* during storage at different temperatures. *J. Appl. Microbiol.* 2004; 96 (1): 154–161.

55. Soner, K.A., Rabe, L.K., Austin, M.N., Meyn, L.A., Hillier, S.L. Quantitative survival of aerobic and anaerobic microorganisms in Port-A-Cul and Copan Transport Systems. *J. Clinic. Micro.* 2008; 46 (8): 2739–2744.

56. Perez-Rodriguez, F., Valero, A., Carrasco, E., Garcia, R.M., Zurera, G. Understanding and modeling bacterial transfer to foods: a review. *Trends Food Sci. Technol.* 2008; 19 (3): 131–144.

57. Kyriakides, A.L., Cosetllo, S.M., Doyle, G., Easter, M.C., Johnson, I. Rapid hygiene monitoring using ATP bioluminescence. In: Bioluminescence and Chemiluminescence: Current Status. (Stanley, P.E., Kricka, L.J., eds.). Chichester, Wiley, 1991: 519–522.

58. Seeger, K., Griffiths, M.W. Adenosine triphosphate bioluminescence for hygiene monitoring in health care institutions. *J. Food Prot.* 1994; 57 (6): 509–512.

59. Bautista, D.A., McIntyre, I., Laleye, L., Griffiths, M.W. The application of ATP bioluminescence for the assessment of milk quality and factory hygiene. *J. Rapid Meth. Auto. Microbiol.* 1996; 1 (3): 179–193.

60. Griffith, C.J., Davidson, C.A., Peters, A.C., Fielding, L.M. Towards a strategic cleaning assessment programme: hygiene monitoring and ATP luminometry, an options appraisal. *Food Sci. Technol. Today.* 1997; 11 (1): 15–24.

61. Poulis, J.A., dePijer, M., Mossel, D.A.A., Dekkers, PPhA. Assessment of cleaning and disinfection in the food industry with the rapid ATP-bioluminescence technique combined with the tissue fluid contamination test and a conventional microbiological method. *Int. J. Food Microbiol.* 1993; 20 (2): 109–116.

62. ISO 29621:2017 Cosmetics – Microbiology – Guidelines for the risk assessment and identification of microbiologically low-risk products, ISO, Geneva, Switzerland.

63. U.S. Food & Drug Administration. 1997. HAACP Principles and Application Guidelines. www.fda.gov/Food/GuidanceRegulation/HACCP/ucm2006801.htm (Updated 2001).
64. Van Scothorst. M.A., Simple Guide to Understanding and Applying the Hazard Analysis and Critical Control Point. ILSI Press, Washington, D.C., 2004.
65. World Health Organization. WHO Technical Report Series. No. 908. Annex 7. Application of Hazard Analysis and Critical Control Point (HACCP) Methodology to pharmaceuticals. 2003.
66. PDA Technical Report # 70. Fundamentals of cleaning and disinfection programs for aseptic manufacturing facilities. Parenteral Drug Association, Bethesda, Md., 2015.

10

Hazard Analysis and Critical Control Point (HACCP) Protocols in Cosmetic Microbiology

Laura M. Clemens and Harry L. Schubert

Introduction

Protocols for microbiological monitoring and control of manufacturing have been established for categories of products regulated by the U.S. Food and Drug Administration (FDA). They are designated the hazard analysis and critical control point (HACCP) protocols (1). Considerable documentation describes appropriate environmental sampling and control of manufacturing systems for drugs (2,3), but cosmetics are not as precisely regulated as foods and drugs. Although guidelines covering cosmetic manufacture exist (4), they do not include functional details for protocols specific to the cosmetics industry. Such details are essential because cosmetics indeed constitute the most unique group of consumer products.

Each cosmetic product has up to hundreds of ingredients combined precisely; manufacture may involve various types of chemical reactions and fermentations conducted at different geographic locations. Although they are not intended to be sterile, cosmetic manufacturing systems involve production demands unrivaled by other categories of consumer products. The unique product forms and packages distinct to cosmetic products are often accompanied by implements (e.g., applicators) of various conformations and compositions. Cosmetic products are distributed and marketed without refrigeration or shelf-life controls. Finally, depending on purpose, they are applied by consumers to all body surfaces and orifices.

Clearly, protocols for foods and drugs are insufficient to serve the cosmetics industry. It is the purpose of this discussion to present new HACCP concepts tailored specifically to serve the cosmetics industry.

What are HACCP protocols? Hazard analysis critical control point is a program for monitoring manufacturing processes to identify potential microbial contamination hazards and ensure the integrity of overall systems. This monitoring program measures the health of a system in its operational entirety and encompasses equipment design, microbiological control procedures, microbiological awareness of operators, operational training, product susceptibility, plant and equipment maintenance, processing parameters, and material flows.

All areas must be in microbiological control to sustain the integrity of the system and prevent microbial contamination. Identifying the hazards and determining the critical control points in order to manage the hazards will be the focus areas of this chapter. A critical control point can be described as any point at which a production control can be applied to minimize, eliminate, or control a hazard. For successful implementation of a HACCP program, operational involvement is key and the program must be integrated among all operations. The seven basic steps to implement a HACCP program are:

1. Conduct an assessment to determine hazards and identify preventative measures to minimize or eliminate each hazard.
2. Identify all critical control points.
3. Establish critical limits for each control point.
4. Establish an ongoing monitoring program.
5. Establish corrective action when a critical control point is outside predetermined limits.
6. Establish a documentation system.
7. Establish an ongoing system to re-evaluate the program and/or verify control.

Why Apply HACCP to Cosmetics?

The ultimate benefit of implementing HAACP is monetary because the program serves as a primary means to avoid microbiological contamination problems that can bring a business to a screeching halt. The cost of a product contamination can be extreme and run well into tens of millions of dollars. Brands have been lost, images tarnished, and manufacturing locations closed as results of product contamination incidents. Potential cost elements include product loss, scrapping costs, and loss of production during the plant operations organization attempts to recover.

Another issue is significant impact on customer service. Most major microbial contamination incidents have involved exposure of an organism to a product preservative system and resistance by the organism as it becomes adapted over time after repeated exposures to a preservative typically in a diluted state. As illustrated in Table 10.1, the ideal state of operation is in the first quadrant where a manufacturer proactively addresses any breaks or trends in integrity. HACCP is a way to maintain an operation in the ideal state of the first quadrant. Product quality is assured by information from the HAACP system followed by confirmation via finished product testing (quality control).

If operations are consistent with the parameters of the second or third quadrant, intervention is a necessity. In the second quadrant, substantial numbers of microbes are present but do not survive due to process controls and product preservation. Most major contaminations of cosmetic products might occur because entry into the third quadrant may not have been detected initially due to certain quality control method parameters (e.g., test sensitivity, preservative neutralization, or sampling frequency) coupled with low microbial numbers. However, once low numbers become detectable, almost any method will recover the organism if it can survive in the product because neutralization effectiveness will not be a barrier to recovery. Under these conditions and with transition into the fourth quadrant, product quality is determined only by finished product testing (quality control).

Areas to be assessed for hazards should include the following at a minimum.

TABLE 10.1

Cycle for building microbial resistance

Ancillary Systems	Formulations	Production Systems
Water system	Raw materials	Hold tanks
Environmental air system	Premixes or intermediates	Delivery and/or transfer lines
Compressed air system	Finished formulations	Processing tanks
Steam system		Bulk storage
Clean-in-place (CIP) system		Packing transfer systems
Wastewater removal system		Filling process systems

Wastewater Removal and CIP Systems

Wastewater removal systems and clean-in-place (CIP) systems are not normally considered when a HACCP program is established, but these can contribute greatly to the integrity of an overall production system and should be evaluated.

Wastewater removal systems pose hazards because they usually maintain populations of organisms adapted to certain concentrations of the preservative systems used at a site. One needs to consider whether to eliminate, kill, or contain organisms when dealing with wastewater removal systems to control operational exposure of a potentially resistant strain. System control must include drain lines from systems, sumps, and associated lines. Control of this ancillary system is critical.

Another factor rarely considered as a risk to microbiological quality is a CIP system by which stand-alone components maintain and deliver cleaning or sanitization medium. These systems are typically seen as tools for cleaning and sanitizing and not as potential hazards or sources of inoculation. Sanitary design may appear as less of a priority; drainability is not seen as a necessity because most systems use some type of cleaning chemical thought to be hostile.

CIP systems can very quickly become inoculation sources rather than means of effective cleaning and sanitization. For this reason, the design and management of these systems can be even more critical than the process systems they support. Inoculation occurs because production systems often remain idle between uses and the last fluid contained is typically purified water. Because such systems are non-drainable and present the risk of building biofilms, they can become ideal sources of organisms adapted to the cleaning and sanitizing media and also to product preservative systems. These biofilms aid the development of resistance to cleaning agents and continue to build protective shields into the process systems they are intended to clean.

Selecting Critical Control Points

In considering the selection of critical control points for a HACCP protocol, validation coupled with assessment (formulation, equipment, process flow) is the key to determining the points within a system and should be based on review of the following factors:

- Areas of low turbulence
- Poor equipment design
- Undrainable sites
- Areas of poor heat penetration (where heat is used for sanitization)
- Human intervention sites
- Low usage or idle pathways.

Parameters of an Effective HACCP Program

Any parameter that directly controls the integrity of the system should be the subject of monitoring and measurement. Examples include temperature of water in hot water storage tanks, ozone concentrations in cold water storage tanks, pH levels of product intermediates, moisture of raw materials, chemical concentrations of sanitizing solutions, equipment surface temperatures during heat sanitization, and the presence of diluted formulation in dead legs.

Not all parameters that can contribute to the control of systems are easy to measure, but they still warrant consideration, for example, execution of process steps that have microbial control significance, maintenance of equipment ("O" ring and gasket replacement), housekeeping, and so on. All physical measurements should be supported with biological monitoring throughout a system to verify that the control parameters are indeed effectively controlling microbiological quality.

Biological examination of systems can involve two approaches based on HACCP objectives:

1. *Maximize product volume without complete neutralization of the formulation.* The objective is to recover organisms capable of surviving in system and product. Basically, this step is intended to

prevent release of product with a potentially adapted organism that could subsequently proliferate in the marketplace.

2. *Optimize product volume to achieve complete neutralization.* The objective is to recover stressed organisms and/or organisms that cannot survive in product. This approach prevents release of product with a non-adapted organism and signals and alerts manufacturing personnel of a potential compromise of the microbial integrity of a system.

In the context of the cycle-for-building resistance diagram (Table 10.1), the first approach will typically result in a window of time of initial contamination during which a product may meet specification because the number of microbes is below the limit of detection determined by typical methods. Upon reanalysis, the product may fail to meet specifications if organisms capable of surviving and growing in the product have had time to grow to detectable levels. Previously tested clean samples may now be confirmed as contaminated. Unfortunately, the saleable product that enjoyed the window of low microbial detection will be typically out on the market, placing both consumers and the manufacturer at risk. The power of the second HACCP approach will eliminate this scenario.

With the second approach, low levels of organisms can be detected before resistance to the product preservative system is established. The source of contamination can be addressed and the risk eliminated. The cycle of resistance will be broken and operations can be maintained in a preventative versus reactive mode. The ultimate result is that both the consumer and the manufacturer are protected against contamination. This approach is consistent with the preventative strategies behind HACCP programs.

When selecting biological sites for monitoring, other areas to be considered include all sites where diluted product and/or preservative is present, areas surrounding functional pieces of equipment such as heat exchangers containing chilled water that can serve as potential sources of contamination, and all other conditions deemed critical based on the principles listed previously. Types of biological samples range from raw materials, product intermediates, final formulations, and cleaning solutions to swabs and/or equipment rinses. Most effective HACCP programs cover a combination of all these types of samples. Swab samples offer the benefits of testing localized areas considered high risk and offer limited surface area accessible to swabbing. Rinse samples offer greater surface area contact, but can dilute a localized contamination source simply by the volume of water passing through the system or subsystem.

Frequency of measurement should be based on the significance of the control point and reflect the executional frequency and control of any related procedure. For example, in a purified water distribution system, microbial control may consist of maintaining 82°C temperatures at all points via recirculation. In this case, monitoring the ongoing temperature and installing alarms to detect malfunctions (temperature drops and/or pump outages) coupled with minimal microbial content monitoring would be appropriate.

If sanitization of a certain piece of equipment is a requirement, the potential monitoring could constitute measurement of microbial contents at all critical points by rotating through them during the sanitization production window. Specific monitoring may be warranted after major maintenance or construction to verify that no microbiological integrity break of the system occurred when the work was carried out.

Critical limits for each control point must be established through assessment and validation data. Once limits are set, an ongoing monitoring program for a continuous determination of control is established and may be modified subsequently if necessary as a function of ongoing observations and change controls. The HACCP program thus becomes a dynamic, data-based system.

A documentation process should be in place to track generated data, aid decision making, allow corrective action, and provide other information relevant to the HACCP program. The HACCP program should also be re-evaluated on an ongoing basis to maintain effectiveness and verify that the systems are under control.

Common manufacturing issues and potential approaches to eliminate or minimize microbiological risk hazards focus on the following areas.

Formulation susceptibility:
- Makes susceptible premix and intermediate materials inherently hostile by maintaining extreme pH levels, lowering water activity, moving preservative additions upstream in the manufacturing process, adding preservatives to premixes and intermediates.

- Maximizes process temperatures of premixes and intermediates.
- Optimizes sanitary equipment design.
- Increases sanitization frequency.

Equipment:
- Optimizes sanitary equipment design and/or eliminates unnecessary equipment or flow paths.
- Optimizes construction materials (chemical or heat tolerance for exposure time required for biological control).
- Increases sanitization time and/or frequency.

Process flow:
- Works toward one common flow path.
- Manages idle equipment and flow paths.
- Plans for major maintenance and/or construction.

Losses Preventable via an Effective HACCP Program

Tri-Blender Operation

A tri-blender is a device that incorporates powders into a liquid product stream using a high-shear mixer. It is much more efficient in dispersing materials than an agitator in a standard mixing tank. The device is particularly useful for incorporation of gelling and suspending agents.

In the sample scenario, powder was introduced through a hopper into a tri-blender and hot purified ingredient water was used to incorporate the powder into the batch. The tri-blender flow path was tied into the recirculation line of the mix tank and retained residual powder diluted in purified water until the next batch of product was produced through this flow path.

The HACCP program identified this as a hazard. The incoming water temperature was a critical control point and the flow path was monitored biologically during normal production and after the longest planned downtime to represent the worst case scenario. This monitoring occurred during the week and then immediately on Monday morning after a prolonged weekend of downtime. The biological monitoring detected sporadic recovery of low levels of *Burkholderia cepacia* on Monday mornings. The hazardous conditions present were:

1. The water temperature could be maintained only prior to the addition and would drop in the tri-blender flow path when the device sat idle.
2. The combination of the residual powder and purified water provided a suitable environment for organisms to grow. This became an inoculation source within the process.
3. The *Burkholderia cepacia* organism acquires resistance very easily and is well known as the causative microbial agent involved in cosmetic product recalls.

The hazard was eliminated by recirculating the final preserved formulation back through the tri-blender pathway to destroy any residual powder diluted in purified water that accumulated when the system was idle. The recirculation step became part of the batch process and was implemented every time a batch was produced.

Retention of Diluted Product in Low-Point Strainer

For pump protection, a basket strainer was located on a transfer line. The basket strainer was the low point of the transfer line and consisted of a ball valve on the bottom of the strainer. The cleaning and sanitization procedure was dependent on the manual cycling of this ball valve.

The filling procedure consisted of the manual purging of product through the low point until full strength product had filled the low-point strainer. The HACCP program identified this as a hazard. The low point was a critical control factor for the operation. It was monitored visually for cleaning rinse water after each cleaning, for temperature during each sanitization, for dilution in the purged product samples, and all these observations were carried out manually through the sanitization window. The visual inspection of the purged product sporadically revealed dilution indicating failure during the filling procedure to purge through the low point valve manually. The hazardous conditions present were:

1. The ball valve was not sanitary and was considered high risk due to its design.
2. The effectiveness of cleaning and sanitization depended on manual intervention by the operator.
3. The elimination of trapped diluted product was dependent on manual intervention by the operator during the purging procedure. The environment allowed organisms to adapt or build resistance to the preservative system.

Hazards were eliminated by the following actions:

1. Short term:
   a. Visual inspections of the purged product after filling the transfer line increased in frequency.
   b. Procedural reviews involved the entire team.
   c. Greater accountability was implemented.
2. Long term:
   a. An in-line strainer was installed.
   b. The low point ball valve was replaced with a more sanitary butterfly valve.
   c. Cleaning, sanitization, and purging procedures were automated to eliminate the need for manual intervention.

Susceptible Premix Operation

Two types of vitamins were mixed with purified water in a premix tank prior to the transfer to the final mix tank. The final formulation became heavily contaminated with *Burkholderia cepacia* and the loss to the company was estimated at $350,000 based on scrapped batches and production time lost while decisions about future production were made. The hazardous conditions present but not identified were:

1. The premix formulation was highly susceptible: the combination of vitamins and water allowed microbial growth.
2. Equipment design was not sanitary for this type of application.
3. The sanitization frequency was inadequate based on the susceptibility of the premix.
4. The premix system was not subjected to biological monitoring to ensure that the overall integrity of the system was maintained.

The hazard was eliminated by process modification. The manufacturing process that caused susceptibility of the vitamin premix to microbial growth was eliminated and the vitamins were added directly to the final mix tank.

Inoculating CIP System and Multiple Processing Flow Paths

A CIP system was utilized to introduce purified water into a process system for purposes of cleaning and sanitization. The CIP system was not drainable, not sanitary, and not monitored for integrity against microorganisms during use. The system became heavily contaminated and was inoculating the process system during cleaning and sanitization.

The process system included multiple flow paths that were not drainable and the cleaning procedure was not effective because diluted formulation was retained within some of the pathways. This provided an environment for *Burkholderia cepacia* organisms to adapt to the final product formula. The contamination resulted in a $20 million loss to the company based on the following factors:

- Packed product containing contamination had to be scrapped.
- A national recall covered product that may have been manufactured during the window of contamination.
- Three contract packing sites were contaminated by materials from the supplying manufacturing site.
- The extent of clean-up to remove the adapted organism from the supplying sites and contract packing sites was massive. Equipment had to be replaced, caustic washes had to be performed, gaskets and other items had to be replaced.
- Equipment at the contract packers' sites was upgraded to sanitary design.
- Moist heat sanitization capability was installed at contract packers' sites.
- The manufacturer paid to have the three contract packing systems put on hold status so that they could start up as soon as the plant sourcing the product was ready.
- The manufacturer lost revenue from more than 30 days of production.
- Product reformulation was required; the manufacturer was out of stock for over 30 days.
- Manufacturing was moved to another site where the adapted organism was not present.

The hazardous conditions that were not identified were as follows:

1. The CIP system was not designed to be sanitary and/or drainable.
2. The CIP system was not sanitized prior to use on the process system; it was not managed via heat and/or recirculation processes that would have maintained the microintegrity of the system when not in use.
3. The cleaning procedure used for the process system was inadequate.
4. Multiple flow paths were not managed when idle and contained diluted product, thus providing an environment in which organisms could adapt.
5. No biological monitoring of the CIP system, the process, or the bulk product was conducted; such monitoring would have ensured acceptable microbial levels prior to packing.

Hazards were eliminated by taking the following actions:

1. Moving production to another site.
2. Designing a sanitary system without multiple flow paths.
3. Implementing a cleaning and sanitization procedure that was effective.
4. Eliminating the need for a separate CIP system.
5. Eliminating dilute product environment within the process.

Conclusion

Cosmetic products are unique in the diversity of formulations, forms, packaging, distribution, and consumer use. Importantly, they are also unique in microbiological risks associated with their manufacture and an effective HACCP program will pay for itself in maintaining control of these risks. Just as preservation measures are intended to cover the life of a product, HACCP programs are perpetual and sustained during active manufacturing and should continue when equipment is idle. With effectively preserved materials, cosmetic HACCP programs provide the ultimate ways to provide microbial quality assurance.

REFERENCES

1. Center for Food Safety and Applied Nutrition, U.S. Food and Drug Administration, HACCP: A State-of-the-Art Approach to Food Safety, 2001, www.cfsan.fda.gov/~lrd/bghaccp.html.
2. Reich, R.R., Miller, M.J., and Reich, H., Developing a viable environmental monitoring program for nonsterile pharmaceutical operations, *Pharm. Technol.*, 27 (3), 92, 2003.
3. Parenteral Drug Association, Fundamentals of an environmental monitoring program, Technical Report 13, Revised, PDA J. Pharm. Sci. Technol., 55 (1), 19. 2001.
4. Center for Food Safety and Applied Nutrition, U.S. Food and Drug Administration, Cosmetic Good Manufacturing Practice Guidelines, 2001, www.cfsan.fda.gov/~dms/cos-gmp.html.

11

Manufacturing Microbiology

A View of the Future

Neil J. Lewis

Introduction

Manufacturing microbiology is fast approaching one of those famous decision points that we are all familiar with from various political and sporting contests. *Decision point* is an expression which is often overused and applied to relatively simple or instinctive choices which must be made during normal life and work. In the case of manufacturing microbiology, the expression may, for the first time, be used correctly and may even be significantly and consistently understated.

The reason for this is simply the fact that for years manufacturing microbiology has been a concept or an idea which has been proposed, discussed and written about, but in reality there has been little motivation or justification from a commercial or a product quality perspective to invest the time and expertise required for the implementation of necessary systems, equipment and training.

For many years, cosmetic products were formulated with high levels of preservatives, with the often-stated intention to enhance and protect consumer's beauty. This not only led to microbiological robustness in use, but indirectly these formulations resulted in relative low levels of manufacturing-induced contamination, even from poorly designed high risk systems or operations. The infrequent number of problems and their relatively small scale were often used as a justification/rationale for the lack of a need for large-scale investment in specific manufacturing control systems, especially in times when capital expenditure or operating costs needed to be reduced or tightly controlled.

From a short-term business perspective, this may well have been an appropriate approach, though it did little to move manufacturing microbiology forward and resulted in a degree of scientific stagnation where the methods and technologies in use at the start of the new century were very similar to those that had been developed in the 1960s and 1970s. It could also be argued that some of this stagnation was also due to a certain amount of reluctance from the microbiological community to move away from some of the classical techniques they were originally trained in. This may be due in part to the perceived additional work, specifications, validation and training that some of the new methodologies would require when there was no visible support or incentive from the business.

The regulators must also take some responsibility for the lack of progress in the development of manufacturing microbiology, in that regulations such as the EU cosmetics directives (1), ISO 22716 (2) or FDA

(Food and Drug Administration) Draft Cosmetic GMPs (Good Manufacturing Practices) (3) are very generic in terms of the microbiological requirements and methodology which does little to encourage innovation or change. However, the real issue came from the long-term and incorrect perception within the industry that the regulators would be unwilling to accept new technologies or methodologies. This often-repeated excuse, along with and a general unwillingness to be the first, has helped reinforce the lack of progress and adoption of new ideas. It may be a recent recognition of this issue that has led to most regulatory bodies implement or reinvigorate their innovation departments, specifically targeted at creating an open door and encouragement for manufacturing companies and suppliers to discuss and present new techniques, equipment and systems for review.

Finally, it must be recognized that the development of novel science and application of alternate sciences to the field of practical microbiological detection, enumeration, and identification has been limited. This is not a reflection on the lack of innovation within the microbiological field, but simply that there has been little reason or incentive for companies to innovate and design practical industry applications without a clear and willing market.

Many will dispute the conclusions mentioned and, will probably argue that microbiology and manufacturing have made significant progress over the past few years in significantly reducing the risks to the consumer. This may very well be true in terms of optimizing and improving the existing systems. We need to recognize that the microbiological monitoring and control systems currently in use depend on methodologies that were first developed over 100 years ago, whereas the manufacturing methodologies have been advancing steadily to the point where it is now possible, in some cases, to 3D print the complete product eliminating the entire traditional making and packing systems. If microbiology and microbiological methods want to keep pace with the rapid development of manufacturing systems, then there is an overwhelming need for these methods to be radically revised, changed, eliminated or completely replaced, along with some of the traditional thinking, risk analysis and management and opinions which have limited this industry for several years.

The Changing Business Demands/Business Model—Speed

We must recognize that both the business model and the consumer needs, for cosmetic products have been changing significantly over the past 20 years. Traditionally companies would develop and market new products at specific times through the year to coincide with the major holidays or fashion changes. These products would be produced to sales forecasts, stored in a warehouse and shipped to the market as orders were received. Product which was not shipped was either discounted or discarded and destroyed when the new season's products were produced. This system has grown up over many years and was as efficient as the logistical and informational flow would permit. When looked at from today's point of view, this system was both inefficient and unsustainable in the long term. Interestingly, the consumer of the time was happy to accept these limitations, or it may be that they did not know that other options were possible, so without clearly defined consumer demands or requests there was very little reason to change or modify the existing business models, other than for cost saving or efficiency.

The situation today is significantly different; today's consumers are much more experimental and more demanding; they are less prepared to wait for the next season's colors or products; brand loyalty or product loyalty is significantly reduced; and they are used to having their needs met in a short space of time. This change in consumer needs has coincided, or maybe has been driven, by the improvement in logistical capability that manufacturing control systems such as SAP® and other MRP 2 systems have provided. In addition, the commercial pressures on supermarkets and stores has pushed them to try and find ways to reduce costs and inventory while still meeting the consumer needs. The result of these different factors has been the development and widespread implementation of produce to demand systems, which has had and will continue to have a profound effect on the microbiological control systems in manufacturing.

If we look at produce to demand systems, they have several components which at first sight may not be fully compatible with the demands and requirements of microbiological testing control. The basic concept of produce to demand is that if a store or supermarket sells a product today, the manufacturer will replace the product tomorrow. This need for rapid reaction means that the manufacturer must either keep significant quantities of the product in inventory to be able to resupply the vendor or have a flexible manufacturing system which allows them to adjust their production schedule to fulfill the customers' demands for products. Keeping significant amounts of inventory near the market is both expensive and difficult, which essentially drives manufacturing sites to be more agile and flexible in their production, planning and execution.

This is where the potential conflict between manufacturing and microbiological control comes together, in that traditional microbiological testing and monitoring usually has incubation periods of 3–5 days, which is inconsistent with the ability to respond rapidly to the market demands. So, the business has a choice to make: does it delay the resupply and potentially lose sales, or does it take the risk of assuming that the product is not microbiologically contaminated and ship to the consumer, neither option is a palatable outcome for the manufacturing operation.

Rapid microbiological methods, which have developed over the past decade or so, have been targeted at trying to resolve this dilemma and provide some means of reassuring the microbiological quality of the product. The application and use of such methods will be discussed later in the chapter, but it must be recognized that the rapid methods, which are currently widely available, usually deliver results in 12–24 hours which is nowhere near the speed demanded by the new consumer requirements.

This contradiction also applies to the receipt and testing of raw materials and packaging. The flexible manufacturing systems also require either extensive inventories of starting materials for the process and packing, which can be expensive to maintain, or very responsive supply chains which allow the materials to be delivered quickly when required. Once again, the need for microbiological control of these materials, which are one of the most common sources of contamination, will be seen as reducing the responsiveness of any supply chain.

These choices are also being limited, by the recent trends in the industry, to reduce inventories significantly, both of finished products and materials in order to release the cash, which is routinely tied up in the purchase and storage of these materials, to provide additional sources of investment of cash flow. This can result in the microbiological requirements and systems, particularly those systems which have been in place for several years, being caught up in the cost, inventory, responsiveness squeeze, which has been a feature of many operations in the current business climate.

This pressure on microbiological systems can also extend into the actual manufacturing operations, where the change in the manufacturing strategies result in significantly shorter, and more frequent production runs. This change results in additional microbiological risk being placed on the systems in terms of more frequent changeovers, resulting in a greater need to clean and sanitize the equipment, as well as introducing a higher level of risk from the increased human interaction with the product and the equipment.

Most manufacturing sites will have usually developed the necessary procedures to accomplish cleaning and sanitization effectively. The issue is that these procedures were not designed to be carried out under the time pressure or frequency which the new business model requires. It is this time pressure which presents the additional risk of contamination or adulteration, as well as prompting manufacturers to either challenge the current processes or ask for better and faster ways to clean the equipment.

The common operational solution to this situation is to challenge either the fundamental need for cleaning and sanitization, usually based on the observed absence of any contamination issues over a specified period, or to simply question the frequency of application. Both options are very easy to suggest as on the surface they are easy to implement and do not require a great deal of investment. They do, however, reflect a fundamental lack of understanding of the role of cleaning and sanitization in the microbiological control program. The cleaning and sanitization program is the only effective preventative controls that can be employed within the manufacturing operations, and just like any other preventative maintenance program, delaying or modifying the frequency can increase the risk of microbiological failure within the system.

Relatively little work has been done over the past 25 years to provide or implement faster methods of cleaning equipment or alternative means of sanitization, which would be necessary to meet the demands of speed and agility which are being placed on the manufacturing system. Once again, the short-term financial view restricts the need for innovation in this area, the time and effort needed to develop the new methods and the potentially more expensive chemicals that could be used instead of water. They are not seen to be productive investments as they are not transparent the benefits which could be delivered to the business operating strategy. In addition, the recent focus that companies have placed on having sustainable operations, both as a part of global citizenship and as a consumer acceptance strategy, means that there is a significant emphasis on reducing water and energy consumption, which are the bedrocks of any effective cleaning and sanitization programs. So just as with the manufacturing operations discussed earlier, there is a three-way conflict: to bring for more frequent changeovers, to introduce more sustainable procedures and to reduce further operating costs. All of which place considerable pressure on the microbiological assurance systems required to satisfy the consumer expectations for clean product. The opportunities and need for improved or alternative cleaning and sanitization strategies in the new business model are discussed later in the chapter.

Changing purchase models have also had an impact on the need for a different microbiological control model; the advent of e-commerce and direct shipment to the consumer has and will have a profound effect on how we think about and implement effective microbiological control. E-commerce, with its ability to customize products for the individual, will require the ability to be confident in the quality of an individual unit versus testing and evaluating several samples to assess a much larger batch. This is going to put much more emphasis on the environment, materials and process rather than the sample and test Quality Control approach which many companies are familiar with.

E-commerce could also have a beneficial effect in simplifying the packaging requirements for the manufacturing systems. In the future if most consumer shopping is done online, there will be no need for elaborate and eye-catching packaging currently used in the supermarkets and stores. Future consumers will select from to the product photographs and simulations which will allow the actual consumer unit to be simplified to allow for easy shipment. This simplification could also bring with it the opportunity to have microbiological controls such as restricting direct access to the product, single use dosing systems or unit dose products.

Along with the changing manufacturing requirements, reducing inventories, frequent changeovers and e-commerce a significant transformation that has to be faced is the consumer awareness brought about by the advent of social media. Many companies are already taking advantage of the opportunities for advertising, product trial and sampling offered by Facebook, Twitter, You Tube and so on. Interestingly, they may not have fully realized how the same global media may work against them, specifically the implications or impact that social media could have when there are issues with a product, which may,

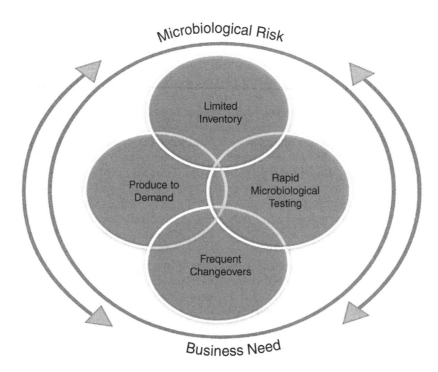

FIGURE 11.1 Microbiological risks and manufacturing requirements.

in the end, drive companies to tighten their specification and control systems to assure the quality and integrity of their products. No company or brand is going to want to have a picture of moldy or degraded product splashed across social media, given the negative impact this can have on a global scale. The historical precedent for such events would show that there is a subsequent reaction to tighten review specifications or systems to reassure the consumer base driven by the industry or the regulators.

So, in summary (Figure 11.1), we face a future with changing business patterns, different consumer practices, conflicting priorities, significantly increased consumer awareness though social media, reducing preservatives, sustainability requirements and an ever present, if not increasing (through bacterial adaptation), risk of contamination. Therefore, if companies are going to remain and become successful in the coming years, it is going to require a significant change in the systems, technology of the microbiological control systems and most importantly the mindset of the generally conservative risk-averse microbiologists.

Microbiological Quality by Design

It is clear that the current microbiological systems are not going to be sufficient for the future demands of the personal care industry, and if companies are to succeed in the coming years, they will have to search out and adapt new technologies or new concepts to their products and processes. In simple terms, the Micro Daily Management systems and programs of the future will need to be fundamentally different from those of today. It will not be sufficient to allow the current programs to evolve over time, to encompass whatever new technology arrives on the market, as this will both be too slow to be effective and is unlikely to meet the overall needs in the end. There will arise a need to develop and design alternate control strategies, which are more compatible with the changing needs of the business.

As with any quality and operating system, the most effective applications are those that are well thought through in their design and implementation. This applies equally to the development of microbiological control systems in the manufacturing, organizations that must carefully consider the approach that not only fits with their business strategy, but also must possesses the capability both in terms of facilities and people to be able to implement. These control strategies will also have to be sufficiently flexible to react appropriately to the development of new technology, regulations and products which will occur in the next 5–10 years.

These operating strategies are likely to fall into the following categories:

- Test faster—An evolution of the current control system based on reaction to rapid microbiological testing methods.
- Eliminate finished product testing—The implementation of microbiological process control and parametric release.
- Remove the need for testing—Process and packing modifications which eliminate the microbiological risks.

All three of these options will require the development, implementation and adoption of a range of new technologies and approaches to be fully effective and practical in meeting the changing needs of the personal care business needs.

Test Faster—The Use of Rapid Microbiological Test Methods

Over the past 20 years or so, there has been a proliferation of rapid microbiological test methods, all aimed at reducing the prolonged incubation period of the traditional test methods, to allow faster release of products and materials and consequently to reduce the overall manufacturing risk. Most currently available rapid methods look to reduce the incubation period by finding an alternate method of detecting or visualizing bacterial growth. The actual test method and technology are discussed at length in technical publications and other chapters of this book, so they will not be repeated here; we will review the benefits and limitations of these technologies in relation to manufacturing microbiological strategy. The intention will be to look at the current common applications of the technology, rather than discuss a specific company, methodology or equipment.

1. **Enhanced visualization methods**—These methods, such as the Growth Direct (Rapid Micro Biosystems; Bedford, MA) or Evisight system (Biomerieux; Marcy L'Etoile, France), utilize advanced optics and computer-aided detection to discover the growth of microorganisms at a much earlier time point than the human eye. The methods have been successfully introduced, applied and validated to products across a range of industries, but as with most of the rapid methods, there are some potential limitations, in this case in terms of colored/particulate materials or slow-growing organisms. In terms of applicability to the needs of the manufacturing systems, the reduced incubation time (approx. 12–24 hours) is an advantage over traditional methods, but it is questionable if this time saving is sufficient to fully meet the potential future challenges, as even a 12-hour testing period would still cause significant delays and costs from demurrage for starting materials, and would still require significant storage space for finished product quarantine or prevent immediate shipment to the customers. The capital cost of these instruments can be relatively high and they also may require specific disposables, which can make the cost per test higher than the traditional methods.

2. **ATP** (adenosine triphosphate) **detection**—Methods such as Celsis (Charles River Laboratories; Wilmington, MA) system rely on the detection of bacterial ATP or ATP enzyme reactions to indicate the presence of microorganisms. These are primarily screening methods that allow the rapid confirmation of the absence any contamination in the product, simplifying the release of product to the market. Organizations are sometimes uncomfortable or unwilling to use a test which simply gives pass/fail results; instead, they prefer to have a numerical value which can be compared (or sometimes debated) against a specification which in many cases lacks a sound technical rationale. In addition, these tests generally require the use of an enrichment broth which increases the sensitivity of detection. This is often perceived as a significant drawback in the test, as it results in so-called false positives, which are detections which cannot be confirmed by subsequent plate count testing. This thinking is driven by the wish or need to demonstrate the equivalence of these new methods to the traditional "gold standard" plate count method, which reflects a profound lack of understanding of the limitations and inaccuracies of the plate count testing. Individuals who favor this point of view are missing one of the key benefits of this technology, which is the very early detection of the initiation of contamination within the system, which could be extremely useful in the future manufacturing microbiology systems.

   As with the visualizing systems described, the initial capital costs, together with the ongoing reagents, mean the cost per test can be 2–3 times the traditional tests, and the need for the enrichment of the sample means there is still a 12–24-hour delay in obtaining the test results with the consequential limitations to the manufacturing systems. There are some applications, such as those used in hygiene monitoring systems, that provide an instantaneous result which may point the way to the future of this type of methodology.

3. **Metabolism-indicating methods**—Systems such as Soleris (Neogen; Lansing, MI) and Greenlight (Mocon Inc.; Minneapolis, MN) utilize the products of microbial metabolism, O_2, CO_2 or pH changes, to rapidly detect the presence or absence of contamination. These methods could combine the ability to screen for contamination quickly and provide a quantitative assessment, but their application and implementation can be limited by the same wish to demonstrate equivalency with current methodology. As with the other methods discussed previously, these also rely on bacterial growth to work effectively. This means that in terms of suitability, for future manufacturing systems, the same limitations of time to obtain a result apply.

All three of these methodologies and the multiple systems they support have a fundamental deficiency in terms of the needs of future manufacturing microbiology, in that they require growth to be able to detect and enumerate the microorganisms. This not only takes time, which will be very limited in the future manufacturing environment, but will also be limited or impacted by the performance of the growth media, the effectiveness of the preservative neutralization and even the variability of the incubation temperatures.

This combination of time and potential inaccuracy will limit the benefits of such growth-based methods in a produce to demand environment.

The need for rapid testing and evaluation in the manufacturing systems of the future will therefore tend to focus on those methods which can give a result instantly or within a very short period. Some of the current methods may have the potential to fulfill this near instantaneous method needs. They are:

1. **Flow cytometry and solid phase laser cytometry**—These methods such as the Chemunex system (Biomerieux) and the Chemscan RDI system (Biomerieux) detect microbial cells in a flowing stream or on a solid matrix via the use of metabolic dyes to differentiate viable cells. This can provide very rapid evaluation of microbial content of the sample/product. This type of testing, as it counts microbial cells, does give a very rapid response to the sample and effectively convert microbiological testing to the speed of normal analytical testing. Capital, reagents, costs and degree of expertise to operate the equipment are similar to the other instruments described. A specific sample preparation is also required; a sample that combines incompatible materials may limit the scope to which this can be applied. Conceptually this type of methodology in terms of speed and applicability could, with an additional development to overcome some of the known issues, such as the accuracy of counting, fit more closely with the future needs.

   One key area which would need to be considered, for all the non-growth methods, is that a fundamental rethink of the product and material specification is a necessity. Currently, specifications are written to match the testing methodology; in traditional methods, where the result is a simple visible count multiplied by the dilution factor, the specifications are stated as less than a maximum number, generally as a factor of 10. With the non-growth methods, where we count individual cells, these specifications may not be appropriate or equivalent, given that it is unlikely that all the cells counted would give rise to colonies when tested using plate counts. This could prompt some fundamental discussion, as to what is an appropriate specification, in terms of risks posed by individual microbial cells or groups of microbial cells which could result in a more precise and scientifically accurate risk-based specification versus the current specifications which could be viewed in some cases as the "conservative sledgehammer" approach to microbiology. There may well be resistance to this new approach to defining specifications, and many people, including the regulators, will see this as simply the industry trying to relax standards or increase risks to fit with the market needs. This will need to be countered by a proactive industry-wide education process supported by the businesses, the equipment manufacturers and the microbiologists for the consumers and the customers to retain confidence in the products and the industry.

2. **Genetic detection**—These types of methods such as the Genedisc system (Pall Corporation; Port Washington, NY) are relatively new to the industry. They rely on gene amplification and counting the number of copies produced to estimate the number of microorganisms in the samples. This technology, as with most DNA/RNA analysis, does depend on having some idea of the nature of the expected contamination, so that the appropriate primers, for example, can be loaded into the system to complete the test. This specification can convey a high degree of accuracy and specificity, but can also limit the overall accuracy of detection if non-routine organisms are encountered. This has been one of the handicaps to this type of technology, as there have been several very specific organism probes or chips developed mainly for objectionable microorganisms, which though are very successful in detecting the target organism have very limited use in general bioburden assays which are usually required to release the product.

   This limitation should not be used to discount the use of this technology in the future manufacturing operations and it brings up the question of a multi-faceted, integrated test. One of the reasons that the traditional plate count has survived for so long, in common use, is that it can meet all three of the key criteria—isolate, enumerate and identify in a single low-cost test. In the future, with the need for speed of analysis, this simplicity is going to have to be replaced by multiple tests to demonstrate that the product meets specifications. This concept has been used in the analytical field for many years and now microbiology might adopt a similar approach to be fully relevant in the 21st century. This has already started over the past 20 years, with the advent of specific identification tools, API, genotypic identification systems, Maldi-ToF (Matrix-assisted laser desorption/

ionization-Time of flight) and so on. However, is very likely that this approach will be disliked or resisted, because of the additional cost and complexity that multiple material/product-specific method/equipment may bring versus the historic simple cheap plate count. However, the holistic benefits that these will deliver to the operation may significantly outweigh the cost question.

3. **Rapid identification methods**—Most of the discussion, so far, has been related to the method to detect and enumerate the bioburden in the product or material of concern, but once a microorganism has been detected, the inevitable question, before deciding the disposition, is "What is it?". So, there is a need for identification methods to keep pace with the development of faster routine analysis methods. In this case, speed is not the only key criteria; in the case of identification, accuracy is also paramount in the provided data for effective decision making. This combination of speed and accuracy has started to become available only recently with the advent of technology such as the Maldi-ToF, using which it is possible to get very accurate identifications in a matter of minutes, allowing very rapid response or decision making to occur. Of course, the accuracy of such systems, which rely on fingerprint or spectral comparison, is only as good as the data base to which it is referenced. The combination of this technology linked to a genomic 16S Identification system can provide additional confidence in the accuracy of the database. In addition, the increasing use of such technology globally will ultimately help build quality and integrity of the database. The one proviso with this system is the need to assure that the scope of the database entries is sufficiently broad, with both clinical and environmental isolates, to assure the appropriate baseline for the identification system to be relevant to the manufacturing operations.

   The reference standard for microbial identifications has over the past few years become the 16S RNA sequencing, which given the database that has been established provides a very accurate identification methodology. This method can provide the result within 12 hours, which may well be sufficient for the future, especially in cases where the product is on hold or quarantined for a bioburden detection. Faster methods will be required where product specification includes the exclusion of specific-objectionable organisms. The development of PCR (polymerase chain reaction) technology, which is the base for this type of testing, is also going forward, which should also help drive simplification of the equipment and cost reduction, allowing this type of technology to become common in microbiology and analytical laboratories.

4. All the methods discussed have required that a sample of the product or material in question is needed to perform the test. Like the traditional test methods, the sampling methodology has not changed or advanced significantly over the past few years other than improved sample valves which can be sanitized prior to use. Recently several companies have been designing automatic sampling devices (Figure 11.2) such as the oasis system (Sentinel Monitoring Systems Inc.; Tucson, AZ 85710), which will not only pull the required sample within a sterile field but will also pass it through a test filter within a single use container. This means that samples could be pulled at preset intervals related to the process requirements, and the only human input would be to collect the sample, place the filter in the media and incubate. These types of devices may not, by themselves, fundamentally change the face of microbiology in manufacturing, but they could be an extremely important transition system as businesses focus on productivity and transition to new production/business systems.

5. **Real-time online methods**—These have long been sought as "The Holy Grail" of microbiology, the ability to detect and count microorganisms in a product or material without the need to sample and grow the organism. This has several profound advantages in terms of product quality maintenance, active microbiological process control and quick and appropriate reaction to prevent out-of-specific situations. Techniques such as flow cytometry, discussed earlier, get closer to this objective, but they still rely on sampling and sample preparation to produce a result, with the associated delay and additional risk and effort.

   The recent development and introduction of systems, which use a matrix of particle size counting, laser-induced microbial auto fluorescence and complex algorithms to identify and count viable microbial cells in a stream or air or liquid, are starting to deliver the promise of the real-time microbiological testing (Figure 11.3). Systems such as the 7000RMS Bioburden analyzer (Mettler Toledo Inc.; Columbus, OH) or the IMD-A or IMD-W (Biovigilant; Tucson, AZ) offer the ability to monitor water and environmental air for microbiological contamination continuously, without

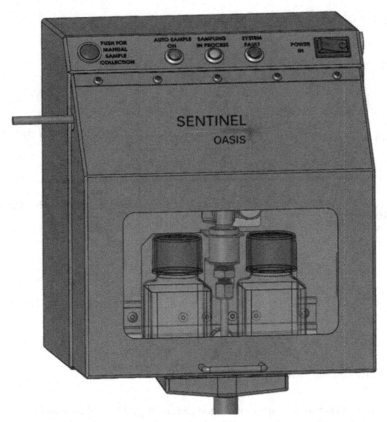

FIGURE 11.2 Automated sampling (sentinel oasis automatic sampling system, by courtesy of Sentinel Systems Inc.).

the need for sampling or other interventions. In addition, the online analysis provides the site about 400 data points a day versus the traditional single sample used to monitor water or the weekly data used for environmental monitoring.

These systems have found an initial home in the pharmaceutical industry in the monitoring of sterile manufacturing areas and water for injection (WFI) systems. This is probably because these systems can be used to monitor/screen the environment and water system for any microorganisms in a very clean medium supplementing the routine sampling and testing.

In this role, there is no pressing requirement or need to have the difficult conversation of changing the specifications, particularly for materials such as water, with the regulators or within the company. This allows the organization to implement, test and become comfortable with the technology while proving out their full capabilities.

While the initial adoption of these technologies has been in the sterile products industries, it is probably the non-sterile manufacturing area that could realize the greatest benefits from these systems if the various industries in this area would be willing to move away from their current specifications or the perceived need to prove equivalence to the traditional methods which is scientifically difficult as they measure different parameters. This is not to say there is no need to validate or prove out the technology, rather it is more a reflection that the regulations, which govern the use of this equipment, have more flexibility and scope to allow the development of new and innovative monitoring programs.

For example, if one of these real-time units, installed on the outlet of a RO water system, detected a higher than normal level of microorganism, it could actuate a valve to send the water it had tested to drain, effectively ensuring that no OOS water reached the storage and distributions system, and removing the reliance on the heat or ozone commonly used to protect the water system. Equally, the airborne monitoring system could predict when the manufacturing areas failed to meet a predefined

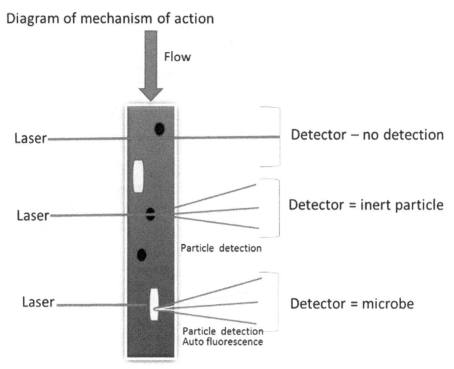

FIGURE 11.3   In-line sampling: an analysis.

hygiene standard before the operation started eliminating the risk of environmentally sourced contamination. The ability to actively control the microbiological risks in the process could present a significant opportunity, both in terms of risk reduction for the consumer and the development and evolution of the production and distribution systems.

The online real-time system represents step change in the non-growth testing systems which can be used in the microbiological control of manufacturing operation. The speed of response, sensitivity and data generation is a good fit for the upcoming needs of the business. Today, the reliability and robustness of this equipment can be a limitation; early models would work very well, but for relatively short period, before requiring adjustment or calibration. This casts doubt on their ability to tolerate the stress and strain of a manufacturing environment. This may have been because the early models were almost all hand built and so suffered from a high degree of variability which has subsequently been rectified in today's systems. These systems may be the blueprint for a completely new way of assuring microbiological integrity of products and materials.

Innovations and New Concepts

The methodologies and techniques discussed can provide data on which release decisions can be made and in this respect, they could be seen as an evolution from what business and operations have historically used as their microbiological control systems—namely testing and releasing finished products. Most microbiologists will argue that the finished product testing is only a confirmatory test for the effectiveness of the whole of the microbiological control systems; it is the in-process monitoring, the preventative cleaning and sanitization, the environmental monitoring, the control procedures and the training of the individuals which provide the actual microbiological integrity.

This concept can be combined with the Quality by Design approach to provide a system whereby the microbiological quality of the finished products is assured and predictable, rather than evaluated and determined by finished product testing. This will not, as some people would like to believe, make testing obsolete or allow manufacturing more flexibility in operations, but if implemented correctly, it would provide the vehicle to meet the customer demand in the future.

This concept is not new: parametric release, controlled state or real-time release has been implemented in the pharmaceutical businesses for several years. The 2006 European Medicine Agency publication on Guidelines for Parametric Release produced one of the better definitions which outlines the scope and scale of the work which could be applied to the cosmetics industry:

> The manufacturer may obtain assurance that the product is of stipulated quality and meets its specification through a system called parametric release. Parametric release is based on evidence of successful validation of the manufacturing process and review of the documentation on the additional process monitoring carried out during manufacture to support parametric release. Consequently, parametric release is used as an operational alternative to routine release testing of certain, specific parameters (4).

This process requires an intentional design of both product and process, specific control limits, rigorous validation, effective monitoring and operational excellence to be effective. This means that it can be difficult to retrofit this process to the existing systems, and partial implementation or sub-optimal design can mean additional risks of undetected contamination occurring in the production systems.

Control Factors for Real-Time Release (RTR)

1. **Raw materials and packaging**—One of the key prerequisites for RTR is that the microbiological quality of incoming materials is assured. The production of these starting materials is effectively outside the control of the manufacturing operation, even with processes to qualify or certify the suppliers. This means that there needs to be effective control steps for the receipt, acceptance and storage of the materials. These control measures usually take two forms:

   a. **Sampling testing and release**—This works for those materials received in discreet containers which can be opened, sampled under very controlled conditions, to preserve the integrity of the sample and the container. Rapid methods can reduce overall inventory and this is an example of the additional sensitivity of the enrichment methods adding to the overall security of the system. Storage of the containers and packaging is also easily controlled with the appropriate conditions and racking and there is no issue with demurrages costs.

   b. **Positive control systems**—This is where a control or kill step, such as filtration, irradiation or pasteurization, is included in the receiving or delivery systems, to assure microbiological integrity of materials. This is an ideal solution for bulk deliveries of materials which, when combined with a rigorous supplier qualification process, can eliminate the need for sampling and testing, which is generally problematic for large bulk deliveries. In addition, it can eliminate the common issue of additional demurrage charges. The unloading and storage systems must be designed to maintain the microbiological integrity after receipt, which is usually via validated cleaning and sanitization systems for the transfer system and isolation of the storage tanks through vent filters or tank blanketing system. The real-time monitoring methods can be used to monitor the control systems during and after validation. This is the approach already used in the process water systems found in most sites, where the treatment systems (Reverse Osmosis or De-ionization) protect the water which meets the specification, ozone or heat is used as a control step to maintain the specification and then the real-time online systems along with temperature or ozone concentration provide data which assures specification compliance.

2. **Utilities**—The utilities present a unique challenge in terms of real-time release, as they are produced continuously on site, which limits the ability to test and control, and they are in constant use by both the manufacturing process and other functions. Systems such as compressed air, steam, HVAC are difficult to sample representatively and there are no specifications shown to deliver the required level of control. This means that the focus in these areas needs to be on the design and installation

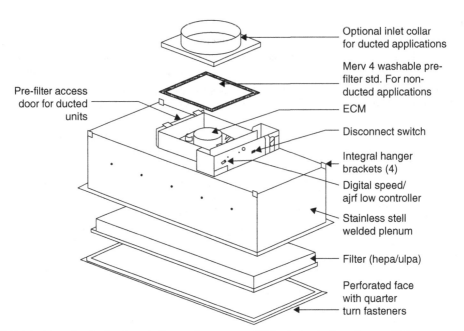

Optional inlet collar
for ducted applications

Merv 4 washable pre-
filter std. For non-
ducted applications

Pre-filter access
door for ducted
units

ECM

Disconnect switch

Integral hanger
brackets (4)

Digital speed/
ajrf low controller

Stainless stell
welded plenum

Filter (hepa/ulpa)

Perforated face
with quarter
turn fasteners

FIGURE 11.4   Example of a filter fan unit diagram (by courtesy of Nailor Industries Inc.; Houston, TX).

of the systems to eliminate the risk; for example, compressed air system can be set to a pressure dew point of –40°C or lower which will prevent microbial growth; steam trap can be designed to be free draining, eliminating the risk of condensate contamination.

HVAC control is often a controversial discussion in the cosmetics industry; there has been a general resistance to the installation of clean rooms or clean room conditions for non-sterile products. The industry perception is that this is not required for the products and the capital costs cannot be justified. From a quality control point of view this may be true, but in a real-time release world removing the environmental contamination risks and the potential for sporadic contamination may be a significant advantage. The advent of filter fan units (Figure 11.4), inexpensive filtration units that can be included in the design of making and packing equipment, can provide a cost-effective localized and controlled environment that may offer an ideal solution for the cosmetic industry that is looking for simple methods to control the environment.

The environment can also be continually monitored by real-time online systems, such as the IMD-A system from Biovigilant. These types of systems have gained increasing acceptance in the sterile products industry with their ability to constantly monitor the operating environment and provide rapid identification of excursions from the required standard.

3. **Environment**—The provision of the appropriate quality of air for the manufacturing units is described in the previous section; however, providing the appropriate environment for a real-time release system requires additional levels of control, many of which must be designed into the process. The key control measures can be summarized as Separation, Segregation, Pressurization and Personnel (SSPP):

a. **Separation**—Specific designated areas for the sensitive manufacturing operations where the product, materials and components are exposed.

b. **Segregation**—Within the manufacturing operations the isolation and control of sensitive operations – material, additions, product filling, and so on.

c. **Pressurization**—The application of differential pressures to maintain the designated conditions through normal operations.

d. **Personnel**—The activities, training and governing of the workforce to minimize the risk of introduced contamination.

In addition to the benefits that the combination of the air quality, design and procedural control can deliver, new technologies are available now that can actively clean the air of microorganisms, allowing the application of these systems to legacy non-ideal designs. Equipment such as the air purifier from Genano (Espoo, Finland), which uses corona discharges to negatively charged particles and microorganisms allowing them to be removed by positively charged collection systems, can be easily installed to supplement the original HVAC design.

4. **Facility design**—The contamination risks from the fit and finish of the manufacturing areas can also be addressed by developing clear design standards for the equipment and facility. The use of impervious materials and anti-bacterial finishes can help reduce both the need for cleaning and the impact of any sporadic contamination. Many academic institutions are already working on the development of omniphobic surfaces, which will help not only reduce the frequency of cleaning but also potentially inhibit microbial attachment. Those that exist today continue to depend on chemical coatings which have a limited lifespan in a manufacturing environment plus may not be compatible with several cosmetic product categories.

   Advances in equipment design with the advent of validated mixed proof valves which allow concurrent cleaning and sanitization, drainable diaphragm pumps which reduce the need for cleaning out of place, filling equipment such as the Ronchi rotary fillers with in-built automatic cleaning and sanitization (Figure 11.5) and the increased use of offline washing machines allow the rigorous validation of both the cleaning and sanitization processes.

   This ability, when combined with the availability and accuracy of digital monitoring devices, such as wireless thermocouples and boroscopes, will deliver significantly more reassured cleanliness in the equipment which is consistent with the needs of real-time release.

5. **Process control**—Consideration for the needs of real-time release design of the manufacturing process during development could also significantly improve the manufacturing sites' capability to meet the future needs. Sequencing additions, wherever possible, to maintain a hostile growth environment as late in the process as possible will reduce the contamination risks, increasing the confidence in the product integrity. To date, preservatives have been perceived to deliver hostility in the process; however, with reducing availability and effectiveness of preservatives, alternative

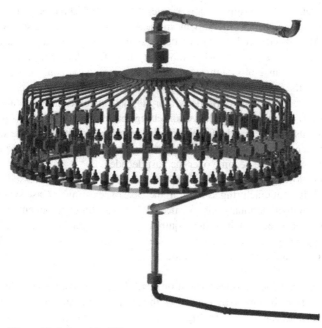

FIGURE 11.5 Rotary fillers with designed-in CIP systems.

strategies using pH, water activity, active concentrations and other potential control measure can be considered and included in determining the microbiological control steps in the overall real-time release process. The process and the key control steps can be designed to assure that the microbiological integrity of the product is maintained. The operating windows for the control steps can be tested and validated as can the process for documenting the process data, which will ultimately be used to "release" the product. In this case, release will be based on the maintenance of validated process parameters, rather than product testing, which could lead to automatic release in the future with integration of digital manufacturing planning, LIMS and process monitoring systems.

Control steps or kill steps can also be an effective consideration for real-time release. This is where this strategy has gained considerable traction in the pharmaceutical industry and where most of the guidelines and information have been published. Historically very few cosmetic products have had defined or have even considered kill steps (pasteurization, E-beam etc.). In the manufacturing process, depending on the nature of the product, this approach applied at the final stages of the filling or packing process, once validated, would eliminate the need for microbiological testing meeting the business requirements for rapid response to the market. For example, surfactant products could be pasteurized effectively at relatively low temperatures (60°C–80°C) with little or no effect on the product performance. A significant watchout with this technology is that it may be perceived as a universal solution to poor hygiene or operating practices though it is actually not the case. These kill steps are designed to deal with relatively low numbers of organism, not remediate contaminated products which are also likely to develop other quality issues because of the contamination.

6. **Cleaning and sanitization**—The manufacturing equipment and facility requires periodic cleaning and sanitization. The effective completion of the process can provide additional assurance that there are no developing microbiological risks in the system. This puts considerable emphasis on the validation of the cleaning and sanitization process and the definition and execution of the process once validated, in a manner similar to the control method of the manufacturing process discussed. The monitoring of the key control parameters and time temperature concentration can with sufficient validation become data used in the real-time release process.

7. **Validation**—The key to confidence in any real-time release process is that the work carried out to prove the control systems are operational and effective. Confidence stems for rigorous and detailed validation, not only of the individual systems but also the interaction between the systems and the transfer of the data to the documentation or release systems. Validation in these types of systems should be viewed as a business investment, in the same way as tangible assets such as equipment and facilities. Also, it will need to be more detailed and extensive than may have historically been required in the cosmetics industry when the safety net of product testing was installed. The validation of the performance of systems such as the environmental control, air quality, air changes, pressurization or the control and storage system for raw materials will be essential part of the microbial process control system. Some will argue that this extensive validation is not necessary for the risks posed by cosmetic products, forgetting that the intention of this process is to try and meet the future business demands. In this respect, effective validation of the various systems and methods will be a critical factor in the operations, in a similar manner as preventative maintenance and digital monitoring have become over the past decade.

Organizations do tend to overthink validation, leading the often-professed need to validate all moving parts of the manufacturing system. In the case of real-time release systems, there is a need to focus clearly on the individual control aspects of each system component and validate the range of setting which consistently deliver the required effect. Once this is completed, the integration of the various components can be validated to confirm the ability to assure microbiological integrity through the process and at the time of shipment.

The future needs of the cosmetics business operations will dictate the manufacturing systems and manufacturing conditions. These in turn will constrain the time, scope and scale of the microbiological systems which can be used. Rapid microbiological methods, real-time online monitoring systems, real-time or parametric release systems backed up with details validation offer the best strategies to make a fundamental shift in microbiological control which will allow full integration with the manufacturing operations. The key question which will remain is cultural—namely, the willingness of the normally risk-averse microbiological organizations to fully embrace and utilize the new technology that are developed inside and outside the microbiological field. It may be that the most significant business advantage will go to the companies willing to adapt or separate science from other fields to deal with microbiological control in manufacturing.

REFERENCES

1. https://ec.europa.eu/growth/sectors/cosmetics_en [accessed February 2020].
2. www.iso.org/standard/36437.html [accessed February 2020].
3. www.fda.gov/regulatory-information/search-fda-guidance-documents/draft-guidance-industry-cosmetic-good-manufacturing-practices [accessed February 2020].
4. European Medicines Agency, Veterinary Medicines and Inspections, EMEA/CVMP/QWP/339588/2005-CONSULTATION, EMA, London 2006.

12

Consumer Safety Considerations of Cosmetic Preservation*

Corie A. Ellison, Alhaji U. N'jai, and Donald L. Bjerke

Introduction

Consumer product safety evaluations of cosmetic products are based on the premise that the product should be safe for consumers under normal and foreseeable use. This means a cosmetics microbiologist must protect the product from significant microbial contamination within the context of a preservative system that is safe for human exposure. The consumer product safety and regulatory assessment can ultimately determine the type of preservative and its level of use in a cosmetic product.

This chapter will provide the cosmetic microbiologist a background in toxicology intended to be helpful for the development of cosmetic preservatives. This information will not, however, prepare the microbiologist to develop his or her own independent preservative safety testing program. Instead, it will provide a basic understanding that will be useful when interacting with toxicologists responsible for preservative safety evaluations.

Use of Existing Information

A microbiologist typically first considers preservatives that are marketed specifically for cosmetic products. He or she will often contact the preservative manufacturer to obtain information about the efficacy of the preservative in question. When obtaining efficacy information, the microbiologist should also specifically request data on toxicological testing that the manufacturer may have available for the preservative. Unnecessary or duplicate preclinical toxicity testing may be avoided by reviewing the data available from the manufacturer. While the types of safety test data vary widely from manufacturer to manufacturer, at a minimum, the information should include systemic toxicity screening, eye irritation, primary skin irritation, skin sensitization, and basic mutagenicity testing data. More extensive safety test data are frequently available from manufacturers of well-established, high sales volume preservatives.

A microbiologist can save considerable time and expense by not performing extensive microbiological evaluations with a preservative that may not be toxicologically suitable for the product application under

---

* This chapter is an update of the 2006 version by S. Heid, A. Kanti, P. McNamee, and W. Apel

consideration. Likewise, if a safety profile provided by a manufacturer is sufficiently robust and indicates no apparent toxicological problems, a microbiologist can commence efficacy testing with a higher degree of confidence that human safety toxicological issues will not preclude the use of the preservative.

Trade Associations

Other sources of information for preservatives and their usage in cosmetics are the various trade associations; for example, the Personal Care Products Council (PCPC), represents member companies who manufacture, distribute, and supply finished personal care products marketed in the United States. Cosmetics Europe is a similar trade association in Europe.

The Cosmetic Ingredient Review (CIR) was established in 1976 as an independent group from industry which reviews the safety of cosmetic ingredients (including preservatives) based on reported uses in cosmetics. The final CIR report is published in the *International Journal of Toxicology*. The conclusion of a CIR report is just a recommendation and is not binding in a regulatory sense; however, PCPC member companies voluntarily sign a Consumer Commitment Code—these are basically the findings of the CIR— by which they are bound. In Europe, the Scientific Committee on Consumer Safety (SCCS) is analogous to the CIR in that it is an independent group of scientists that advises the European Commission Scientific Committee for Consumer Products (SCCP) in accordance with their published guidelines for the safety evaluation of cosmetic ingredients and cosmetic products (1).

Regulatory Considerations

The use of preservatives as ingredients in finished products is subject to stringent regulatory supervision in different regions. Regulations can involve specified physicochemical and toxicity tests for certain ingredients, with implications for safety evaluations of finished products. Examples of relevant legislation and regulatory bodies that monitor cosmetic products include the European Commission's Cosmetics Regulation 1223/2009, the Food and Drug Administration (FDA) in the United States, and the Ministry of Health, Labor, and Welfare (MHLW) in Japan.

Some of the most specific legislation related to cosmetic preservatives is defined in the European Commission's Cosmetics Regulation 1223/2009 which states that cosmetics should be free of harmful levels of microorganisms. The US FDA has published similar recommendations in their draft guidance for industry on cosmetic good manufacturing practices (CGMP) which indicate that finished products should be tested for adequate preservation against microbial contamination under reasonable conditions of storage and use (2).

Annex V of the European Commission's Cosmetics Regulation 1223/2009 provides a list of all preservatives that may be used in cosmetic products sold in the EU along with any restrictions of use such as the level in product, product form (aerosol vs. cream), and product type (leave-on product vs. rinse-off product). Entry into Annex V of the directive is dependent upon a safety review (subsequently published on the agency's Web site) by the SCCS (3). Other regions of the world may have a separate list of preservatives allowed for use in cosmetics, as illustrated by Japan's Standards for Cosmetics (Ministry of Health and Welfare Notification No. 331 of 2000) which requires preservatives to be among those listed in Appendix 3 of the Regulation.

External and Technical Considerations

The rapid spread of information over the Internet and other media has enhanced education about preservative safety but also in certain circumstances perpetuated misinformation about safety to the public. Both peer-reviewed scientific journal articles and rumors generated by certain special interest groups are available to consumers today, often without the appropriate context or framework that would allow the public to assess the information.

For cosmetic products, the human health effect that receives the most external attention is contact allergy. Several well-known cosmetic preservatives have been identified as having the ability to induce contact allergy and/or elicit allergic contact dermatitis (ACD) under certain exposure conditions. For many of the preservatives known to be contact allergens, use of appropriate risk assessment approaches can assure that they are used safely and effectively in formulations. Nevertheless, the literature contains well-documented information about situations in which the use of preservatives in cosmetic products caused concern about contact allergy.

The concerns regarding contact allergy can sometimes be the main factor in determining what is a safe and supportable level of a preservative is in a finished product. The SCCS has published opinions for multiple preservatives where the end decision was based on the contact allergy potential of the preservative. Such examples include the usage limits determined for methylisothiazolinone (one trade name is Neolone 950®) and methylchloroisothiazolinone/methylisothiazolinone (one trade name is Kathon CG®), the labeling requirement for chloroacetamide, and the usage bans for methyldibromoglutaronitrile (one trade name is Tektamer®) and benzisothiazoline (4–8).

Great care has been taken to demonstrate that preservatives can be safely used in cosmetic products at certain lower levels (9). For preservatives to be considered both safe and efficacious, strong collaboration involving the cosmetics industry, external scientific groups, and the dermatology community is essential. Strengthening this collaboration will help in the development and the continued safe and effective use of preservatives.

In the early 21st century, the paraben family of preservatives came under special external scrutiny because of concern over their potential estrogenicity or endocrine disruption capabilities and possible links of paraben-containing underarm cosmetics to breast cancer. Although this issue attracted a great deal of public attention, no objective evidence has demonstrated any significant risk from current cosmetic usage of these preservatives (10). The SCCP published an extended opinion specifically focused on the breast cancer question and stated that, "in light of the present knowledge, there is no evidence of demonstrable risk for the development of breast cancer caused by the use of paraben-containing underarm cosmetics" (11). Additional opinions from the SCCP and SCCS further reviewed the paraben family and established usage limits for methyl- ethyl- propyl and butylparaben (12).

Consumers have shown a growing trend and desire for products that are natural or naturally derived. This trend provoked a strong push by the cosmetics industry to identify natural ingredients that have antimicrobial efficacy and can potentially replace existing preservatives. An important consideration to this trend is that natural should not be implied as safe. A natural preservative should undergo the same considerations and safety evaluation as a synthetic preservative.

Consumer Safety Considerations for Preservatives

When developing a new preservative system or choosing an existing preservative system for a cosmetic product, four primary areas related to consumer safety evaluation and risk assessment must be addressed:

1. *Hazard identification*: The potential toxic effects associated with a given material in preclinical and clinical evaluations.
2. *Dose–response assessment*: Understanding the relationship between dose and the nature, severity and incidence of adverse effects.
3. *Exposure*: Exposure to the preservative from actual use of the product, based on habits and practices data.
4. *Risk characterization*: Combines the assessments of exposure and response under various exposure conditions to estimate the probability of specific harm to exposed an exposed individual or population.

These concepts are developed further in the rest of this chapter. If safety test data are insufficient, it may be necessary to begin microbial efficacy testing of a preservative at the same time as safety testing is conducted. This is acceptable if no human exposure during the efficacy testing is anticipated or if the available safety data support the requested human exposure. Explanations of typical safety tests conducted with cosmetic preservatives together with fundamental background in the principles of toxicology are outlined in the sections that follow.

Fundamentals of Toxicology

Toxicology is the study of deleterious effects of chemical, physical, or biological agents on living organisms. The degree to which these deleterious effects are manifested is dependent on several factors such as species or strain of the organism exposed, stage of development of the organism when tested, compound or physical effect to which the organism is exposed, duration of exposure, frequency of exposure, route of exposure, and site of exposure.

"The dose makes the poison" is a true statement made by Paracelsus, one of the founders of modern toxicology, in that every chemical has both a safe exposure level and a hazardous exposure level (13). The central premise of toxicology is to define both the hazardous and safe exposure levels of a compound to the species of interest and to ensure that exposure of a particular chemical as a cosmetic ingredient is well within the range of safety.

Traditionally, toxicological data relevant for humans have been obtained by investigating the toxicological profile of the chemical using experimental animals. More recently, there have been substantial efforts to minimize the use of animals and to rely more on animal alternative methods. There are several areas in the toxicological assessment where health protective decisions for an ingredient can be made in the absence of any animal data. Even though significant progress has been made toward developing and validating animal alternative methods, more research is needed in multiple areas. Validated test guidelines for historical, animal-based test as well as animal alternative approaches have been developed and published by the Organization for Economic Co-operation and Development (OECD) (14).

Some of the most impactful legislation related to the use of animals in the toxicological assessment of a cosmetic is defined in the 7th Amendment to the EU Cosmetic Directive (Regulation 1223/2009). The European cosmetic legislation prohibits the marketing of finished products containing ingredients or combinations of ingredients that have been subject to acute animal toxicity testing after March 2, 2009, and any animal testing after March 11, 2013, thus making it necessary to use validated alternative replacement methods in the toxicological assessment.

Hazard Identification

The purpose of a hazard identification is to determine whether exposure to the ingredient of interest can cause an increase in the incidence of adverse health effects. For example, does exposure to the ingredient result in damage to the major organs of the body (e.g., liver, kidney, lung, reproductive), or can it cause diseases such as cancer or birth defects? This type of information has historically been generated using experimental animals but the move toward animal-alternative approaches has enabled hazard identification in ways which don't rely on utilizing animals, as discussed later in this chapter.

Dose–Response Assessment

Dose–response assessment is the process of quantitatively evaluating toxicity information for an ingredient. The process involves characterizing the relationship of the dose of the ingredient delivered in a toxicity study and the nature, severity and incidence of adverse health effects following a given route of administration in the exposed population (15). The dose–response is intended to distinguish the highest dose that does not cause an adverse effect from the lowest dose that does cause an adverse effect.

Exposure Considerations

The magnitude, duration, frequency, and route of exposure can all dramatically influence the toxicity exhibited by a compound. Major routes of exposure are dermal (a particularly important exposure route for cosmetics), inhalation, oral, intravenous, intraperitoneal, and subcutaneous. For the dermal route, an additional consideration is the thickness of the skin, which can impact the likelihood of the absorption of a chemical. For example, an ingredient may be more likely to cross the skin and become systemically available at a site where the skin is thin (e.g., the post-mandibular area) than it would at a site where the skin is thicker and less subject to absorption (e.g., the soles of the feet). Other important considerations for topical products like cosmetics include: whether the area of application is open, semi-occluded or fully occluded; whether there is damage to the skin barrier. The formula matrix can also potentially impact systemic exposure by enhancing or limiting permeation of an ingredient.

Other factors that impact an exposure assessment include the dose, frequency of application, duration of exposure and surface area of application for which there is published guidance for appropriate values to use (16).

Risk Characterization

Risk characterization is the final step in the risk assessment process. In this step, the hazard identification and exposure assessments are summarized and integrated into quantitative and qualitative expressions of risk (Risk = Hazard × Exposure). Extrapolations of toxicity data from the model on which the compound was tested (an animal model or alternative validated in vitro model) to humans are made. In this process of extrapolation, uncertainty factors are commonly used. A typical risk assessment utilizes an allowable daily exposure that is determined by taking the highest dose that is not associated with any adverse effects (NOAEL) and dividing it by the total uncertainty factors to arrive at a reference dose or an allowable daily intake. This value is then compared to the consumer exposure to determine the margin of safety.

Extrapolating from an animal model to a human typically requires a factor of 10 and extrapolation to sensitive populations within species requires an additional factor of 10 (17). Additional uncertainty factors may be required and are specific to each case. Risk characterization serves as a bridge between risk assessment and risk management and is therefore a key step in the ultimate decision-making process (18,19).

Toxicity Studies Grouped by Exposure Duration

Acute Toxicity Studies

An acute toxicity study involves either a single administration of a test chemical or several administrations within a 24-hour period. The animals are then observed for signs of toxicity for a defined period, often 14 days. Most acute toxicity studies are designed to determine the median lethal dose (LD_{50}) of a toxicant. Acute toxicity testing is less important for modern-day risk assessments.

Guidelines for acute oral (OECD 420, 423, 425), dermal (OECD 402), and inhalation (OECD 403) toxicity studies have been published. Currently, they are used more for classification and labeling purposes, not for risk assessment purposes.

Subacute and Subchronic Toxicity Studies

Historically, repeated dose animal toxicity studies were done to determine the safety profile of ingredients, preferably with animals that can metabolize chemicals in a manner similar to biotransformation in humans. The rat is most often the species of choice.

Chemicals are usually administered by routes of exposure intended for human use. The preferred exposure is oral (incorporating the chemical into the diet of the animal or administered by oral gavage). The dermal and inhalation routes may also be considered, depending upon the ingredient or type of cosmetic product in which it is to be used.

Because these studies aim to determine NOAEL, at least three doses are typically selected: (1) a dose high enough to induce toxic effects in the animals, (2) a medium dose, and (3) a low dose that does not cause any adverse effects. Observations made during and immediately following testing include mortality, body weight, food consumption rate, blood and serum chemistries, hematology, clinical observations, gross pathology observations, organ weights, and histology. These tests yield information about toxicity with respect to target organs, types of effects, and reversibility of effects (if the study includes a recovery group) and help define dose–response relationships.

Subacute tests are usually conducted for short durations (7–14 days) as dose range–finding studies to assist in dose selection for longer-term studies and 28-day studies for understanding the dose–response safety profile of the ingredient. Subchronic toxicity testing is of intermediate duration; a typical test lasts about 90 days and is preferred to subacute testing for understanding extended exposure to a given chemical.

Chronic Toxicity Studies

The definition of *chronic* depends on the species, but is intended to cover at least a very significant portion of the lifespan of an animal—if not its entire lifetime. Test duration may vary from 6 months up to 2 years or more in animals, thus mimicking lifetime exposure in humans. The study considerations are similar to those for subchronic toxicity tests.

In some cases, lifetime exposure bioassays in rodents may be helpful for detecting carcinogenicity potential.

Toxicity Studies Grouped by Toxic Endpoint

Ocular Irritation Tests

The eyes may be exposed to cosmetic products and their ingredients via use of products meant to be used around the eyes (e.g., mascaras and eye creams) or through accidental exposure to products that may enter the eyes in diluted form during normal use (e.g., shampoos). The evaluation of eye irritation potential of a cosmetic product and its ingredients is essential to obtain reassurance that a product is safe for consumers to use through intended and foreseeable uses and accidental exposures. The preservative used in a formulation can impact the irritation profile, depending upon the type of preservative, its use level, and the specific cosmetic of interest.

Historically, the best-known method of assessing ocular irritation was the Draize test (OECD 405) that involves instilling the test compound into rabbit eyes and then grading the eyes for irritancy (20). However, efforts to minimize the use of animals in cosmetic testing combined with advances in animal alternative methods has made it possible to assess an ingredient or product's ocular irritation potential using validated OECD in vitro assays. Examples of such validated target organ–based in vitro assays for evaluating ocular irritation are the Bovine Corneal Opacity and Permeability (BCOP) test method (OECD 437) and the Isolated Chicken Eye (ICE) test method (OECD 438). Both BCOP and ICE may be used to identify test chemicals (substances or mixtures) that have potential to cause serious eye damage and those not requiring classification as eye hazard. Other well-known and OECD-validated organotypic, cell-based or tissue construct based in vitro assays for evaluating ocular irritation are Fluorescence Leakage test method (OECD 460), Short-Term Exposure test method (OECD 491), and Reconstructed Human Cornea-Like Epithelium test method (OECD TG 492). Such assays have proven useful for the evaluation of cosmetic product formulations. The use of these validated in vitro assays is restricted to domains of applicability from mild to extremely irritating ingredients or products. For example, certain assays are more predictive for surfactant-oriented products such as shampoos and others are more robust indicators of irritation for other types of cosmetics. Hence, these animal alternative methods are not stand-alone assays for evaluating ocular irritation potential of a range of chemicals but should be part of an integrated testing approach for ocular irritation (21,22).

Introduction to Skin

Since most cosmetic products are directly applied to the skin, a brief overview of skin anatomy and function is presented. The skin is the largest organ of the body and serves as a barrier to protect the organism from external insult. Thus, the skin is exposed to a wide variety of chemicals, cosmetics, topical medications, and industrial pollutants. Topical exposure coupled with dermal penetration is the most common route of exposure. The skin is composed of the epidermis and the dermis, a structure that rests on the subcutaneous tissue.

The living layer of the epidermis consists of a basal cell layer (stratum basale/germinativum), which provides the outer layers with new cells. The epidermis also contains melanocytes that produce pigments and also contains cells such as macrophages and lymphocytes involved in the immune process. The outermost layer of the epidermis is the stratum corneum, which provides a protective outer cover of squamous epithelial cells.

The dermis is mainly composed of collagen and elastin that form important matrices to support the skin. The dermis layer contains several types of cells; the most abundant are the fibroblasts that aid the biosynthesis of fibrous proteins. Subcutaneous tissue lies underneath the dermis. In addition, the skin contains sweat glands, hair follicles, and small blood vessels. These components are commonly known as skin "appendages".

The absorptive characteristics of a chemical are often significant factors in determining whether it will produce dermal toxicity. Many non-polar, lipophilic compounds readily diffuse across the skin barrier (23). Diffusion of hydrophilic polar compounds is highly influenced by the hydration state of the stratum corneum. Depending on environmental conditions, the stratum corneum can be hydrated with 10–70% water. As the stratum corneum becomes hydrated, hydrophilic compounds diffuse more easily across the barrier. Therefore, the conditions under which skin testing (e.g., closed patch, open patch, etc.) is conducted can significantly affect the outcome of the test.

Skin Responses to Preservatives

In general, two categories of skin responses should be thoroughly investigated for preservative agents: irritant responses and immunologically mediated allergic responses. The mechanisms for these responses are different and they will be discussed separately.

Irritant Responses

Preservatives are evaluated against two potential irritant responses: (1) corrosion and (2) irritation. Corrosion results from the direct necrotic action of a chemical on skin with an irreversible disintegration of the skin tissue that often results in scarring. Chemical burns, such as those produced by strong acids or bases, are classic examples of corrosion. Irritation is typically divided into three categories: (1) acute irritation, (2) cumulative irritation, and (3) photoirritation.

Acute irritation occurs as a localized response to a single application of a compound and typically involves erythema (i.e., skin redness) but could also involve inflammation or edema.

Cumulative irritation results from repeated exposures to compounds that, upon initial application, do not elicit acute irritation. The difference in the development of acute versus cumulative irritation may be simply a function of exposing the skin to a certain concentration of a compound in a formulation or the bioaccumulation of the compound in the skin.

Photoirritation results from light-induced chemical changes in a compound that cause the compound to become an irritant after it is applied to the skin. Photo-cytotoxicity potential and susceptibility to photochemical degradation can be evaluated using the validated tests: in vitro 3T3 NRU phototoxicity test (OECD 432) and UV-VIS absorption spectra test (OECD 101).

In practice, preservatives that elicit irritation responses act as either acute or cumulative irritants, and a toxicologist should test for this type of irritancy with patch tests that involve placing varying concentrations of the preservative under patch on the skin.

Most patch testing in humans is conducted on the arms or backs of volunteers. For acute irritancy testing, toxicologists often use a 24- or 48-hour patch testing protocol (24). The amount of erythema and edema of the skin is evaluated for irritation initially and up to 48 or 72 hours after patch removal.

The International Contact Dermatitis Research Group Scoring Scale can be used to score the skin responses (25). Table 12.1 summarizes this 4-point scale grading. Toxicologists use the cumulative

TABLE 12.1

International contact dermatitis research group scoring
scale for irritation testing

Description	Score
No reaction	0
Erythema	1+
Erythema and edema	2+
Marked erythema and edema	3+

TABLE 12.2

Potential contact sensitizers used for preservative
applications in cosmetics

Formaldehyde
Isothiazolinones
Organic mercurial compounds
Phenolics (e.g., hexachlorophene)

irritancy patch test to test chemicals for irritancy over time following repeated exposure (26). This test is a variation on the single 24- or 48-hour patch test outlined earlier except that testing typically continues for 14–21 days with repeated daily applications of the test material (27). The interval for this type of test is a matter of choice and relevance to the cosmetic of interest.

Skin Sensitization

Skin sensitization, also known as delayed contact hypersensitivity, is an immunologically mediated allergic response and is classified as a type IV response according to the scheme of Combs and Gell (28). The key factors characterizing type IV reactions are typically delayed onset of symptoms that get worse over a 24–72-hour timeframe. The symptoms typically involve pruritis, erythema, and edema and can progress to vesicle formation. These symptoms can also spread beyond the site of application of the product. Type IV reactions are associated with IgG antibodies. Poison ivy allergic contact dermatitis is a classic example of delayed type IV hypersensitivity. One way type IV sensitization can be distinguished from the irritation responses discussed is that the poison ivy rash-like sensitization, intense itching, and vesiculation response will likely spread beyond the site of exposure of the chemical insult, while the irritation response (typically with less edema than sensitization) tends to be localized to the initial area of the insult, and the skin response will typically persist for a longer period. In addition, induction of skin sensitization is a permanent change because memory cells within the immune system will remember the original exposure and the individual may react to any future exposures to the allergen that are above the threshold for elicitation of allergic contact dermatitis.

From a simplistic standpoint, a type IV skin reaction has two stages: (1) induction in which the individual becomes sensitized to a chemical; (2) elicitation in which the skin reacts to the chemical upon subsequent exposure. In addition to catechols from poison ivy, many other compounds are known to have the potential to cause induction when the exposure scenario exceeds the induction threshold. Table 12.2 lists these sensitizers (29,30).

Historically, the test of choice for toxicologists who wanted to understand the sensitization potentials of materials including preservatives was the in vivo mouse local lymph node assay (LLNA) (31,32). Advances in animal alternative methods have now made it possible to evaluate a chemical's sensitization potential through in vitro assays. An example of an in vitro assay for skin sensitization is the Direct

Peptide Reactivity Assay (OECD 442C). This method measures the ability of a chemical to react with proteins, a determinant step in the induction of sensitization (33). Other validated in vitro methods for sensitization include the in vitro skin sensitization ARE-Nrf2 luciferase test (OECD 442D) and the human cell line activation test (OECD 442E). The alternative methods are not intended to be utilized as a stand-alone assay but rather as an integrated testing strategy that informs on skin sensitization potential (34).

After the contact allergy hazard of a material has been identified, a quantitative risk assessment is conducted as previously described (16). Confirmatory human tests may be conducted to confirm the lack of sensitizing potential of the specific ingredient of interest or in the context of a finished product containing the preservative. It must be noted that such human tests are always confirmatory and not intended for hazard identification purposes. One example of such a confirmatory step is the human repeat insult patch test (HRIPT). Important details regarding experiments of the HRIPT have been published previously and are beyond the scope of this chapter (35). The study design of a HRIPT includes two basic stages. The first is the induction period when patches containing the test material are applied typically for 24 hours to the upper arms or backs of 100 or more subjects 9 times over the course of 3 weeks. The second stage is elicitation. This phase is conducted after a brief rest period of about 2 weeks after the final induction patch application. It consists of reapplying a challenge patch containing the same test material to the same site and/or an alternative skin site. After removal of the challenge patch, the skin grader evaluates the responses of the subjects at several time intervals (24, 48, 72, and 96 hours) for signs of positive or negative sensitization responses. The skin reactions evaluated include erythema, edema, pruritis, and in some cases vessiculation or bullae. Defined criteria exist for the determination of sensitization responses based on the observed skin reactions (35).

Provocative Use Testing for Sensitization

Human patch testing, while confirmatory in nature, occasionally produces equivocal results. The technique employed to resolve equivocal results is provocative use testing. This type of testing is conducted typically at exposure levels that more closely relate to the exposure that would be experienced by a consumer in normal use of the product rather than under the highly exaggerated exposure conditions of a patch test. This technique can be particularly useful in evaluating the elicitation potential of a preservative in a pre-sensitized test population. An informed volunteer is given the product of interest and instructed to use it the same way he or she would typically use it in a personal (no-test) situation.

At the beginning of the test, panel members are told to report any erythema, edema, or unusual itching. Panelists are periodically examined during the test for signs of skin responses suggestive of skin sensitization. If the product containing the preservative elicits a response, it is likely that a substitute preservative with less sensitization potential will be needed. If no response is seen under actual test conditions with a large test population, then supporting evidence demonstrates that the preservative as used in the product is acceptable from the human safety viewpoint of contact allergy.

Genotoxicity and Carcinogenicity Testing

Mutagenicity or mutation is defined as a permanent change in the content or structure of the genetic material of an organism that may result in a heritable change in the characteristics of the organism. These changes may involve many aspects of the genetic structure including a gene or gene segment, a block of genes, or whole chromosomes.

Genotoxicity is a broader term and includes harmful effects on genetic materials such as DNA strand breaks and DNA adducts that do not necessarily lead to mutagenicity. Genotoxic effects can occur in both somatic and germ cells. Malformation, death, or a permanent heritable change in the resulting embryo can occur in germ cells, while somatic cell mutations could result in cancer since cancer often arises from a mutagenic occurrence. Thus, genotoxicity testing is important for evaluating the ability of a preservative to interact with genetic material and cause adverse effects that could produce cancer or heritable changes in the offspring.

Although hundreds of genotoxicity assays exist, several standard in vitro and in vivo tests can detect chemically induced mutations. Many of these tests are indirect evaluations of mutational events. They detect phenotypic changes due to mutations versus the actual alterations of the DNA. Perhaps the most common mutagenesis assay is the in vitro Ames test (OECD 471), which identifies gene mutations. The in vitro Micronucleus test (OECD 487) is another commonly used assay and detects changes in the structure and number of chromosomes, an endpoint not evaluated by the Ames test. Since the different in vitro assays for mutagenicity and genotoxicity evaluate different aspects of the mechanism involved in this endpoint, it is necessary to utilize a battery of assays.

The 2-year rodent carcinogenicity bioassay was historically used to evaluate the carcinogenicity potential of a chemical. Today, these tests are typically not done for cosmetics, especially following the animal testing/marketing ban of the EU. Instead, a decision on the carcinogenic potential of a chemical is made based on the in vitro mutagenicity test battery. A favorable genotoxicity profile and repeated dose toxicity study can indicate a lack of carcinogenicity potential while a positive result in a mutagenicity test is seen as indicative of carcinogenic potential unless a scientific justification can be provided.

The SCCS has published some of the most detailed guidance on mutagenicity and genotoxicity testing for cosmetic products (3). The committee recommends hazard evaluation using tests for gene mutation (mutagenicity), chromosome breakage and/or rearrangements (clastogenicity), and numerical chromosome aberrations (aneugenicity). Since no single validated test is capable of addressing all these endpoints, the recommended in vitro battery consists of the Ames assay (OECD 471) and the in vitro micronucleus test (OECD 487). Bacterial assays, like the Ames assay, may not be suitable for preservatives due to their biocidal activity and it may be more appropriate to utilize a gene mutation test in mammalian cells such as the hypoxanthine phosphorybosyl transferase (HPRT) test or mouse lymphoma assay.

Reproductive and Developmental Toxicity Testing

Reproductive toxicity refers to the wide variety of toxicological effects of a substance on different phases of the reproductive cycle. Any agent that causes an adverse effect in a developing embryo or fetus at doses that are not toxic to the mother is a developmental toxicant or teratogen. The number of known developmental toxicants is extensive and includes biological entities (rubella virus), physical entities (x-rays), and a diversity of chemicals including pharmaceuticals like thalidomide and diethylstilbestrol; however, ingredients at current use concentrations in cosmetics are not teratogens (36–40).

Those agents that do cause developmental effects do so under very specific conditions of exposure duration and during windows of sensitivity of the species being tested. For the evaluation of potential adverse effects of a cosmetic ingredient, where data suggest significant systemic absorption, an in vivo developmental toxicity study in the rat (OECD TG 414) submitted by the manufacturer was deemed sufficient by SCCS. In a few cases, additional safety data from a 1- or 2-generation study (OECD TG 415 and 416) are included in the submission. In additional cases, some indication of adverse effects on the fertility could be obtained from repeat dose toxicity studies that indicate, for example, histopathologic effects on reproductive organs or endocrine system.

Manson et al. (1982) provided a thorough review of teratogenic or developmental toxicity testing procedures (41). This type of testing is usually conducted in three parts, although for cosmetics, segment two alone or an extended segment one study is deemed sufficient:

1. Female animals are dosed before and during mating with continued dosing during pregnancy and lactation. They are then sacrificed during pregnancy and the unborn offspring are examined for abnormalities. Other animals are allowed to deliver and the delivered offspring are weaned and examined for abnormalities.
2. Pregnant females are dosed only during organogenesis and sacrificed just before delivery. The unborn offspring are examined for abnormalities.
3. Pregnant females are dosed during the final trimester of pregnancy and through the lactation period. Offspring may be examined for abnormalities immediately following weaning or be allowed to reach adulthood prior to examination. By modifying dosing, investigators may compensate for effects of exposure timing on the teratogenic potential of the test compound.

To evaluate the effects of longer-term exposures to potential teratogenic agents, multiple generation studies proceeding through at most two generations or an extended one generation are used. They are conducted much like single generation studies except that a portion of each generation is retained and mated to produce the next study generation. In this way, the potential of the test compound to provoke congenital abnormalities as well as affect fertility, litter size, viability, and growth may be determined.

Since the developmental toxicity endpoint is very complex, there has yet to be any validated in vitro assays that can address this endpoint. One potential alternative approach to cover this endpoint is to rely on existing historical developmental toxicity data as illustrated by Structural Activity Relationship and/or decision tree–based approaches (42,43).

Post-Marketing Surveillance

After a new cosmetic formulation has been launched on the market, post-marketing surveillance to ensure that no unexpected safety issues have arisen is very important. This surveillance is performed in a passive sense, through consumers who might contact the company that launched the product, but it also involves active collaborations with members of the dermatological community. Many dermatologists in Europe and elsewhere patch test their patients with various preservatives as part of their standard allergy-testing protocols.

This testing works to monitor sensitization levels to various preservatives in patients with skin reactions who present themselves at a dermatologist's clinic. A dermatologist then extrapolates these clinical data to the public at large and determines whether preservative allergy incidence rates are increasing.

Conclusion

Current toxicological and risk assessment methods, as partially described in this chapter, are applied to cosmetic ingredients and formulas to assure safe use in the marketplace. Each ingredient, including preservatives, in the cosmetic formulation are assessed to ensure the safety profile is favorable with respect to standard toxicity endpoints, including eye irritation, skin irritation, and sensitization; and for ingredients that are absorbed across the skin, consideration is also given to systemic toxicity endpoints. The overall assessment considers the general toxicological profile of the ingredients, their chemical structure, and their level of exposure in products based on consumer habits and practices data. The finished cosmetic product is also evaluated to ensure a favorable safety profile when used under normal and reasonably foreseeable conditions of use, considering the product's presentation, labelling, any instructions for its use and disposal as well as any other indication or information provided by the manufacturer through a post-market surveillance process. Given the complexity of the safety assessment, the on-going evolution of the science and the dynamic regulatory environment, it is critical for the microbiologist and other members of the product development team to partner early with a qualified toxicologist and regulatory manager.

REFERENCES

1. Scientific Committee on Consumer Safety (SCCS; Adopted 24-25 October 2018). The SCCS Notes of Guidance for the Testing of Cosmetic Ingredients and Their Safety Evaluation 10th Revision. SCCS/1602/18 Final Version.
2. U.S. Department of Health and Human Services, Food and Drug Administration, Center for Food Safety and Applied Nutrition, Guidance for industry: Cosmetic good manufacturing practices, June 2013.
3. The Scientific Committee on Consumer Safety (SCCS), Notes of guidance for the testing of cosmetic ingredients and their safety evaluation, 9th revision, September 29, 2015, SCCS/1564/15
4. The Scientific Committee on Consumer Safety (SCCS), Opinion on methylisothiazolinone (MI) (P94), submission III (sensitisation only), December 15, 2015, SCCS/1557/15.

5. The Scientific Committee on Consumer Safety (SCCS), Opinion on the mixture of 5-chloro-2-methylisothiazolin-3(2H)-one and 2-methylisothiazolin-3(2H)-one, December 8, 2009, SCCS/1238/09.
6. The Scientific Committee on Consumer Safety (SCCS), Opinion on Chloroacetamide, March 22, 2011, SCCS/1360/10.
7. The Scientific Committee on Consumer Products (SCCP), Opinion on methyldibromoglutaronitrile (sensitisation only), June 20, 2006, SCCP/1013/06.
8. The Scientific Committee on Consumer Safety (SCCS), Opinion on benzisothiazolinone, June 26–27, 2012, SCCS/1482/12.
9. Gray, J.E., McNamee, P.M., *Scientific Review Series – Preservatives – Their Role in Cosmetic Products*, Munksgaard, Copenhagen, 2000.
10. CTFA Response Statement concerning Parabens, November 2003.
11. European Commission – The Scientific Committee on Consumer Products (SCCP), Extended opinion on parabens, underarm cosmetics, and breast cancer, January 28, 2005, SCCP/0874/05.
12. The Scientific Committee on Consumer Safety (SCCS), Opinion on parabens, May 3, 2013. SCCS/1514/13.
13. *Casarett and Doull's, Toxicology: The Basic Science of Poisons*, 6th ed., McGraw-Hill, New York, 2001.
14. OECD Guidelines for the Testing of Chemicals. www.oecd.org/chemicalsafety/testing/oecdguidelinesforthetestingofchemicals.htm Accessed August 10, 2017.
15. Environmental Protection Agency, EPA approach to assessing the risk associated with exposure to environmental carcinogens: Appendix B to the integrated risk information system, 1989.
16. Api, A.M., Basketter, D.A., Cadby, P.A., Cano, MF., Ellis, G., Gerberick, G.F., Griem, P., McNamee, P.M., Ryan, C.A., Safford R., Dermal sensitization quantitative risk assessment (QRA) for fragrance ingredients, *Reg. Toxicol. Pharmacol.*, 52, 1, 2008.
17. EPA, Health effects test guidelines, hazard evaluation, *Code of Federal Regulations*, Title 40, Part 792 and 798, 1989.
18. Environmental Protection Agency, Guidelines for carcinogen risk assessment, *Fed. Reg.*, 51, 33992, 1986.
19. Environmental Protection Agency, Guidelines for exposure assessment, *Fed. Reg.*, 51, 34042, 1986.
20. Draize, J.H., Kelley, E.A., Toxicity to eye mucosa of certain cosmetic preparations containing surfactant active agents, *Proc. Sci. Sect. Toilet Goods Assoc.* 17, 1, 1952.
21. McNamee, P., Hibatallah, J., Costabel-Farkas, M., Goebel, C., Araki, D., Dufour, E., Hewitt, N.J., Jones, P., Kirst, A., Le Varlet, B., Macfarlane, M., Marrec-Fairley, M., Rowland, J., Schellauf, F., Scheel, J., A tiered approach to the use of alternatives to animal testing for the safety assessment of cosmetics: Eye irritation, *Regul. Toxicol. Pharmacol.*, 54, 2, 2009.
22. Scott, L., Eskes, C., Hoffmann, S., Adriaens, E., Alepée, N, Bufo, M., Clothier, R., Facchini, D., Faller, C., Guest, R., Harbell, J., Hartung, T., Kamp, H., Varlet, B.L., Meloni, M., McNamee, P., Osborne, R., Pape, W., Pfannenbecker, U., Prinsen, M., Seaman, C., Spielmann, H., Stokes, W., Trouba, K., Berghe, C.V., Goethem, F.V., Vassallo, M., Vinardell, P., Zuang, V., A proposed eye irritation testing strategy to reduce and replace in vivo studies using bottom-up and top-down approaches, *Toxicol. In Vitro*, 24, 1, 2010.
23. Scheuplein, R.J., Blank, I.H., Permeability of the skin, *Physiol. Rev.* 51, 702, 1971.
24. Schwartz, L., Peck, S.M., The patch test and contact dermatitis, *Pub. Heal. Rep.* 59, 2, 1944.
25. International Contact Dermatitis Research Group, Terminology of contact dermatitis, *Acta. Dermatol.*, 50, 287, 1970.
26. Lanman, B.M., Zelvers, W.V., Howard, C.S., The role of human patch testing the product development program, in *Proceedings of the Joint Conference of Cosmetic Science*, The Toilet Goods Association, Washington, D.C., 1968.
27. Berger, R.S., Bowman, J.P., Early appraisal of the 21 day cumulative irritation test in man, *J. Toxicol. Cut. Ocular Toxicol.*, 1, 109, 1982.
28. Combs, R.R.A., Gell, P.G.H., Classification of allergic reactions responsible for clinical hypersensitivity and disease, in *Clinical Aspects of Immunology*, Gell, P.G.H., Coombs, R.R.A., Lachman, P.J., Eds., Blackwell, England, 1975.
29. Schorr, W.F. Cosmetic allergy: A comprehensive study of the many groups of chemical antimicrobial agents. *Arch. Dermatol.*, 104, 459, 1971.

30. Bauer, R.L., Ramsey, D.L., Bondi, E., The most common contact allergens, *Arch. Dermatol.*, 108, 74, 1973.
31. Dean, J.H, Twerdok, L.E., Tice, R.R., Sailstad, D.M., Hattan, D.G., Stokes, W.S., ICCVAM evaluation of the murine local lymph node assay: Conclusions and recommendations of an independent scientific review panel, *Reg. Tox. Pharmacol.*, 34, 258, 2001.
32. Haneke, K.E., Tice, R.R., Carson, B.L., Margolin, B.H., Stokes, W.S., ICCVAM evaluation of the murine local lymph node assay: Data analyses completed by the National Toxicology Program Interagency Center for the evaluation of alternative toxicological methods, *Reg. Toxicol. Pharmacol.*, 34, 274, 2001.
33. Gerberick, G.F., Vassallo, J.D., Bailey, R.E., Chaney, J.G., Morrall, S.W., Lepoittevin, J.P., Development of a peptide reactivity assay for screening contact allergens, *Toxicol. Sci.*, 81, 2, 2004.
34. Jaworska, J., Integrated testing strategies for skin sensitization hazard and potency assessment – State of the art and challenges.,*Cosm.*, 3, 16, 2016.
35. McNamee, P.M., Api, A.M., Basketter, D.A., Gerberick, G.F., Gilpin, D.A., Hall, B.M., Jowsey, I., Robinson, M.K., A review of critical factors in the conduct and interpretation of the human repeat insult patch test, *Regul. Toxicol. Pharmacol.*, 52, 1, 2008.
36. Alford, C.A., Rubella, in *Infectious Diseases of the Fetus and Newborn Infant*, Remington, J.S., Klein, J.O., Eds., Saunders, Philadelphia, 1976. p. 894–926.
37. Gregg, N.M., Congential cataract following German measles in the mother, *Trans. Ophthalmol.*, 3, 35, 1941.
38. Warkany, J., Wilson, J.G., Warkany, J., Eds., University of Chicago Press, Chicago, 1965. p. 1–11.
39. McBride, W.G., Thalidomide and congenital anomalies, *Lancet*, 2, 1358, 1961.
40. Postkanzer, D., Herbst, A., Epidemiology of vaginal adenosis and adenocarcinoma associated with exposure to stilbestrol in utero, *Cancer*, 39, 1892, 1977.
41. Manson, J.M., Zenick, H., Costlow. R., Teratology test methods for laboratory animals, in *Principles and Methods of Toxicology*, Hayes, A.W., Ed., Raven Press, New York, 1982. p 141–184.
42. Blackburn, K., Bjerke, D., Daston, G., Felter, S., Mahony, C., Naciff, J., Robison, S., Wu, S., Case studies to test: A framework for using structural, reactivity, metabolic and physicochemical similarity to evaluate the suitability of analogs for SAR-based toxicological assessments, *Regul Toxicol Pharmacol.* 60, 1, 2011.
43. Wu, S., Fisher, J., Naciff, J., Laufersweiler, M., Lester, C., Daston, G., Blackburn, K., Framework for identifying chemicals with structural features associated with the potential to act as developmental or reproductive toxicants, *Chem Res Toxicol.*, 26, 12, 2016.

13

Global Regulation of Preservatives and Cosmetic Preservatives

David C. Steinberg

Introduction

All countries require that cosmetics sold inside their borders be safe. Part of the safety issue for a cosmetic is freedom from microbial contamination when it is placed on the market and the ability to remain free from contamination during normal and foreseeable use by consumers. Preservatives are chemicals added to cosmetics to prevent the growth of and destroy microbes arising from contamination. Although the primary purpose of a preservative is to maintain a cosmetic in "clean" condition and keep it free from contamination during consumer use, the true purpose of adding preservatives is to eliminate accidental contamination during production.

Because preservatives are biologically active chemicals, they have the potential to injure users in addition to killing microbes. This potential for injury has resulted in their regulation by governments. Japan and the European Union have developed lists of permitted or positive preservatives and it is illegal in Japan or Europe to use a preservative that is not permitted or listed as approved by the respective governments. The U.S. Food and Drug Administration (FDA) does not have a similar positive list because the agency does not preapprove preservatives. Instead, the FDA utilizes a list of banned (or negative) preservatives. This chapter will review the regulations of these three major markets.

United States Regulations

Regulation of Preservatives

As noted earlier, the FDA does not approve preservatives for use in cosmetics or topical cosmetic drugs. However, the agency has prohibited the use of bithionol (1) and halogenated salicylanilide (2) preservatives, and the use of hexachlorophene and Mercury are restricted. The maximum allowed level of hexachlorophene is 0.1%, provided no other preservative has been shown to be effective, and not be used in cosmetics that may be applied to mucous membranes (3). Mercury compounds (4) are limited to

65 ppm as the free metal, may be used in eye-area cosmetics only, provided no other effective and safe preservative is available. The State of Minnesota prohibits this application totally.

The Personal Care Products Council (PCPC)—formerly the Cosmetic, Toiletry, and Fragrance Association (CTFA)—with the support of the FDA and the Consumer Federation of America established the Cosmetic Ingredient Review (CIR) system in 1976. Although funded by PCPC, CIR assessments are independent of PCPC and the cosmetics industry. The CIR thoroughly reviews and assesses the safety of ingredients used in cosmetics in an open, unbiased, and expert manner and the results are published in peer-reviewed scientific publications (5). The CIR system has issued assessments on most preservatives used in cosmetics. A CIR opinion may conclude that an ingredient is (1) safe to use, (2) safe at maximum concentrations, (3) unsafe to use, or (4) data submitted are insufficient to allow a determination. Ingredients found unsafe through this review process are not used in the U.S. because no one would market or buy an unsafe product. Where review data are found to be insufficient, an ingredient is given a certain time to supply the requested safety data or it will be changed to being unsafe (6).

The CIR process determined that chloroacetamide is unsafe for use in cosmetics. The following preservatives presented problems and as of this writing have insufficient data status:

- Benzylparaben (2019)
- Sodium iodate (1995—no reported uses)
- Glutaral
- 2-Bromo-2-nitropropane-1,3-diol and 5-bromo-5-nitro-1,3 dioxane when used where amines and nitrosamines could be formed
- Formaldehyde in aerosols

Regulation of Biocides

Chemicals used as preservatives in non-FDA-regulated industries must be preapproved for their respective applications by the U.S. Environmental Protection Agency (EPA) through authority granted by the Federal Insecticide, Fungicide, and Rodenticide Act (FIFRA). It is important to note that the majority of cosmetic preservatives are *not* EPA registered and their use is not permitted in non-FDA-regulated applications. It is important to know that all disinfectants must be approved by the EPA.

Regulation of Antimicrobial Ingredients

Antimicrobial compounds can be active ingredients in drugs in the U.S. Drugs sold without prescriptions (known as over-the-counter [OTC] drugs) are regulated under a monograph system published by the FDA. The other method for antimicrobial drug approval is by submission and approval via a New Drug Application (NDA). It should be noted that a NDA approval is for the formulation that was submitted. Changes in this formulation require FDA approval before being allowed on the market.

Monographs for the compounds listed in Table 13.1 are in effect; permitted levels are listed where appropriate.

When the final monograph is issued for a Category III ingredient, the ingredient must be permitted or disallowed. Until that time, it may still be used. Three types of applications were permitted for healthcare antiseptic drugs:

1. Patient preoperative skin preparations
2. Antiseptic handwashes or healthcare personnel handwashes
3. Surgical hand scrubs

The PCPC and Soap & Detergent Association (now called the American Cleaning Institute) have been urging the FDA to allow additional applications and have proposed the following uses:

- Preoperative skin preparations
- Surgical scrubs

TABLE 13.1

Healthcare antiseptic drugs

Category I (Safe and Effective)[a]	Category III (Either Insufficient Safety or Efficacy Data Is Needed)
Alcohol, 60–95% by volume	Benzalkonium chloride
Povidone–iodine, 5–10%	Chlorhexidine gluconate
Iodine tincture, USP	Chloroxylenol
Iodine topical solution, USP	Chloroxylenol
Isopropyl alcohol, 70–91.3% by volume	Hexylresorcinol
	Cloflucarban
	Hexylresorcinol
	Undecoylium chloride–iodine complex
	Mercufenol chloride
	Methylbenzethonium chloride
	Phenol
	Secondary amylcresols
	Sodium oxychlorosene
	Triclocarban
	Triclosan

[a] See Federal Register, Vol. 59, No. 116, pp. 31402–31452, June 17, 1994.

- Healthcare personnel handwash
- Food handler handwash
- Antimicrobial handwash
- Antimicrobial bodywash

In 2010, the Natural Resources Defense Council filed a complaint against the FDA (and Health and Human Services [HHS]) for not issuing a final monograph (FM) for products containing triclosan. This was settled in a consent decree of 11/21/13. The FDA agreed to a timeline for the completion of FM for healthcare antiseptics washes and handrubs with triclosan. The agreement's timeline was that by 12/21/2013 a TFM for products used with water (handwashes, bodywashes, etc.) had to be issued. An FM was required to be issued one year later. On 12/17/2013, the FDA issued the TFM which moved all Category I and Category III to Category III status requiring new standardizations for safety and efficacy. They are:

Efficacy Tests

The old method was laboratory testing to show it kills microbes. The new requirement is similar to NDA-preclinical and placebo tests on thousands of subjects which will take a long time to complete and will involve significant costs. They had to compare infection rates of the placebo group to active users. This is more stringent than what is required for a new drug!

Safety Tests

This involves animal pharmacokinetic absorption, distribution, metabolism, and excretion, human pharmacokinetics, carcinogenicity, development toxicity, and reproductive toxicity.

As these involve animal testing, it will eliminate their use in the EU (and all other countries that prohibit animal testing for safety determination in cosmetics or ingredients used in cosmetics) as they have an animal testing ban of cosmetic ingredients (note that the EU regulates these types of products as cosmetics, medicines, or biocides, depending on the claims, while these are regulated as drugs in the U.S.).

The FDA allowed a one-year comment period which lasted until 2/17/2015. They issued the FM draft on 8/31/2016 and an FM on 9/15/16. The FM placed all actives in Category II and effectively abolished antiseptic consumer washes. To sell one, an NDA is now necessary.

The FDA had similar deadlines for two other antiseptic drugs: those that were rubbed onto the skin (leave-on) and a new category called Instant Hand Sanitizers. The deadlines for these TFMs were combined on 6/30/2016 and all actives were moved to Category III. Comments had a 12/27/2016 deadlines. On 04/12/2019, the FDA issued their FM for Antiseptic Rubs (AKA Hand Sanitizers). It is effective as of 4/13/2020.

This FM deferred status on three active ingredients to allow for submission of additional safety/efficacy data. These are:

1. Alcohol 60–95% (must be denatured alcohol)
2. Isopropyl alcohol 70–91.3%
3. Benzalkonium chloride (no level is listed; however, previous levels allowed are 0.1–0.13%)

With the outbreak of the pandemic of Covid-19 in December 2019 in China and the U.S. in January 2020, the FDA issued a document on the Policy for Temporary Compounding of Certain Alcohol-Based Hand Sanitizer Products (https://www.fda.gov/media/136118/download). The FDA allowed compounders to prepare alcohol-based hand sanitizers for consumer and healthcare professionals under these conditions for the duration of the public health emergency declared by the Secretary of Health and Human Services on January 31, 2020:

1. The hand sanitizer is compounded using only the following ingredients in the preparation of the product:
   a. *(Select one of two options)* (1) Alcohol (80%) that is not less than 94.9% ethanol by volume; *OR* (2) Isopropyl alcohol (75%)
   b. Glycerin (1.45%) (glycerol) United States Pharmacopeia (USP) or Food Chemical Codex (also known as "food grade")
   c. Hydrogen peroxide (0.125%)
   d. Sterile water (e.g., by boiling, distillation, or other process that results in water that meets the specifications for Purified Water USP). Water should be used as quickly as possible after it is rendered sterile or purified.

The compounder does not add other active or inactive ingredients (e.g., to improve the smell or taste) due to the risk of accidental ingestion by children. Different or additional ingredients may impact the quality and potency of the product.Note-it is a requirement that all OTC drugs intented for topical use, must be denatured according ATF regulations.

This policy does not extend to other types of products, such as products that use different active ingredients, whose potency falls above or below the formulation described, that are marketed with claims that do not conform to the "Topical Antimicrobial Drug Products for Over-the-Counter Human Use; Tentative Final Monograph for Health-Care Antiseptic Drug Products," Proposed Rule, 59 FR 31402 (June 17, 1994) (e.g., pathogen-specific disease claims), that are surgical hand rubs, or whose advertising or promotion is false or misleading in any particular manner.

FDA encourages consumers and health care professionals to report adverse events experienced with the use of hand sanitizers to FDA's MedWatch Adverse Event Reporting program:

- Complete and submit the report online: www.accessdata.fda.gov/scripts/email/oc/buyonline/english.cfm
  or
- Download and complete the form, then submit it via fax at 1-800-FDA-0178.

TABLE 13.2

First aid antiseptic drugs

Category I (Approved Active Ingredients)[a]	Category III (Active Ingredients)
Alcohol, 48–95% by volume	Benzyl alcohol
Benzalkonium chloride, 0.1–0.13%	Calomel
Benzethonium chloride, 0.1–0.2%	Chlorobutanol
Hexylresorcinol, 0.1%	Merbromin
Hydrogen peroxide topical solution USP	Mercufenol chloride
Iodine tincture USP	Phenylmercuric nitrate
Iodine topical solution USP	Secondary amytricresols
Isopropyl alcohol, 50–91.3%	Triclocarban
Methylbenzethonium chloride, 0.13–0.5%	Triclosan
Phenol, 0.5 to 1.5%	

Category I Combination

Eucalyptol 0.091%, menthol 0.042%, methyl salicylate 0.055%, and thymol 0.063 percent in 26.9% alcohol.

Category I Complexes

Camphorated metacresol (3–10.8% camphor and 1–3.6% metacresol) in a ration of 3:1

Camphorated phenol (10.8% camphor and 4.7% phenol) in a light mineral oil; U.S.P. vehicle

Povidone-Iodine complex 5–10%

Category III Combinations/Complexes

Iodine complex (ammonium ether sulfate and polyoxyethylene sorbitan monolaurate)

Iodine complex (phosphate ester of alkylaryloxypolyoxyethylene glycol)

Mercufenol chloride and secondary amylticresols

Nonylphenoxypoly (ethyleneoxy) ethanol iodine

Poloxamer-Iodine complex

Triple dye

Undecoylium chloride Iodine complex

[a] See Federal Register, Vol. 56, No. 140, pp. 33644–33680, July 22, 1991.

When the final monograph is issued for a Category III ingredient, the ingredient must be permitted or disallowed. Until that time, it may still be used in a first aid antiseptic application (see Table 13.2) (7).

Topical Acne Drugs

The chemicals listed in Table 13.3 are permitted for use to treat acne under a final monograph issued on August 16, 1991. Benzyl Peroxide was changed from Category III to Category I in 2010.

TABLE 13.3

API's permitted for topical acne drug products

Benzoyl Peroxide 2.5–10%
Resorcinol, 2%, with 3–8% sulfur
Resorcinol monoacetate, 3%, with 3–8% sulfur
Salicylic acid, 0.5–2%
Sulfur, 3–10%

Topical Antifungal Drugs

Antifungal Drugs (see Table 13.4) (8)

TABLE 13.4

API's permitted for topical antifungal drug products

Clioquinol, 3%
Haloprogin, 1%
Miconazole nitrate, 2%
Povidone–iodine, 10%
Tolnaftate, 1%
Undecylenic acid or its calcium, copper, or zinc salts, individually or in any ratio with a total concentration of 10 to 25%
Clotrimazole, 1%

Dandruff, Seborrheic Dermatitis, and Psoriasis Drugs (see Table 13.5) (9)

TABLE 13.5

API's permitted for external drug products for over-the-counter human use: dandruff, seborrheic dermatitis, and psoriasis drug products

---

Coal tar, 0.5–5%[a]
Pyrithione zinc, 0.3–2% when formulated to be applied, then washed off after brief exposure
Pyrithione zinc, 0.1–0.25% when formulated to be applied and left on skin or scalp
Salicylic acid, 1.8–3%
Selenium sulfide, 1%
Selenium sulfide, micronized, 0.6%
Sulfur, 2–5%

---

[a] When a coal tar solution, derivative, or fraction serves as the source of the coal tar, labeling shall specify the identity and concentration of the coal tar source and the concentration of coal tar present in the final product.

Regulation of Cosmetic Microbiology

The FDA prohibits the distribution of adulterated or misbranded cosmetics. It also prohibits production of cosmetics under conditions that could cause contamination. Cosmetics should preferably be manufactured in conformity with current good manufacturing practices (cGMPs). The *Cosmetic Handbook* issued by the FDA lists these guidelines (10,11).

The FDA states that cosmetics and topical cosmetic drugs need not be sterile; however, they must not be contaminated with pathogenic microorganisms, and the density of non-pathogenic organisms must be low. The FDA requires that:

1. Each batch of a cosmetic that is not self-preserving must be tested for microbial contamination before it is released for interstate shipment.
2. Each cosmetic, particularly each eye-area cosmetic, must be tested during product development for adequacy of preservation against microbial contamination that may occur under reasonably foreseeable conditions of consumer use.

Because the FDA does not specify acceptable levels, the cosmetics industry generally follows CTFA guidelines with regard to microbial levels and the absence of pathogens:

1. For eye area and baby products, not more than 500 CFU/mL
2. For all other products, not more than 1000 CFU/mL

Generally, most companies set their own internal limits of less than 10 CFU/mL for all aqueous-based products and oil-in-water emulsions and set higher levels for atypical cosmetics.

European Union Regulations

Cosmetics in the European Union (EU) are regulated by Regulation 1223/2009. This Regulation consists of 40 articles and 10 annexes. Article 4 requires that only preapproved preservatives listed on Annex V may be used in cosmetics. Article 7a, Part 1(b) requires microbiological specifications for each ingredient used in finished cosmetic products.

Annex I Part A

#1 requires the qualitative and quantitative composition (including chemical name, INCI, CAS, and EINECS/ELINCS) and the function of each ingredient, in the cosmetic.

#3 requires the microbiological specifications of all raw materials and the cosmetic. It also requires the results of a preservative challenge test.

Annex II is the list of prohibited chemicals in cosmetics.

Annex V is the list of permitted preservatives.

Annex V–Approved Preservatives

Annex V is a list of preservatives that cosmetic products may contain. Each listing for a permitted preservative includes its reference number, chemical name, INCI, CAS, EINECS/ELINCS, maximum permitted concentration, limitations, and conditions of use and warnings that must be printed on the label in all languages.

The salts are sodium, potassium, calcium, magnesium, ammonium, and ethanolamine. The anions are chlorides, bromides, sulfates, and acetates. The esters are methyl, ethyl, propyl, isopropyl, butyl, isobutyl, and phenyl.

The list can be found at https://ec.europa.eu/growth/sectors/cosmetics/legislation_en

Requirements for Annex V Submissions

The Scientific Committee for Consumer Safety (SCCS) examines the safety of new preservatives. The committee's requirements can be accessed at https://ec.europa.eu/health/sites/health/files/scientific_committees/consumer_safety/docs/sccs_o_224.pdf. After a positive opinion is issued, a preservative is referred to the European Union Commission. If the commission concurs, a document known as an adaptation to technical progress (ATP) is issued and the new preservative is added to Annex V.

Prohibited Preservatives

Annex II of the EU Regulations lists ingredients prohibited from use in cosmetics. The following preservatives are listed (Table 13.6):

TABLE 13.6

Preservatives prohibited in the EU

Number	INCI*
221	Mercury compounds except those listed in Annex V
348	Tetrachlorosalicylanilides
349	Dichlorosalicylanilides

(continued)

TABLE 13.6

Preservatives prohibited in the EU (Continued)

Number	INCI*
350	Tetrabromosalicylanilides
351	Dibromosalicylanilides
352	Bithionol
369	Sodium pyrithione
370	Captan
371	Hexachlorophene
373	Tribromosalicylanilide
1175	Phenol
1374	Isopropylparaben
1375	Isobutylparaben
1376	Phenylparaben
1377	Benzylparaben
1378	Pentylparaben
1387	Chloroacetamide
1396	Boric acid and its salts
1528	Ketoconazole
1577	Formaldehyde
1578	Paraformaldehyde
1579	Methylene Glycol

* International Nomenclature Cosmetic Ingredient

Japan Regulations

Approved Preservatives for Cosmetics

In 2001, Japan changed its cosmetic regulations to eliminate the need for preapproval of most cosmetic ingredients (see Table 13.7). The exceptions for which preapproval is still required are UV filters, colors, preservatives, and a few miscellaneous items. It is important to note that the change covers only cosmetics and does not include quasi-drugs.

Requirements for New Preservatives

Obtaining approval and placement on the list requires a formal submission to the Japanese Minister of Health, Labor, and Welfare (MHW), Examination and Administration Section, who, after reviewing a submission will approve or reject it or request additional data. A submission must include data on the chemistry of the preservative, method of production, purity, and efficacy. If the preservative has been approved in any other market, this information must be included along with maximum use levels and any restrictions. If the chemistry is similar to the chemistries of other preservatives, a comparison is also required.

Safety testing data should cover single administration toxicity, repetitive administration toxicity, reproductive development toxicity, skin primary irritation, continuous skin irritation, sensitivity, phototoxicity, photosensitization, eye irritation, genetic toxicity, human patch tests on Japanese subjects, absorption, distribution, metabolism, and excretion. All data must be submitted on official forms in the Japanese language.

TABLE 13.7

Preservatives approved for use in Japan

Preservative	Maximum Concentrations for All Cosmetics %	Rinse-Off; No MM %	Leave-On; No MM %	Use On MM %
Benzoic acid and its salts	0.2 as acid 1.0 as salts as total			
Salicylic acid and its salts	0.2 as acid 1.0 as salts as total			
Sorbic acid and its salts	0.5 as total			
o-Phenylphenol and its salts		∞	0.3	0.3
Zinc pyrithione		0.1	0.01	0.01
Chlorobutanol	0.1			
p-Hydroxy Benzoic acid esters and salts (parabens)	1.0 as total			
Dehydroacetic acid and its salts	0.5 as total			
Triclocarban		∞	0.3	0.3
Triclosan	0.1			
Chloroxylenol		0.3	0.2	0.2
Imidazolidinyl urea		0.3 with warning[a]	NA	NA
Phenoxyethanol	1.0			
DMDM hydantoin		0.3 with warning[a]	NA	NA
Methylchloroisothi-azolinone and methylisothiazoli-none		0.1 (as sold)	NA	NA
Chlorhexidine and salts		0.1 (gluconate ∞)	0.05 (chloride 0.1)	0.05 (chloride 0.001)
Chlorphenesin		0.3	0.3	NA
Benzethonium chloride			0.05	0.05
Benzalkonium chloride		0.5	0.2	NA
----------------------		==========	------------------	-------------
Iodopropynyl butylcarbamate		0.02	0.02%	0.02

Notes: MM = mucous membrane. NA = not allowed. ∞ = any amount.

[a] Warning required for imidazolidinyl urea and DMDM hydantoin: should not be used on infants or by people who are hyper-sensitive to formaldehyde.

Prohibited Preservatives

Japan now has a list of 31 ingredients that are prohibited from use in cosmetics. The list includes these preservatives:

- Dichlorophen
- Mercury and its compounds
- Halogenated salicylanides
- Bithionol
- Hexachlorophene
- Formalin

Non-Regulatory Considerations

Formaldehyde Issues—Formaldehyde may be used as a preservative everywhere in the world except in Japan and the EU. However, due to consumer pressure, certain countries including Germany and Denmark do not permit the use of formalin or the so-called formaldehyde releasers.

"Green" Party Issues—The environmentalist or green political parties are generally against all preservatives but they especially dislike formaldehyde and all halogen-containing products. These groups also do not approve of the use of ethylene oxide and ingredients such as ethylenediaminetetraacetic acid (EDTA) that are not readily biodegradable.

Triclosan Issues—In addition to green political party objections to halogenated compounds, a very strong movement in the EU seeks to limit or even prohibit new uses for triclosan.

Biodegradation Issues—The non-biodegradability of EDTA has become an issue in the EU. Although currently not restricted, this could become a critical issue in the future.

Non-Preservative Preservatives

When is a preservative not a preservative? Rationally, when a product acts as a preservative but is not listed in Annex V of the EU Cosmetics Regulations, it cannot be a preservative! Therefore, it must have a different function in the formulation. This principle does not include the addition of high levels of glycols, polyols, or salts or lower water activity levels. Non-preservative preservatives must show microbicidal properties and function as one of three chemical entities: essential oils, emulsifiers, and humectants.

Essential oils—We have known for years that many essential oils found in fragrances have antimicrobial properties. In general, the level of essential oil needed to preserve a product far exceeds the levels used in fragrances and formulations. Sometimes simple emulsification of the oil will eliminate most microbial activity. For example, tea tree (INCI: *Melaleuca alternifolia*) leaf oil at 100% shows good activity. After emulsification, its activity cannot be measured. The critical issue for formulators is that their fragrances may have microbial activities and this can mean that smaller amounts of additional chemical preservatives are required.

Emulsifiers—One of the earliest emulsifiers promoted for its antimicrobial properties is the 90% monoester of glyceryl monolaurate (INCI: glyceryl laurate). This compound never achieved great popularity because its antimicrobial action and emulsifying activity were both weak.

Humectants or hydroxy-containing compounds—Although high concentrations of propylene glycol can act as preservatives, the safety of products that contain them would prevent their marketing. The esthetics of products with glycol levels high enough to reduce water activity to sufficiently low levels to prohibit microbial growth are unacceptable to consumers. Certain products are antimicrobial and fulfill this function when used as humectants in cosmetics. They include:

Farnesol, a long-chained unsaturated hydrocarbon with a terminal hydroxyl group; frequently found in fragrances; also shows activity against Gram-positive bacteria.
- Pentylene glycol, a 5-carbon 1,2-diol, shows good broad-spectrum activity when used at levels over 2%; functions as an excellent humectant at that level.
- Caprylyl glycol, an 8-carbon 1,2-diol, exerts major activity against bacteria.
- 1,2 Hexanediol, a 6-carbon 1,2-diol, has been shown to be synergistic with pentylene and caprylyl glycol to offer broad-spectrum coverage and adequate humectancy.

Concluding Comments

Regulatory constraints on global preservative use are varied, complex, and costly, and they will further constrain preservative choices in the future. Requirements for increasingly diverse formulations and packaging, consumer use and price pressures from cosmetic manufacturers, and limited market sizes for cosmetic preservatives are factors that restrain producers from developing and qualifying new cosmetic preservatives. These constraints may make the effective global preservative system an obsolete concept. Clearly, cosmetic manufacturers will be faced with efforts to develop multiple formulations in order to satisfy various requirements based on geographic markets and regulatory activities. A company that can satisfy all these requirements with the least duplication of effort will maintain a significant competitive edge.

REFERENCES

1. 21 CFR 700.11.
2. 21 CFR 700.15.
3. 21 CFR 250.250.
4. 21 CFR 700.13.
5. www.cir-safety.org
6. 21 CFR 740.10.
7. 21 CFR 333.310.
8. 21 CFR 333.210.
9. 21 CFR 358710.
10. www.FDA.gov
11. U.S. Food and Drug Administration, Cosmetic Handbook, Washington, D.C., 1992. p. 10. (www.cfsan.fda.gov/~dms/cos-hdbk.html)

Index

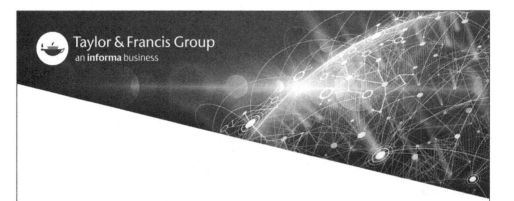
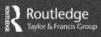
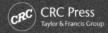